Advances in Cardiac Mapping and Catheter Ablation: Part II

Editors

MOHAMMAD SHENASA
AMIN AL-AHMAD

CARDIAC ELECTROPHYSIOLOGY CLINICS

www.cardiacEP.theclinics.com

Consulting Editors
RANJAN K. THAKUR
ANDREA NATALE

December 2019 • Volume 11 • Number 4

ELSEVIER

1600 John F. Kennedy Boulevard • Suite 1800 • Philadelphia, Pennsylvania, 19103-2899

http://www.theclinics.com

CARDIAC ELECTROPHYSIOLOGY CLINICS Volume 11, Number 4
December 2019 ISSN 1877-9182, ISBN-13: 978-0-323-68349-4

Editor: Stacy Eastman
Developmental Editor: Donald Mumford

Cardiac Electrophysiology Clinics (ISSN 1877-9182) is published quarterly by Elsevier Inc., 360 Park Avenue South, New York, NY 10010-1710. Months of issue are March, June, September, and December. Subscription prices are $224.00 per year for US individuals, $366.00 per year for US institutions, $249.00 per year for Canadian individuals, $413.00 per year for Canadian institutions, $303.00 per year for international individuals, $442.00 per year for international institutions and $100.00 per year for US, Canadian and international students/residents. To receive student/resident rate, orders must be accompanied by name of affiliated institution, date of term, and the signature of program/residency coordinator on institution letterhead. Orders will be billed at individual rate until proof of status is received. Foreign air speed delivery is included in all Clinics subscription prices. All prices are subject to change without notice. **POSTMASTER:** Send address changes to Cardiac Electrophysiology Clinics, Elsevier Health Sciences Division, Subscription Customer Service, 3251 Riverport Lane, Maryland Heights, MO 63043. **Customer Service: 1-800-654-2452 (US and Canada). From outside of the US and Canada, call 314-477-8871. Fax: 314-447-8029. E-mail: JournalsCustomerService-usa@elsevier.com (for print support);** JournalsOnlineSupport-usa@elsevier.com (for online support).

Reprints. For copies of 100 or more of articles in this publication, please contact the Commercial Reprints Department, Elsevier Inc., 360 Park Avenue South, New York, NY 10010-1710. Tel.: 212-633-3874; Fax: 212-633-3820; E-mail: reprints@elsevier.com.

Cardiac Electrophysiology Clinics is covered in *MEDLINE/PubMed (Index Medicus)*.

Contributors

CONSULTING EDITORS

RANJAN K. THAKUR, MD, MPH, MBA, FHRS
Professor of Medicine and Director, Arrhythmia
Service, Thoracic and Cardiovascular Institute,
Sparrow Health System, Michigan State
University, Lansing, Michigan, USA

ANDREA NATALE, MD, FACC, FHRS
Executive Medical Director, Texas Cardiac
Arrhythmia Institute, St. David's Medical
Center, Austin, Texas; Consulting Professor,
Division of Cardiology, Stanford University,
Palo Alto, California; Adjunct Professor of
Medicine, Heart and Vascular Center, Case
Western Reserve University, Cleveland, Ohio;
Director, Interventional Electrophysiology,
Scripps Clinic, San Diego, California; Senior
Clinical Director, EP Services, California Pacific
Medical Center, San Francisco, California, USA

EDITORS

**MOHAMMAD SHENASA, MD, PhD, FACC,
FESC, FAHA, FHRS**
Department of Cardiovascular Services, Heart
and Rhythm Medical Group, O'Connor
Hospital, San Jose, California, USA

AMIN AI-AHMAD, MD, FHRS
Texas Cardiac Arrhythmia Institute, St David's
Medical Center, Austin, Texas, USA

AUTHORS

AMIN AL-AHMAD, MD, FHRS
Texas Cardiac Arrhythmia Institute,
St. David's Medical Center, Austin, Texas,
USA

CLEMENTINE ANDRÉ, MD
Electrophysiology and Cardiac Stimulation,
Bordeaux University Hospital, IHU LIRYC,
Electrophysiology and Heart Modeling
Institute, Bordeaux, France

HUSEYIN AYHAN, MD
Texas Cardiac Arrhythmia Institute, St. David's
Medical Center, Austin, Texas, USA,
Department of Cardiology, Ankara Yildirim
Beyazit, Ankara, Turkey

MOHAMED BASSIOUNY, MD
Texas Cardiac Arrhythmia Institute, St. David's
Medical Center, Austin, Texas, USA

TINA BAYKANER, MD
Instructor, Department of Medicine/
Cardiovascular Medicine, Stanford University,
Stanford, California, USA

OLIVIER BERNUS, PhD
IHU LIRYC, Electrophysiology and Heart
Modeling Institute, Univ Bordeaux, CRCTB,
U1045, Bordeaux, France

JOHN DAVID BURKHARDT, MD
Texas Cardiac Arrhythmia Institute, St. David's
Medical Center, Austin, Texas, USA

UGUR CANPOLAT, MD
Texas Cardiac Arrhythmia Institute, St. David's
Medical Center, Austin, Texas, USA;
Arrhythmia and Electrophysiology Unit,
Department of Cardiology, Hacettepe
University, Ankara, Turkey

DOMENICO GIOVANNI DELLA ROCCA, MD
Texas Cardiac Arrhythmia Institute, St. David's
Medical Center, Austin, Texas, USA

HANY DEMO, MD, FACC, FHRS
Electrophysiology Laboratory Director,
Swedish Covenant Hospital, Chicago, Illinois,
USA

NICOLAS DERVAL, MD
Electrophysiology and Cardiac Stimulation,
Bordeaux University Hospital, IHU LIRYC,
Electrophysiology and Heart Modeling
Institute, Bordeaux, France

SUBODH R. DEVABHAKTUNI, MD
Indiana University, Indianapolis, Indiana, USA

LUIGI DI BIASE, MD, PhD
Texas Cardiac Arrhythmia Institute, St. David's
Medical Center, Department of Biomedical
Engineering, University of Texas, Austin,
Texas, USA; Montefiore Medical Center,
Albert Einstein College of Medicine, Bronx,
New York, USA; Department of Clinical and
Experimental Medicine, University of Foggia,
Foggia, Italy

REMI DUBOIS, PhD
IHU LIRYC, Electrophysiology and Heart
Modeling Institute, Bordeaux, France

JOSSELIN DUCHATEAU, PhD, MD
Electrophysiology and Cardiac Stimulation,
Bordeaux University Hospital, IHU LIRYC,
Electrophysiology and Heart Modeling
Institute, Bordeaux, France

JOSEPH G. GALLINGHOUSE, MD
Texas Cardiac Arrhythmia Institute, St. David's
Medical Center, Austin, Texas, USA

FERMIN C. GARCIA, MD
Assistant Professor of Clinical
Electrophysiology, Cardiac Electrophysiology,
Hospital of the University of Pennsylvania,
Philadelphia, Pennsylvania, USA

CAROLA GIANNI, MD, PhD
Texas Cardiac Arrhythmia Institute, St. David's
Medical Center, Austin, Texas, USA

MICHEL HAÏSSAGUERRE, MD
Electrophysiology and Cardiac Stimulation,
Bordeaux University Hospital, IHU LIRYC,

Electrophysiology and Heart Modeling
Institute, Univ Bordeaux, CRCTB, U1045,
Bordeaux, France

MÉLÈZE HOCINI, MD
Electrophysiology and Cardiac Stimulation,
Bordeaux University Hospital, IHU LIRYC,
Electrophysiology and Heart Modeling
Institute, Univ Bordeaux, CRCTB, U1045,
Bordeaux, France

RODNEY P. HORTON, MD
Texas Cardiac Arrhythmia Institute,
St. David's Medical Center, Austin, Texas,
USA

HENRY H. HSIA, MD, FHRS
Cardiac Electrophysiology Service, University
of California, San Francisco, San Francisco,
California, USA

PIERRE JAIS, MD
Electrophysiology and Cardiac Stimulation,
Bordeaux University Hospital, IHU LIRYC,
Electrophysiology and Heart Modeling
Institute, Bordeaux, France

MOHAMMAD-ALI JAZAYERI, MD
Chief Cardiology Fellow, Department of
Cardiovascular Medicine, University of
Kansas Medical Center, Kansas City, Kansas,
USA

SURAJ KAPA, MD
Assistant Professor of Medicine, Department
of Cardiovascular Diseases, Mayo Clinic
College of Medicine, Rochester, Minnesota,
USA

JOSEF KAUTZNER, MD, PhD
Department of Cardiology, Institute for Clinical
and Experimental Medicine (IKEM), Prague,
Czech Republic

SANTHISRI KODALI, MD
Fellow, Cardiac Electrophysiology, Hospital of
the University of Pennsylvania, Philadelphia,
Pennsylvania, USA

DENNIS H. LAU, MBBS, PhD
Department of Cardiology, Centre for Heart
Rhythm Disorders, University of Adelaide,
Royal Adelaide Hospital, Adelaide, South
Australia, Australia

CARLO LAVALLE, MD
Department of Cardiovascular, Respiratory, Nephrological, Anesthesiological and Geriatric Sciences, "Sapienza" University of Rome, Policlinico Umberto I, Rome, Italy

THOMAS LAVERGNE, MD
IHU LIRYC, Electrophysiology and Heart Modeling Institute, Bordeaux, France

ANTHONY LI, MD
Cardiology Clinical Academic Group, St. George's University of London, London, United Kingdom

DOMINIK LINZ, MD, PhD
Department of Cardiology, Centre for Heart Rhythm Disorders, University of Adelaide, Royal Adelaide Hospital, Adelaide, South Australia, Australia

BRYAN MACDONALD, MD
Texas Cardiac Arrhythmia Institute, St. David's Medical Center, Austin, Texas, USA

MARCO VALERIO MARIANI, MD
Department of Cardiovascular, Respiratory, Nephrological, Anesthesiological and Geriatric Sciences, "Sapienza" University of Rome, Policlinico Umberto I, Rome, Italy

JOHN M. MILLER, MD
Professor of Medicine, Indiana University School of Medicine, Director, Clinical Cardiac Electrophysiology, Indiana University, Indianapolis, Indiana, USA

SANGHAMITRA MOHANTY, MD
Texas Cardiac Arrhythmia Institute, St. David's Medical Center, Austin, Texas, USA

WEE NADEMANEE, MD
Bumrungrad Hospital, Bangkok, Thailand

SANJIV M. NARAYAN, MD, PhD
Professor, Department of Medicine/ Cardiovascular Medicine and Cardiovascular Institute, Stanford University, Stanford, California, USA

ANDREA NATALE, MD, FACC, FHRS
Texas Cardiac Arrhythmia Institute, Center for Atrial Fibrillation at St. David's Medical Center, Department of Biomedical Engineering, University of Texas, Austin, Texas, USA;

Interventional Electrophysiology, Scripps Clinic, La Jolla, California, USA; MetroHealth Medical Center, Case Western Reserve University School of Medicine, Cleveland, Ohio, USA; Division of Cardiology, Stanford University, Stanford, California, USA

THOMAS PAMBRUN, MD
Electrophysiology and Cardiac Stimulation, Bordeaux University Hospital, IHU LIRYC, Electrophysiology and Heart Modeling Institute, Bordeaux, France

PETR PEICHL, MD, PhD
Department of Cardiology, Institute for Clinical and Experimental Medicine (IKEM), Prague, Czech Republic

AGOSTINO PIRO, MD
Department of Cardiovascular, Respiratory, Nephrological, Anesthesiological and Geriatric Sciences, "Sapienza" University of Rome, Policlinico Umberto I, Rome, Italy

SUNNY S. PO, MD, PhD
Department of Medicine, Heart Rhythm Institute, University of Oklahoma Health Sciences Center, Oklahoma City, Oklahoma, USA

MARK POTSE, PhD
IHU LIRYC, Electrophysiology and Heart Modeling Institute, Bordeaux, France

SEYED-MOSTAFA RAZAVI, MD
Department of Cardiovascular Services, Heart and Rhythm Medical Group, O'Connor Hospital, San Jose, California

MANSOUR RAZMINIA, MD
Electrophysiology Laboratory Director, Amita Health-Elign Campus, Elgin, Illinois, USA

MAGDI M. SABA, MD
Cardiology Clinical Academic Group, St. George's University of London, London, United Kingdom

FREDERIC SACHER, MD
Electrophysiology and Cardiac Stimulation, Bordeaux University Hospital, IHU LIRYC, Electrophysiology and Heart Modeling Institute, Bordeaux, France

JAVIER SANCHEZ, MD
Texas Cardiac Arrhythmia Institute, St. David's
Medical Center, Austin, Texas, USA

PRASHANTHAN SANDERS, MBBS, PhD
Department of Cardiology, Centre for Heart
Rhythm Disorders, University of Adelaide,
Royal Adelaide Hospital, Adelaide, South
Australia, Australia

PASQUALE SANTANGELI, MD, PhD
Assistant Professor of Clinical
Electrophysiology, Cardiac Electrophysiology,
Hospital of the University of Pennsylvania,
Philadelphia, Pennsylvania, USA

HOSSEIN SHENASA, MD, FHRS
Department of Cardiovascular Services, Heart
and Rhythm Medical Group, O'Connor
Hospital, San Jose, California, USA

**MOHAMMAD SHENASA, MD, PhD, FACC,
FESC, FAHA, FHRS**
Department of Cardiovascular Services, Heart
and Rhythm Medical Group, O'Connor
Hospital, San Jose, California, USA

JONATHAN T. SHIRAZI, MD
Indiana University, Indianapolis, Indiana, USA

MASA TAKIGAWA, MD
Electrophysiology and Cardiac Stimulation,
Bordeaux University Hospital, Bordeaux,
France

AHMED KARIM TALIB, MD, PhD
Head of Cardiac Electrophysiology Division,
Najaf Center for Cardiac Surgery and Trans-
catheter Therapy, Najaf city, Iraq;
Cardiovascular Division, Faculty of Medicine,
University of Tsukuba, Tsukuba, Japan

NICOLA TARANTINO, MD
Montefiore Medical Center, Albert Einstein
College of Medicine, Bronx, New York, USA

CHINTAN TRIVEDI, MD, MPH
Texas Cardiac Arrhythmia Institute, St. David's
Medical Center, Austin, Texas, USA

RODERICK TUNG, MD
Associate Professor of Medicine, Department
of Medicine, Section of Cardiology, The
University of Chicago Medicine, Center for
Arrhythmia Care, Pritzker School of Medicine,
Chicago, Illinois, USA

GEORGE F. VAN HARE, MD
Professor of Pediatrics, Washington
University School of Medicine, St Louis,
Missouri, USA

ED VIGMOND, PhD
IHU LIRYC, Electrophysiology and Heart
Modeling Institute, Bordeaux, France

RICK WALTON, PhD
IHU LIRYC, Electrophysiology and Heart
Modeling Institute, Bordeaux, France

YUHONG WANG, MD
Department of Cardiology, Renmin Hospital of
Wuhan University, Cardiovascular Research
Institute, Wuhan University, Hubei Key
Laboratory of Cardiology, Wuhan, Hubei,
China

CAMERON WILLOUGHBY, DO
Electrophysiology Laboratory Director,
McLaren Health-Macomb Campus, Clinton
Township, Michigan, USA

NANQING XIONG, MD
Department of Cardiology, Husham Hospital
Furan University, Shanghai, China

LILEI YU, MD, PhD
Department of Cardiology, Renmin Hospital of
Wuhan University, Cardiovascular Research
Institute, Wuhan University, Hubei Key
Laboratory of Cardiology, Wuhan, Hubei,
China

JUNAID ZAMAN, MD, PhD
Honorary Research Fellow, Stanford
University, Stanford, California, USA;
Imperial College London, London, United
Kingdom

Contents

> This review focusses on novel findings in atrial fibrillation mechanisms derived from mapping studies. Recent panoramic mapping techniques have identified 2 arrhythmic mechanisms of interest, namely, rotational (rotors) and ectopic focal activations as drivers of atrial fibrillation. Epicardial adipose tissue and fatty infiltration into the myocardium have been described as novel substrates for atrial fibrillation. There is increasing appreciation that the thin atrial walls harbor a complex 3-dimensional electrostructural substrate to contribute to atrial fibrillation sustenance. Further research is warranted to advance the field toward more targeted therapy.

> Atrial arrhythmias, including atrial tachycardia and atrial flutter, are not uncommon after prior ablation. Mechanisms for arrhythmogenesis may vary and include recurrent conduction through sites of ablation, leading to recurrence of prior ablated arrhythmias and creation of new substrate. Incidence of postablation atrial arrhythmias varies across studies and may relate to the approach to ablation, including extent of ablation performed, or to extent of substrate identified at the time of prior ablation and how that relates to the lesion set. In addition, postablation atrial arrhythmias may be more common in certain types of cardiomyopathy, including hypertrophic cardiomyopathy.

> Drivers are increasingly studied ablation targets for atrial fibrillation (AF). However, results from ablation remain controversial. First, outcomes vary between centers and patients. Second, it is unclear how best to perform driver ablation. Third, there is a lack of practical guidance on how to identify critical from secondary sites using different AF mapping methods. This article addresses each of these issues.

> Arrhythmias arising from the ventricular outflow tracts are commonly encountered. Although largely benign, they can also present with heart failure and sudden cardiac death. Mapping and ablation of these arrhythmias is commonly performed in the

electrophysiology laboratory with a high success rate, but occasionally can prove challenging to abolish. This article discusses the mapping and ablation of outflow tract arrhythmias and the challenges that can be overcome by a systematic approach.

Fascicular ventricular tachycardia (FVT) usually involves the left fascicular system; namely the left posterior fascicle, anterior fascicle, and rarely the upper septal fascicle. It may also involve the right Purkinje arborization. This tachycardia can be seen in normal heart or in the setting of structural heart diseases. Monomorphic FVT can be reentrant or nonreentrant and verapamil-sensitive left FVT is the second most common type of idiopathic ventricular tachycardia (VT) after right ventricular outflow tract VT. This article focuses on the practical approach for both reentrant and nonreentrant FVT, explaining the mechanism, electrocardiographic features, and electrophysiologic features of FVT.

Ventricular tachycardia (VT) remains a common cause of sudden cardiac death. It is widely accepted that VTs are strongly associated with autonomic imbalance with reduced vagal and increased sympathetic activities. Pharmacologic therapy remains the first-line therapy, but antiarrhythmic agents may not be effective or carry significant side effects. Sympathetic denervation is an emerging therapy to prevent or treat VTs by rebalancing the sympathetic and parasympathetic activity. This article focuses on the role of sympathetic activation in VT, and the mapping and ablation of sympathetic nervous system in patients with VT.

Mapping and ablation of ventricular arrhythmias in patients with nonischemic cardiomyopathies remain a major challenge. The electroanatomic abnormalities are frequently inaccessible to conventional endocardial ablations. Diagnostic diligence with a thorough understanding of the potential mechanisms/substrate, coupled with detailed electroanatomic mapping, is essential. Careful procedural planning, advanced imaging, and unipolar recordings help to formulate ablation strategy, facilitate work flow, and improve outcomes. Inaccessibility of arrhythmogenic substrate and disease progression are important causes of ablation failure. Early intervention may help to improve outcome and minimize complications. Several novel adjunctive ablation techniques are capable of serving as alternative options in refractory cases.

Ventricular tachycardia is typically hemodynamically unstable. Strategies to target the arrhythmogenic substrate during sinus rhythm are essential for therapeutic ablation. Electroanatomic mapping is the cornerstone of substrate-based strategies; ablation can be directed within a delineated scar region defined by low voltage. Bipolar voltage mapping has inherent limitations. Specific electrogram characteristics may improve the specificity of localizing the most arrhythmogenic regions within the substrate. Deceleration zones during sinus rhythm are niduses for reentry and can be identified by isochronal late activation mapping, which is a functional analysis of substrate propagation with local annotation to electrogram offset.

Despite advances in our understanding of the relevant anatomy and mapping and catheter ablation techniques of idiopathic outflow tract ventricular arrhythmias, challenging sites for catheter ablation remain the aortic cusps, pulmonary artery, and notably the left ventricular summit. A systematic approach should be used to direct mapping efforts efficiently between endocardial, coronary venous, and epicardial sites. Foci at the left ventricular summit, particularly intraseptal and at the inaccessible epicardial region, remain difficult to reach and when percutaneous techniques fail, surgical ablation remains an option but with risk of late coronary artery stenosis.

In stable ventricular tachycardia (VT), activation mapping and entrainment mapping are the most important strategies to describe the reentrant circuit and its critical components. In many patients, however, VT is noninducible or hemodynamically unstable and unmappable. Several technological advances have broadened ablation options in unmappable VTs. Preprocedural imaging and intraprocedural imaging play an important role in location and extent of the substrate. Electroanatomic mapping with several technological improvements allows more precise electrical assessment of the substrate. A combination of imaging and electroanatomic mapping allows substantial modification of arrhythmogenic substrate in sinus rhythm or during device pacing without hemodynamic compromise.

Ventricular arrhythmias (VA) constitute well-known problems in patients with left ventricular assist devices (LVADs), with incidence ranging from 18% to as high as 52%. Catheter ablation has become a common therapeutic intervention to treat drug-refractory VA, particularly with the increase and more widespread use of durable LVADs to bridge patients to transplantation or as destination therapy. In this article, we focus on etiology, mechanisms, periprocedural management, and mapping and ablation techniques in patients with LVADs and VA.

Idiopathic ventricular fibrillation and J-wave syndromes are causes of sudden cardiac death (SCD) without any identified structural cardiac disease after extensive investigations. Recent data show that high-density electrophysiological mapping may ultimately offer diagnoses of subclinical diseases in most patients including those termed "unexplained" SCD. Three major conditions can underlie the occurrence of SCD: (1) localized depolarization abnormalities (due to microstructural myocardial alteration), (2) Purkinje abnormalities manifesting as triggering ectopy and inducible reentry; or (3) repolarization heterogeneities. Each condition may result from a spectrum of pathophysiologic processes with implications for individual therapy.

The field of congenital cardiac electrophysiology is growing rapidly due to the rapid growth in the population of survivors of childhood critical congenital heart disease surgery. Chronic arrhythmias pose one of the biggest challenges in this patient population, and catheter ablation, despite its challenges, is still the most desirable and acceptable approach when successful. Clinicians who propose catheter ablation in such patients need to understand the congenital anatomy, should carefully review the details of all prior cardiac surgery, and should be prepared to deal with the various challenges posed by lack of normal cardiac access and the possibility of poor hemodynamics. Still, experienced laboratories can achieve excellent results in this difficult patient population.

Fluoroless catheter ablation of all endocardial cardiac arrhythmias is feasible using current, and often standard, electrophysiology laboratory equipment. This article lays out a road map for performing fluoroless ablations, safely and efficaciously. We outline optimizing intracardiac echocardiography, performing complex ablations with radiofrequency and cryoballoon technology.

Atrial fibrillation catheter ablation has emerged as the most effective strategy to restore and maintain sinus rhythm. The cornerstone of atrial fibrillation ablation is elimination of triggers from the pulmonary veins by pulmonary vein isolation. Nevertheless, some patients may experience atrial tachyarrhythmia recurrences even with permanent pulmonary vein antral isolation. Whether and in which patients pulmonary vein antral isolation should be considered as the only ablation strategy remains a matter of debate. This review aims to summarize the rationale and effectiveness of different ablation approaches and identify key points for a uniform atrial fibrillation ablation strategy.

Cardiac mapping has witnessed significant and unprecedented progress over more than a century. At present, several mapping/imaging technologies are commercially available, alone or in combination. This article briefly discusses the advantages and limitations (disadvantages) of each technique

CARDIAC ELECTROPHYSIOLOGY CLINICS

Foreword
Mapping the Heart

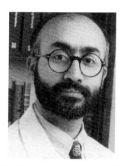 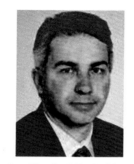

Ranjan K. Thakur, MD, MPH, MBA, FHRS   Andrea Natale, MD, FACC, FHRS

Consulting Editors

Cardiac mapping is simply the correlation of the electrical activity of the heart to the underlying anatomy. In its simplest form, placement of multipolar intracardiac catheters and induction of sustained arrhythmias are a form of mapping to determine the location of an accessory pathway or the site of origin of ventricular tachycardia, and such. Since interventional electrophysiology began in the 1980s, more and more sophisticated cardiac mapping tools as well as electrophysiologic concepts have been developed to pinpoint the mechanisms and the exact anatomic localization of susceptible arrhythmic substrates. Cardiac mapping has not been fully automated, but requires detailed electrophysiology study, the use of electrophysiologic maneuvers, and deductive reasoning.

Dr Shenasa has been active for over 2 decades in summarizing the advancements in cardiac mapping periodically. His current book, *Cardiac Mapping* is in its fifth edition. We are grateful to Drs Shenasa and Al-Ahmad for their effort of providing a summary of contemporary issues of interest in cardiac mapping for the clinical electrophysiology community. They have assembled an international panel of experts to discuss everything from anatomical

considerations in mapping, the fundamentals of cardiac mapping, and unipolar mapping, all the way to the comparative advantages of the commercially available mapping systems. This issue contains useful information for electrophysiology fellows, associated professionals in electrophysiology as well as the practicing electrophysiologist.

We hope the readership will find this issue useful and informative.

Ranjan K. Thakur, MD, MPH, MBA, FHRS
Sparrow Thoracic and Cardiovascular Institute
Michigan State University
1200 East Michigan Avenue, Suite 580
Lansing, MI 48912, USA

Andrea Natale, MD, FACC, FHRS
Texas Cardiac Arrhythmia Institute
Center for Atrial Fibrillation at
St. David's Medical Center
1015 East 32nd Street, Suite 516
Austin, TX 78705, USA

E-mail addresses:
thakur@msu.edu (R.K. Thakur)
andrea.natale@stdavids.com (A. Natale)

Card Electrophysiol Clin 11 (2019) xiii
https://doi.org/10.1016/j.ccep.2019.09.002
1877-9182/19/© 2019 Published by Elsevier Inc.

Preface
Advances in Cardiac Mapping Part 2

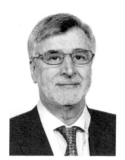

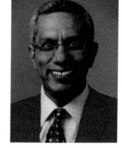

Mohammad Shenasa, MD, PhD, FACC, FESC, FAHA, FHRS

Amin Al-Ahmad, MD, FHRS

Editors

Cardiac mapping has come a long way, and it has been an integral part of interventional cardiac electrophysiology. Cardiac mapping started with direct single-analogue point-by-point registration of cardiac electrical activity to its utmost complex online multimodality mapping and imaging. Technological advances in cardiac mapping and ablation allowed rhythmologists and interventional electrophysiologists to better understand the mechanisms and management of arrhythmias. Despite the unprecedented technological advances in the diagnosis and management of cardiac arrhythmias, such as atrial fibrillation, epicardial ventricular tachycardias, and arrhythmias in congenital heard disease, challenges remain ahead.

The future lies in the noninvasive mapping and imaging in the diagnosis of cardiac arrhythmias, such as electrocardiographic imaging, in even a single cardiac beat to the noninvasive ablation techniques, such as noninvasive cardiac radiation and zero to near-zero fluoroscopy, to avoid radiation exposure.

We are pleased that the consulting editors of *Cardiac Electrophysiology Clinics*. Ranjan K. Thakur, MD, and Andrea Natale, MD, invited us to serve as editors for this important topic. In addition, we are delighted that a group of pioneers in the field of cardiac mapping and ablation has unanimously accepted our invitation to contribute their state-of-the-art articles for this and the next issue of *Cardiac Electrophysiology Clinics*, both on advances in cardiac mapping.

We initially planned to have a single issue dedicated to this topic. However, due to important topics that needed to be covered, we were obliged to include a 2-issue comprehensive review. Part 1 covers the basic concepts, including cardiac embryology and anatomy relevant to cardiac mapping and ablation, followed by novel mapping and imaging techniques, such as cardiac computed tomography and MRI, and catheter and energy sources. Part 2 discusses mapping and ablation of particular arrhythmias in specific substrates, such as atrial fibrillation, ventricular tachycardia, and fibrillation.

We are confident that these 2 issues on advances in cardiac mapping will be useful to clinical cardiac electrophysiologists, fellow trainees, attending, and allied professionals who participate in the management of patients with complex arrhythmias, and we hope that it improves patients' quality of life and survival.

Mohammad Shenasa, MD, PhD, FACC, FESC, FAHA, FHRS
Department of Cardiovascular Services
O'Connor Hospital
Heart and Rhythm Medical Group
105 North Bascome Avenue
San Jose, CA 95128, USA

Amin Al-Ahmad, MD, FHRS
Texas Cardiac Arrhythmia Institute
St David's Medical Center
Austin, TX 78705, USA

E-mail addresses:
mohammad.shenasa@gmail.com (M. Shenasa)
aalahmadmd@gmail.com (A. Al-Ahmad)

Card Electrophysiol Clin 11 (2019) xv
https://doi.org/10.1016/j.ccep.2019.09.001
1877-9182/19/© 2019 Published by Elsevier Inc.

cardiacEP.theclinics.com

New Findings in Atrial Fibrillation Mechanisms

Dennis H. Lau, MBBS, PhD, Dominik Linz, MD, PhD, Prashanthan Sanders, MBBS, PhD*

KEYWORDS

• Atrial fibrillation • Mechanism • Drivers • Catheter ablation • Remodeling

KEY POINTS

- Panoramic mapping studies of atrial fibrillation has unraveled drivers thought to sustain the arrhythmia; however, there are divergent findings on the electrophysiological properties of atrial fibrillation drivers.
- There has been increasing focus on epicardial adipose tissue as a novel substrate for atrial fibrillation with direct fatty infiltration in the contiguous atrial myocardium and paracrine effects leading to increased fibrosis.
- Simultaneous endo-epicardial mapping has shown a 3-dimensional atrial fibrillation substrate with dissociated electrical activations between the 2 layers that may account for most of the focal sources.
- Ongoing research on the complex electrostructural remodeling underlying atrial fibrillation will advance the field toward individualized and targeted therapy to modify the substrate responsible for atrial fibrillation perpetuation.

INTRODUCTION

The pathophysiologic mechanisms underlying atrial fibrillation (AF) are highly complex and variable among sufferers of this arrhythmia.[1,2] This can be attributable to the different risk factors fueling the adverse atrial remodeling process in the given individual to result in AF.[3] Yet, our current classification of AF remains rudimentary with focus on the clinical presentation according to the duration of AF episodes and the mode of termination, that poorly reflect the severity of the underlying atrial disease.[2] Beyond the traditional concept of reentry and multiple wavelet hypothesis as key AF sustaining mechanisms, our understanding of this complex arrhythmia has progressed significantly over the last decades. One important breakthrough was the identification of AF triggers originating from the myocardial sleeves of the pulmonary veins by Haissaguerre and colleagues.[4] Indeed, isolation of the pulmonary veins has remained as the cornerstone of catheter ablation procedures for AF, although the long-term success rates in patients with more advanced atrial remodeling remain suboptimal.[2,5]

Disclosure Statement: Dr Lau reports that the University of Adelaide has received on his behalf lecture and/or consulting fees from Abbott Medical, Bayer, Biotronik, BMS Pfizer, Boehringer Ingelheim and Medtronic. Dr Linz reports having served on the advisory board of LivaNova and Medtronic. Dr Linz reports having received lecture and/or consulting fees from LivaNova, Medtronic, and ResMed. Dr Linz reports having received research funding from Sanofi, ResMed and Medtronic. Dr Sanders reports having served on the advisory board of Boston Scientific, CathRx, Medtronic, Abbott Medical and Pacemate. Dr Sanders reports that the University of Adelaide has received on his behalf lecture and/or consulting fees from Medtronic, Boston-Scientific, and Abbott Medical. Dr Sanders reports that the University of Adelaide has received on his behalf research funding from Medtronic, Abbott Medical, Boston Scientific, and Microport.
Department of Cardiology, Centre for Heart Rhythm Disorders, University of Adelaide, Royal Adelaide Hospital, 1 Port Road, Adelaide, South Australia 5000, Australia
* Corresponding author.
E-mail address: prash.sanders@adelaide.edu.au

The progressive nature of AF calls for earlier intervention to improve outcomes and reduce complications.[6] Recent work on aggressive lifestyle and risk factor management has shown promising results in reversing AF progression and improved sinus rhythm maintenance, and the use of an integrated care approach in AF has been shown to decrease cardiovascular hospitalizations and all-cause mortality.[3,7–10] Current armamentarium to combat AF with antiarrhythmic drugs are limited by suboptimal efficacy and toxicity concerns, whereas invasive catheter ablation remains resource intensive with attrition in success over time despite decreasing complication rates.[11,12] Hopefully, advances in our understanding of AF mechanisms will pave the way toward more targeted and individualized therapy to modify the substrate responsible for AF perpetuation.[13] Here, we aim to focus on the novel findings in AF mechanisms derived from recent advances in cardiac mapping both from the bench and the bedside.

PANORAMIC MAPPING OF DRIVERS OF ATRIAL FIBRILLATION

It has long been recognized that pulmonary vein isolation alone is insufficient in patients with more advanced atrial remodeling. However, electrophysiologists have been confronted by the lack of efficacy of additional substrate-based ablation by means of linear lines and targeting of complex fractionated atrial electrograms (CFAE) in those with a persistent form of AF.[14] The demise of CFAE-based ablation may be attributed to inadequacy of the semiautomated CFAE algorithms and limitations of point-by-point CFAE mapping of a temporally unstable arrhythmia in AF.[15–17] Similarly, other efforts in identifying AF drivers, such as spectral analysis and dominant frequency mapping from AF electrograms obtained via point-by-point mapping, have shown promise from an initial retrospective study.[18] However, a prospective randomized trial using real-time frequency analysis to guide targeting of AF drivers failed to demonstrate incremental success.[19] It remains unclear if novel index that identifies temporally stable AF driver sites may yield different outcomes.[20]

Over the last decade, the field has shifted focus to panoramic mapping techniques that have identified 2 arrhythmic mechanisms of interest, namely, rotational (rotors) and ectopic focal activations as drivers of AF. However, these mapping techniques are not yet widely available or ready for prime time. The divergent mapping techniques and phase-based signal analysis algorithms used in these panoramic mapping studies have produced different findings and ablation outcomes as detailed elsewhere in this article (**Fig. 1**). Further, recent work demonstrated rotors detected by phase mapping to be of low specificity for identifying rotating wavefronts when compared with activation time mapping in high-density epicardial AF electrograms, because most of these rotors were found to be within close proximity to a line of conduction block.[21]

Focal Impulse Rotor Modulation

The focal impulse and rotor modulation (FIRM) technique uses 64-pole basket-type endocardial catheters (FIRMap, Abbott Electrophysiology, CA) to provide panoramic mapping of the atria (see **Fig. 1**).[22] It uses a proprietary phase-based signal processing algorithm to identify up to 3 rotors or focal sources in each patient that lasted for thousands of cycles.[23] Additional FIRM-guided ablation was shown to improve 3-year freedom from AF recurrence as compared with conventional pulmonary vein isolation alone after a mean of 1.2 procedures (77.8% vs 38.5%) in the initial series.[24] However, recent systematic reviews and meta-analyses of AF rotor and driver ablation have shown high variability in success rates that seem to be nonsuperior to conventional pulmonary vein ablation alone, whereas acute termination of AF to sinus rhythm or atrial tachycardia rate was less than 40%.[25–27] The discrepancy of these findings suggest several challenges with the FIRM-guided approach that may require a steeper operator-dependent learning curve, including electrode contact or coverage, low-density mapping, and analytical assumptions that the electrodes are evenly spaced over a 2-dimensional grid as opposed to the actual spread in 3-dimensional spatial orientation.[28–30] Larger, multicenter, prospectiv randomized, controlled trials are needed to delineate its utility in our armamentarium against AF.

Electrocardiographic Imaging

This mapping technique uses a body surface array of 252 electrodes to derive virtual potentials on the atrial epicardium with inverse-solution electrocardiographic imaging and geometric localization with thoracic computed tomography.[31,32] It identified up to 5 drivers in each persistent AF patient with predominance of such sources in the left atrium but the rotors were transient for several cycles only.[31,33] Electrocardiographic imaging-guided ablation of rotors and focal sources was shown to achieve similar results as pulmonary vein plus electrogram-guided ablation with advantage of shorter radiofrequency ablation time.[31] Subsequent multicenter experience demonstrated

	FIRM	ECGI
	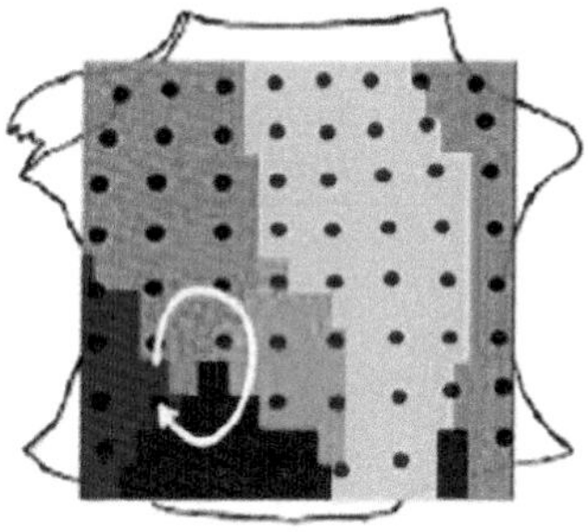	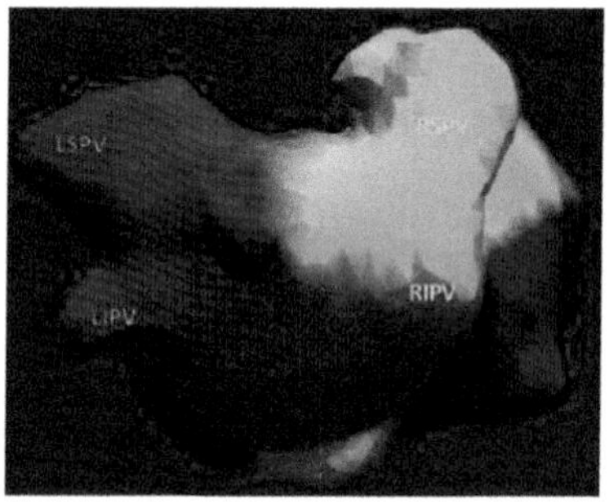
Mapping tool	64-electrode basket type catheter	252-electrode body surface vest
Contact mapping, Surface	Yes, Endocardial	No, Epicardial
Mapping window, Electrogram	Unknown, Unipolar and Bipolar	9s, Unipolar surface potentials
Signal processing algorithm	Phase mapping (proprietary)	Wavelet and phase mapping (proprietary)
No. of persistent AF patients studied (n)	>600	>200
Key Findings	• AF rotors/foci are sustained • Variable outcomes from meta-analysis • <40% acute AF termination	• AF Rotors/foci are transient • Favorable outcomes from multi-centre experience • 60–70% acute AF termination

Fig. 1. Panoramic mapping of AF. Differences between FIRM and electrocardiographic imaging mapping. (FIRM map image from Narayan SM, Baykaner T, Clopton P, et al. Ablation of rotor and focal sources reduces late recurrence of atrial fibrillation compared with trigger ablation alone: extended follow-up of the CONFIRM trial (Conventional Ablation for Atrial Fibrillation With or Without Focal Impulse and Rotor Modulation). J Am Coll Cardiol. 2014;63(17):1761-1768; with permission; and ECGI map from Lim HS, Hocini M, Dubois R, et al. Complexity and Distribution of Drivers in Relation to Duration of Persistent Atrial Fibrillation. J Am Coll Cardiol. 2017;69(10):1257-1269; with permission.)

77% of the patients with persistent AF were free from AF at the 1-year follow-up.[33] Interestingly, this modality was able to terminate AF in 60% to 70% of the cases.[33,34] However, there remain several limitations with this technique, including the inability to map regions such as the interatrial septum and the left atrial appendage ridge, as well as a decreased sensitivity to detect low-amplitude signals.

Other Mapping Techniques

The CARTOFINDER mapping technique uses the CARTO 3-D electroanatomic mapping system (Biosense, Webster, CA), where unipolar electrograms acquired with a mapping catheter (64-electrode basket-type or PentaRay) were automatically annotated to determine focal activation using QS patterns and rotational activations using sequential activation gradients.[35] Several earlier reports also used Hilbert phase-based or dominant frequency analysis.[36,37] This technique yielded up to 6 AF drivers per patient, but such sources were found to be transient and lasting only several cycles.[35,37] This technology remains in the development phase with outcome data awaited. There is limited experience with panoramic endocardial noncontact mapping using the Ensite multielectrode array catheter (St Jude Medical, MN).[38,39] This technique allows recording of virtual unipolar electrograms that are superimposed onto the 3-dimensional (3-D) atrial geometry to display wavefront propagation as animated isopotential color maps. Investigators using this setup were able to record transient rotors in 1 study; no focal sources were seen in another.[38,39]

MAPPING THE ATRIAL FIBRILLATION SUBSTRATE

A large body of translational research over more than a century has helped to shape the current clinical practice in cardiac electrophysiology.[40] Here, we highlight key research studies in the mapping of AF mechanisms in relationship to the underlying atrial substrate.

Atrial Fibrosis

Atrial structural remodeling has been recognized to contribute to the perpetuation of AF since the description of atrial fibrosis and the resultant conduction slowing and increased conduction heterogeneity in experimental model of heart failure at the turn of the century.[41] These changes have subsequently been reported to occur in both experimental and clinical studies of various AF risk factors, including hypertension, obesity, obstructive sleep apnea, diabetes mellitus, metabolic syndrome, heart failure, valvular heart disease, and endurance training.[42–55] Despite several positive experimental studies on antifibrotic drug therapy, there remains a lack of translational work to advance this treatment paradigm to clinical use.[56] The atrial fibrosis contributes to AF persistence through discontinuous conduction that favors reentry or preferential conduction as well as anchoring of AF drivers.[57] Advances in late gadolinium-enhanced (LGE) MRI have afforded a noninvasive mean of assessing atrial fibrosis. Initial studies in small numbers of patients failed to demonstrate a significant association between AF drivers and the extent or location of LGE detected fibrosis.[58,59] However, in a more recent study with more included subjects and a different phase mapping algorithm, electrocardiographic imaging detected AF drivers were found to cluster around the borders of fibrotic areas as detected by LGE-MRI and the driver regions demonstrated higher density of LGE than nondriver regions.[60] The contrasting results may also be accounted for by the technical challenges with LGE-MRI, including spatial resolution, motion artifact, and the quantitation of LGE, which can be algorithm dependent.[61] Nevertheless, atrial fibrosis quantified by LGE-MRI has been associated with increased AF recurrence in those undergoing catheter ablation.[62] A large prospective randomized trial is underway to examine whether additional targeting of LGE-MRI detected atrial fibrotic regions by catheter ablation will improve ablation outcome (DECAAF-II, NCT02529319).

Epicardial Adipose Tissue and Fatty Infiltration

The epicardial adipose tissue (EAT) is closely approximated to the myocardium without fascia separation and in recent years there has been an increasing focus on its role in AF pathogenesis.[63] Computed tomography or MRI-derived EAT volume has been associated with increased risk of developing AF, AF persistence, and post-ablation recurrences independent of other measures of adiposity.[64–66] Notably, the strength of the association between AF and EAT seems to be stronger than with abdominal or overall adiposity.[67] The pathogenicity of EAT on adverse atrial structural remodeling can be a result of its paracrine effects, leading to increased fibrosis or direct fatty infiltration in the contiguous atrial myocardium (**Fig. 2**).[46,68,69] Electroanatomic mapping has confirmed more pronounced changes with larger low-voltage areas in the posterior and inferior left atrium that are adjacent to the posteriorly located increased EAT seen on MRI (**Fig. 2**D).[47] Further, left atrial EAT demonstrated a better correlation with electrogram fractionation and conduction slowing than body mass index.[47] These mounting evidence on the role of EAT and fatty infiltration on atrial electrostructural remodeling call for further studies to evaluate targeted ablation strategy, such as posterior left atrial isolation and to delineate the pathobiology of EAT to guide development of novel therapeutics.

Endoepicardial Dissociation

Simultaneous mapping of the endocardium and epicardium in isolated atrium has elegantly demonstrated discordant activation times that correlated with the underlying anatomic heterogeneity decennia ago.[70] Subsequent in vivo simultaneous endo-epicardial mapping confirmed significant electrical dissociation that constitute a complex 3-D atrial substrate during experimental AF.[71] Similarly, endo-epicardial dissociation has been shown in human AF that are thought to sustain the arrhythmia with breakthrough waves from the opposite layers.[72] Importantly, these studies have shown that majority of focal sources during AF are not due to ectopic activity and can be explained by endo-epicardial activation that increases with increasing underlying substrate complexity.[72,73] Further, advanced multimodality

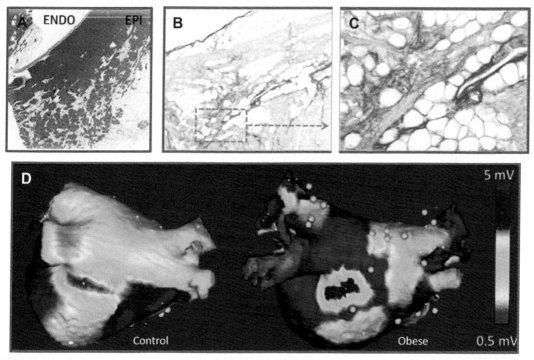

Fig. 2. Epicardial adipose tissue and atrial remodeling. (A) Hematoxylin and eosin staining of posterior left atrial wall in obese sheep showing fatty infiltration from epicardial adipose tissue (*blue arrow* shows fat cell infiltration). (B, C) Picrosirius red staining of human atrial myocardium. Magnified section in C shows adipocytes infiltration surrounded with fibrosis. (D) Human left atrial voltage maps from control (*left*) and obese subjects (*right*). The obese atrium demonstrates increased low voltage areas in the posterior and inferior walls (*red*) as well as more sites with electrogram fractionation (*pink*) and double potentials (*blue*). (*From* [A] Mahajan R, Lau DH, Brooks AG, et al. Electrophysiological, Electroanatomical, and Structural Remodeling of the Atria as Consequences of Sustained Obesity. *J Am Coll Cardiol.* 2015;66(1):1-11; [B, C] Hatem SN, Sanders P. Epicardial adipose tissue and atrial fibrillation. *Cardiovasc Res.* 2014;102(2):205-213; and [D] Mahajan R, Nelson A, Pathak RK, et al. Electroanatomical Remodeling of the Atria in Obesity: Impact of Adjacent Epicardial Fat. *JACC Clin Electrophysiol.* 2018;4(12):1529-1540; with permission.)

mapping using near-infrared optical mapping, FIRM contact mapping, and 3-D contrast-enhanced MRI scans in coronary-perfused explanted human hearts have demonstrated that intramural micro-entry may account for the rotors and focal sources seen with clinical panoramic mapping.[74] However, the challenge remains on how sophisticated endo-epicardial substrate mapping is clinically feasible to guide specific ablation strategy at sites with endo-epicardial dissociation.

Electrogram-Based Substrate Mapping: Technical Considerations

The current standard mapping approach involves 3-D electroanatomic voltage mapping to identify areas of low voltage or regions with increased electrogram fractionation. Low-voltage areas (typically <0.5 mV during sinus rhythm) in the atrium have been associated with endocardial

scar and/or structural defects although the threshold can vary with rhythm change. Several multielectrode mapping catheters are currently in use for detailed high density electroanatomic mapping (**Fig. 3**). These catheters have 16 to 64 electrodes and different interelectrode spacing. Generally, local bipolar electrogram are used as they are less prone to far-field potentials but naturally depend on bipolar vector orientation and interelectrode spacing.[16] Additionally, contact force may impact electrogram characteristics, although this information is unavailable in multipolar mapping catheters.[75] Owing to the layout and design of the respective catheters in relation to the atrial size, some anatomic regions can be difficult to access for mapping (see **Fig. 3**). Finally, clinical mapping is often limited by a relatively short recording time periods (often for 5–10 seconds), which may be insufficient to characterize the dynamic nature of the arrhythmia.

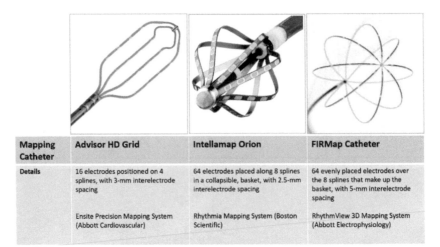

Mapping Catheter	Advisor HD Grid	Intellamap Orion	FIRMap Catheter
Details	16 electrodes positioned on 4 splines, with 3-mm interelectrode spacing	64 electrodes placed along 8 splines in a collapsible, basket, with 2.5-mm interelectrode spacing	64 evenly placed electrodes over the 8 splines that make up the basket, with 5-mm interelectrode spacing
	Ensite Precision Mapping System (Abbott Cardiovascular)	Rhythmia Mapping System (Boston Scientific)	RhythmView 3D Mapping System (Abbott Electrophysiology)

Fig. 3. Multipolar mapping catheters. (Advisor™ HD Grid Mapping Catheter, Sensor Enabled™ image courtesy of Abbott Electrophysiology, Abbott Park, IL; Intellamap Orion image provided courtesy of Boston Scientific. ©2019 Boston Scientific Corporation or its affiliates. All rights reserved; and FIRMap®, RhythmView® image courtesy of Abbott Electrophysiology, Abbott Park, IL.)

SUMMARY

Recent advances in cardiac mapping technology have unraveled new understandings of the complex substrate and drivers underlying AF. The ability to identify new putative mechanisms amenable to more focal catheter ablation approaches is highly attractive. Ongoing research efforts will hopefully bring to fruition individualized and targeted therapy to modify the substrate responsible for AF perpetuation. Meanwhile, electrophysiologists must integrate aggressive lifestyle and risk factor management as the fourth pillar of AF care given the established evidence of its role in improving AF outcomes, underpinned by reverse atrial remodeling.

ACKNOWLEDGMENTS

Sources of Funding: Dr Lau is supported by a Fellowship from The Hospital Research Foundation. Dr Linz is supported by a Beacon Fellowship from the University of Adelaide. Dr Sanders is supported by a Practitioner Fellowship from the National Health and Medical Research Council of Australia and the National Heart Foundation of Australia.

REFERENCES

1. Schotten U, Verheule S, Kirchhof P, et al. Pathophysiological mechanisms of atrial fibrillation: a translational appraisal. Physiol Rev 2011;91(1): 265–325.
2. Lau DH, Linz D, Schotten U, et al. Pathophysiology of paroxysmal and persistent atrial fibrillation: rotors, foci and fibrosis. Heart Lung Circ 2017;26(9): 887–93.
3. Lau DH, Nattel S, Kalman JM, et al. Modifiable risk factors and atrial fibrillation. Circulation 2017; 136(6):583–96.
4. Haissaguerre M, Jais P, Shah DC, et al. Spontaneous initiation of atrial fibrillation by ectopic beats originating in the pulmonary veins. N Engl J Med 1998;339(10):659–66.
5. Clarnette JA, Brooks AG, Mahajan R, et al. Outcomes of persistent and long-standing persistent atrial fibrillation ablation: a systematic review and meta-analysis. Europace 2018;20(FI_3): f366–76.
6. Nattel S, Guasch E, Savelieva I, et al. Early management of atrial fibrillation to prevent cardiovascular complications. Eur Heart J 2014;35(22):1448–56.
7. Gallagher C, Elliott AD, Wong CX, et al. Integrated care in atrial fibrillation: a systematic review and meta-analysis. Heart 2017;103(24):1947–53.
8. Pathak RK, Middeldorp ME, Lau DH, et al. Aggressive risk factor reduction study for atrial fibrillation and implications for the outcome of ablation: the ARREST-AF cohort study. J Am Coll Cardiol 2014; 64(21):2222–31.
9. Pathak RK, Middeldorp ME, Meredith M, et al. Long-term effect of goal-directed weight management in an atrial fibrillation cohort: a long-term follow-up study (LEGACY). J Am Coll Cardiol 2015;65(20): 2159–69.
10. Middeldorp ME, Pathak RK, Meredith M, et al. PREVEntion and regReSsive Effect of weight-loss and risk factor modification on Atrial Fibrillation: the REVERSE-AF study. Europace 2018;20(12): 1929–35.

11. Gupta A, Perera T, Ganesan A, et al. Complications of catheter ablation of atrial fibrillation: a systematic review. Circ Arrhythm Electrophysiol 2013;6(6): 1082–8.

12. Ganesan AN, Shipp NJ, Brooks AG, et al. Long-term outcomes of catheter ablation of atrial fibrillation: a systematic review and meta-analysis. J Am Heart Assoc 2013;2(2):e004549.

13. Lau DH, Schotten U, Mahajan R, et al. Novel mechanisms in the pathogenesis of atrial fibrillation: practical applications. Eur Heart J 2016;37(20):1573–81.

14. Verma A, Jiang CY, Betts TR, et al. Approaches to catheter ablation for persistent atrial fibrillation. N Engl J Med 2015;372(19):1812–22.

15. Lau DH, Maesen B, Zeemering S, et al. Stability of complex fractionated atrial electrograms: a systematic review. J Cardiovasc Electrophysiol 2012; 23(9):980–7.

16. Lau DH, Maesen B, Zeemering S, et al. Indices of bipolar complex fractionated atrial electrograms correlate poorly with each other and atrial fibrillation substrate complexity. Heart Rhythm 2015;12(7): 1415–23.

17. Stiles MK, Sanders P, Lau DH. Targeting the substrate in ablation of persistent atrial fibrillation: recent lessons and future directions. Front Physiol 2018;9: 1158.

18. Sanders P, Berenfeld O, Hocini M, et al. Spectral analysis identifies sites of high-frequency activity maintaining atrial fibrillation in humans. Circulation 2005;112(6):789–97.

19. Atienza F, Almendral J, Ormaetxe JM, et al. Comparison of radiofrequency catheter ablation of drivers and circumferential pulmonary vein isolation in atrial fibrillation: a noninferiority randomized multicenter RADAR-AF trial. J Am Coll Cardiol 2014;64(23): 2455–67.

20. Kimata A, Yokoyama Y, Aita S, et al. Temporally stable frequency mapping using continuous wavelet transform analysis in patients with persistent atrial fibrillation. J Cardiovasc Electrophysiol 2018;29(4): 514–22.

21. Podziemski P, Zeemering S, Kuklik P, et al. Rotors detected by phase Analysis of filtered, epicardial atrial fibrillation electrograms colocalize with regions of conduction block. Circ Arrhythm Electrophysiol 2018;11(10):e005858.

22. Narayan SM, Krummen DE, Shivkumar K, et al. Treatment of atrial fibrillation by the ablation of localized sources: CONFIRM (conventional ablation for atrial fibrillation with or without focal impulse and rotor modulation) trial. J Am Coll Cardiol 2012; 60(7):628–36.

23. Swarup V, Baykaner T, Rostamian A, et al. Stability of rotors and focal sources for human atrial fibrillation: focal impulse and rotor mapping (FIRM) of AF sources and fibrillatory conduction. J Cardiovasc Electrophysiol 2014;25(12):1284–92.

24. Narayan SM, Baykaner T, Clopton P, et al. Ablation of rotor and focal sources reduces late recurrence of atrial fibrillation compared with trigger ablation alone: extended follow-up of the CONFIRM trial (Conventional Ablation for Atrial Fibrillation with or without Focal Impulse and Rotor Modulation). J Am Coll Cardiol 2014;63(17):1761–8.

25. Parameswaran R, Voskoboinik A, Gorelik A, et al. Clinical impact of rotor ablation in atrial fibrillation: a systematic review. Europace 2018;20(7):1099–106.

26. Baykaner T, Rogers AJ, Meckler GL, et al. Clinical implications of ablation of drivers for atrial fibrillation: a systematic review and meta-analysis. Circ Arrhythm Electrophysiol 2018;11(5):e006119.

27. Mohanty S, Mohanty P, Trivedi C, et al. Long-term outcome of pulmonary vein isolation with and without focal impulse and rotor modulation mapping: insights from a meta-analysis. Circ Arrhythm Electrophysiol 2018;11(3):e005789.

28. Pathik B, Kalman JM, Walters T, et al. Absence of rotational activity detected using 2-dimensional phase mapping in the corresponding 3-dimensional phase maps in human persistent atrial fibrillation. Heart Rhythm 2018;15(2):182–92.

29. Walters TE, Lee G, Spence S, et al. The effect of electrode density on the interpretation of atrial activation patterns in epicardial mapping of human persistent atrial fibrillation. Heart Rhythm 2016; 13(6):1215–20.

30. Kuklik P, Zeemering S, van Hunnik A, et al. Identification of rotors during human atrial fibrillation using contact mapping and phase singularity detection: technical considerations. IEEE Trans Biomed Eng 2017;64(2):310–8.

31. Haissaguerre M, Hocini M, Denis A, et al. Driver domains in persistent atrial fibrillation. Circulation 2014; 130(7):530–8.

32. Cuculich PS, Wang Y, Lindsay BD, et al. Noninvasive characterization of epicardial activation in humans with diverse atrial fibrillation patterns. Circulation 2010;122(14):1364–72.

33. Knecht S, Sohal M, Deisenhofer I, et al. Multicentre evaluation of non-invasive biatrial mapping for persistent atrial fibrillation ablation: the AFACART study. Europace 2017;19(8):1302–9.

34. Lim HS, Hocini M, Dubois R, et al. Complexity and distribution of drivers in relation to duration of persistent atrial fibrillation. J Am Coll Cardiol 2017;69(10): 1257–69.

35. Verma A, Sarkozy A, Skanes A, et al. Characterization and significance of localized sources identified by a novel automated algorithm during mapping of human persistent atrial fibrillation. J Cardiovasc Electrophysiol 2018;29(11):1480–8.

36. Calvo D, Rubin J, Perez D, et al. Ablation of rotor domains effectively modulates dynamics of human: long-standing persistent atrial fibrillation. Circ Arrhythm Electrophysiol 2017;10(12) [pii:e005740].

37. Honarbakhsh S, Schilling RJ, Dhillon G, et al. A novel mapping system for panoramic mapping of the left atrium: application to detect and characterize localized sources maintaining atrial fibrillation. JACC Clin Electrophysiol 2018;4(1):124–34.

38. Yamabe H, Kanazawa H, Ito M, et al. Prevalence and mechanism of rotor activation identified during atrial fibrillation by noncontact mapping: lack of evidence for a role in the maintenance of atrial fibrillation. Heart Rhythm 2016;13(12):2323–30.

39. Lee G, McLellan AJ, Hunter RJ, et al. Panoramic characterization of endocardial left atrial activation during human persistent AF: insights from noncontact mapping. Int J Cardiol 2017;228:406–11.

40. Lau DH, Volders PG, Kohl P, et al. Opportunities and challenges of current electrophysiology research: a plea to establish 'translational electrophysiology' curricula. Europace 2015;17(5):825–33.

41. Li D, Fareh S, Leung TK, et al. Promotion of atrial fibrillation by heart failure in dogs: atrial remodeling of a different sort. Circulation 1999;100(1): 87–95.

42. Lau DH, Mackenzie L, Kelly DJ, et al. Hypertension and atrial fibrillation: evidence of progressive atrial remodeling with electrostructural correlate in a conscious chronically instrumented ovine model. Heart Rhythm 2010;7(9):1282–90.

43. Lau DH, Shipp NJ, Kelly DJ, et al. Atrial arrhythmia in ageing spontaneously hypertensive rats: unraveling the substrate in hypertension and ageing. PLoS One 2013;8(8):e72416.

44. Medi C, Kalman JM, Spence SJ, et al. Atrial electrical and structural changes associated with long-standing hypertension in humans: implications for the substrate for atrial fibrillation. J Cardiovasc Electrophysiol 2011;22(12):1317–24.

45. Abed HS, Samuel CS, Lau DH, et al. Obesity results in progressive atrial structural and electrical remodeling: implications for atrial fibrillation. Heart Rhythm 2013;10(1):90–100.

46. Mahajan R, Lau DH, Brooks AG, et al. Electrophysiological, electroanatomical, and structural remodeling of the atria as Consequences of sustained obesity. J Am Coll Cardiol 2015;66(1):1–11.

47. Mahajan R, Nelson A, Pathak RK, et al. Electroanatomical remodeling of the atria in obesity: impact of adjacent epicardial fat. JACC Clin Electrophysiol 2018;4(12):1529–40.

48. Dimitri H, Ng M, Brooks AG, et al. Atrial remodeling in obstructive sleep apnea: implications for atrial fibrillation. Heart Rhythm 2012;9(3):321–7.

49. Iwasaki YK, Kato T, Xiong F, et al. Atrial fibrillation promotion with long-term repetitive obstructive sleep apnea in a rat model. J Am Coll Cardiol 2014;64(19): 2013–23.

50. Linz D, Hohl M, Dhein S, et al. Cathepsin A mediates susceptibility to atrial tachyarrhythmia and impairment of atrial emptying function in Zucker diabetic fatty rats. Cardiovasc Res 2016;110(3): 371–80.

51. Hohl M, Lau DH, Muller A, et al. Concomitant obesity and metabolic syndrome add to the atrial arrhythmogenic phenotype in male hypertensive rats. J Am Heart Assoc 2017;6(9) [pii:e006717].

52. Lau DH, Psaltis PJ, Mackenzie L, et al. Atrial remodeling in an ovine model of anthracycline-induced nonischemic cardiomyopathy: remodeling of the same sort. J Cardiovasc Electrophysiol 2011;22(2): 175–82.

53. Sanders P, Morton JB, Davidson NC, et al. Electrical remodeling of the atria in congestive heart failure: electrophysiological and electroanatomic mapping in humans. Circulation 2003;108(12):1461–8.

54. John B, Stiles MK, Kuklik P, et al. Electrical remodelling of the left and right atria due to rheumatic mitral stenosis. Eur Heart J 2008;29(18):2234–43.

55. Guasch E, Benito B, Qi X, et al. Atrial fibrillation promotion by endurance exercise: demonstration and mechanistic exploration in an animal model. J Am Coll Cardiol 2013;62(1):68–77.

56. Thanigaimani S, Lau DH, Agbaedeng T, et al. Molecular mechanisms of atrial fibrosis: implications for the clinic. Expert Rev Cardiovasc Ther 2017;15(4): 247–56.

57. Maesen B, Zeemering S, Afonso C, et al. Rearrangement of atrial bundle architecture and consequent changes in anisotropy of conduction constitute the 3-dimensional substrate for atrial fibrillation. Circ Arrhythm Electrophysiol 2013;6(5):967–75.

58. Chrispin J, Gucuk Ipek E, Zahid S, et al. Lack of regional association between atrial late gadolinium enhancement on cardiac magnetic resonance and atrial fibrillation rotors. Heart Rhythm 2016;13(3): 654–60.

59. Sohns C, Lemes C, Metzner A, et al. First-in-Man analysis of the relationship between electrical rotors from noninvasive panoramic mapping and atrial fibrosis from magnetic resonance imaging in patients with persistent atrial fibrillation. Circ Arrhythm Electrophysiol 2017;10(8) [pii:e004419].

60. Cochet H, Dubois R, Yamashita S, et al. Relationship between fibrosis detected on late gadolinium-enhanced cardiac magnetic resonance and Re-entrant activity assessed with electrocardiographic imaging in human persistent atrial fibrillation. JACC Clin Electrophysiol 2018;4(1):17–29.

61. Karim R, Housden RJ, Balasubramaniam M, et al. Evaluation of current algorithms for segmentation of scar tissue from late gadolinium enhancement cardiovascular magnetic resonance of the left

atrium: an open-access grand challenge. J Cardiovasc Magn Reson 2013;15:105.

62. Marrouche NF, Wilber D, Hindricks G, et al. Association of atrial tissue fibrosis identified by delayed enhancement MRI and atrial fibrillation catheter ablation: the DECAAF study. JAMA 2014;311(5): 498–506.

63. Hatem SN, Sanders P. Epicardial adipose tissue and atrial fibrillation. Cardiovasc Res 2014;102(2): 205–13.

64. Batal O, Schoenhagen P, Shao M, et al. Left atrial epicardial adiposity and atrial fibrillation. Circ Arrhythm Electrophysiol 2010;3(3):230–6.

65. Thanassoulis G, Massaro JM, O'Donnell CJ, et al. Pericardial fat is associated with prevalent atrial fibrillation: the Framingham Heart Study. Circ Arrhythm Electrophysiol 2010;3(4):345–50.

66. Wong CX, Abed HS, Molaee P, et al. Pericardial fat is associated with atrial fibrillation severity and ablation outcome. J Am Coll Cardiol 2011; 57(17):1745–51.

67. Wong CX, Sun MT, Odutayo A, et al. Associations of epicardial, abdominal, and overall adiposity with atrial fibrillation. Circ Arrhythm Electrophysiol 2016; 9(12) [pii:e004378].

68. Venteclef N, Guglielmi V, Balse E, et al. Human epicardial adipose tissue induces fibrosis of the atrial myocardium through the secretion of adipo-fibrokines. Eur Heart J 2015;36(13):795–805a.

69. Haemers P, Hamdi H, Guedj K, et al. Atrial fibrillation is associated with the fibrotic remodelling of adipose tissue in the subepicardium of human and sheep atria. Eur Heart J 2017;38(1):53–61.

70. Schuessler RB, Kawamoto T, Hand DE, et al. Simultaneous epicardial and endocardial activation sequence mapping in the isolated canine right atrium. Circulation 1993;88(1):250–63.

71. Eckstein J, Maesen B, Linz D, et al. Time course and mechanisms of endo-epicardial electrical dissociation during atrial fibrillation in the goat. Cardiovasc Res 2011;89(4):816–24.

72. de Groot N, van der Does L, Yaksh A, et al. Direct proof of endo-epicardial asynchrony of the atrial wall during atrial fibrillation in humans. Circ Arrhythm Electrophysiol 2016;9(5) [pii:e003648].

73. Eckstein J, Zeemering S, Linz D, et al. Transmural conduction is the predominant mechanism of breakthrough during atrial fibrillation: evidence from simultaneous endo-epicardial high-density activation mapping. Circ Arrhythm Electrophysiol 2013;6(2): 334–41.

74. Hansen BJ, Zhao J, Li N, et al. Human atrial fibrillation drivers resolved with integrated functional and structural imaging to benefit clinical mapping. JACC Clin Electrophysiol 2018;4(12): 1501–15.

75. Ullah W, Hunter RJ, Baker V, et al. Impact of catheter contact force on human left atrial electrogram characteristics in sinus rhythm and atrial fibrillation. Circ Arrhythm Electrophysiol 2015;8(5): 1030–9.

Postablation Atrial Arrhythmias

Suraj Kapa, MD

KEYWORDS

- Atrial fibrillation • Atrial arrhythmias • Cardiac mapping • Cardiac ablation • Atrial tachycardia
- Atrial flutter

KEY POINTS

- Atrial arrhythmia recurrence after prior atrial fibrillation ablation may include recurrent fibrillation, focal tachycardia, or microreentrant or macroreentrant atrial flutters.
- Mechanism of recurrent arrhythmias may include new substrate created by prior ablation or already present substrate associated with atrial myopathy.
- Mapping and ablation of postablation arrhythmias includes induction of arrhythmias, recognition of mechanism, and correlation with activation/substrate mapping.
- Ablation of postablation atrial arrhythmias can be highly successful but needs to be balanced against potential risk of stiff left atrial syndrome.

INTRODUCTION

Atrial fibrillation ablation has become a mainstay of therapy since its first description in the 1980s. The approach to ablation generally consists of pulmonary vein isolation but may include targeting of nonpulmonary vein triggers. Depending on the underlying disease state, initial success rates for ablation may vary from 40% to 80%, according to most studies over intermediate term (3–5 year) follow-up.[1] The most common cause of recurrence after prior ablation presents as atrial fibrillation, although incident atrial tachycardia or atrial flutter related to both previously existing and newly created substrate also may be seen. The mechanisms for such arrhythmias may include focal tachycardias not identified at prior ablation, microreentrant atrial flutters, and macroreentry engaging larger areas of scar.

The approach to recognition, treatment, and mapping may vary between patients. Furthermore, the approach to treatment may vary between arrhythmia type (focal vs reentrant) as well as the underlying substrate (extensive vs limited) and nature of coexisting myopathies (such as hypertrophic cardiomyopathy vs structurally normal heart). This review focuses on the incidence and mechanisms for such postablation arrhythmias, the approach to nonablative and ablative treatment, and current considerations in approach to mapping and ablation.

INCIDENCE AND MECHANISM OF POSTABLATION ATRIAL ARRHYTHMIAS

In the first 6 weeks to 3 months after prior atrial fibrillation ablation (also referred to as the blanking period), it is not uncommon to have arrhythmia recurrence. Mechanisms for recurrence vary and are thought to include in part the gradual reduction in inflammation incurred by the prior ablation procedure. Thus, generally, incident arrhythmias are treated conservatively via a combination of cardioversion, β-blockers/calcium channel blockers, and antiarrhythmic drugs. In cases of organized arrhythmias that are recurrent, persistent, and

Disclosure Statement: The author has no disclosures relevant to this article.
Department of Cardiovascular Diseases, Mayo Clinic College of Medicine, 200 First Street Southwest, Rochester, MN 55905, USA
E-mail address: kapa.suraj@mayo.edu

Card Electrophysiol Clin 11 (2019) 573–582
https://doi.org/10.1016/j.ccep.2019.08.008
1877-9182/19/© 2019 Elsevier Inc. All rights reserved.

thought to reflect a potentially more persistent substrate, however, it may be reasonable to consider earlier ablation. Early reablation has been associated with reduced likelihood of future recurrences, although studies are limited.[2,3] Decisions to reablate early often are case dependent and require careful consideration of the ablation previously performed, the clinical condition of the patient, and whether there are single or multiple arrhythmia foci on the basis of electrocardiographic follow-up.

Long-term postablation (ie, >3 months) patients may present with recurrent atrial fibrillation, atrial tachycardia, or atrial flutter. Rates of recurrence may vary depending on patient-specific considerations, with higher recurrence seen in those with more extensive atrial fibrosis at baseline, with persistent atrial fibrillation, or with more underlying comorbidities or specific myopathic processes, such as hypertrophic cardiomyopathy, sarcoidosis, amyloidosis, and so forth.[4-8] These 3 considerations overlap considerably, because those patients with underlying comorbidities, such as diabetes or hypertension, or other myopathic processes as well as those with more persistent atrial fibrillation generally have more extensive atrial fibrosis. Thus, counseling on likelihood of recurrence of an atrial arrhythmia may be directly impacted by preablation patient characteristics or testing, including magnetic resonance imaging (MRI).

Reasons for postablation atrial arrhythmias beyond the blanking period may include arrhythmias previously present but not specifically targeted, recurrence of prior targeted arrhythmias due to procedural failure or recurrent conduction across previous areas of ablation, new substrate created from prior ablation, and progression in the underlying atrial myopathy leading to new proarrhythmic substrate. Differentiating these mechanisms may be difficult due to changes in normal cardiac activation that may lead to the inability to use P-wave morphology alone to localize arrhythmia site of origin.[9] Postablation atrial arrhythmias may be less, similarly, or more symptomatic, however, than the previously ablated atrial fibrillation, depending on ventricular rate.

APPROACH TO NONABLATIVE MANAGEMENT

In the blanking period postablation, it is not uncommon to use antiarrhythmic drugs due to their efficacy in suppressing incident arrhythmias that may not necessarily predict long-term recurrence. Prospective clinical trials and large, observational retrospective studies have supported the use of antiarrhythmic drugs early postablation in reducing these incident postablative arrhythmias.[10,11] Decisions to use a drug may vary, however, and be considered in the context of a patient's ability to tolerate the medication. Often, medications that previously failed to offer sufficient arrhythmia control may be more effective postablation. In cases of atrial fibrillation, tachycardia, or flutter recurring in the blanking period and a patient not yet on an antiarrhythmic drug or already on 1 drug, adjustment of pharmacologic therapy may be warranted. In cases of persistent arrhythmias, however, adjustment of pharmacologic therapy may need to be coupled with cardioversion.

In the long-term postablation, pharmacologic therapy may be approached similarly to prior to ablation, with special considerations given to potential differences in arrhythmia mechanism. Although class IC antiarrhythmics may be more effective for triggered atrial fibrillation, postablation, substrate-related arrhythmias, including microreentrant and macroreentrant atrial flutters, may be more effectively treated with class III antiarrhythmics. Consideration of patient tolerance and need for hospitalization may inform the selection of a specific agent.

PATHOPHYSIOLOGIC CONSIDERATIONS

Incident postablation arrhythmias may be due to any number of causes, as discussed previously. This article considers several different mechanisms and how they may inform decisions on therapy:

1. Previously existing arrhythmias not targeted at ablation: due to limitations of monitoring, coexisting arrhythmias (such as atrial fibrillation with atrial tachycardia and atrial flutter with atrial fibrillation) may not necessarily be identified prior to ablation. Anesthesia and ablation approach may be informed, however, by the type of arrhythmia being ablated—for example, general anesthesia and pulmonary vein isolation for atrial fibrillation or mild to moderate sedation with targeted ablation for atrial flutter or atrial tachycardia. Deeper anesthesia or not performing an induction protocol may make coexisting arrhythmias inapparent at the time of atrial fibrillation ablation, and lack of preoperative recognition may lead to not targeting that specific arrhythmia.[12] This is of particular importance in focal atrial tachycardias, which may not be easily inducible at the time of electrophysiology study.

2. Arrhythmogenic sites not identified at the time of index ablation: although pulmonary vein isolation is the mainstay of atrial fibrillation ablation, nonpulmonary vein triggers are not uncommon.[13,14] Trigger protocols (including isoproterenol, burst pacing, and programmed stimulation) may be used at the time of ablation but nonpulmonary vein arrhythmogenic sites may not manifest. In general, clinical studies have not supported empiric isolation of other structures, such as the superior vena cava, left atrial appendage, and ligament of Marshall.[15]

3. Recurrence of targeted arrhythmias: one of the main limitations in current ablation is durability of the lesion set. Specifically, even in the presence of acute isolation, it is not uncommon to experience recurrent conduction across previous lines of block leading to arrhythmia recurrence. This reconduction may be seen in greater than 40% of patients, although not always associated with arrhythmia recurrence.[16] Mechanisms for reconnection across lines of block may include myocardial stunning or edema that may settle over the course of hours to weeks after ablation.

4. Creation of new substrate postablation: the hallmark of any ablation procedure is the creation of scar to isolate or eliminate proarrhythmic sites or sources. In this process, however, scar is created. Depending on the nature of the surrounding atrial substrate, proximity of lesion sets, and extent of ablation performed, new slow conduction zones may be created that may facilitate microreentrant or macroreentrant flutters. Identification of proarrhythmic substrate may be facilitated by postablation mapping at the time of the index ablation but is not universally productive.

5. Evolution of atrial substrate over long-term follow-up: although substrate may be created by the ablation procedure itself, it also is possible for the atrial substrate to evolve over long-term follow-up. This nonfixed nature of atrial fibrosis may contribute to future new sites of origin, which could not have been appreciated at the time of prior ablation.[17]

CONSIDERATIONS PRIOR TO REPEAT ABLATION

In addition to considering the duration since prior ablation, the following should be considered:

1. Extent of prior ablation: after multiple prior ablations or after extensive ablation, the risk of stiff left atrial syndrome increases.[18] Thus, the ability to successfully eliminate all possible arrhythmia sources should be balanced against the complication risk of causing such extensive left atrial injury as to impair normal contractility. The likelihood of stiff left atrial syndrome is generally low after limited prior ablation, such as with pulmonary vein isolation alone. Preablative discussion of this possibility, however, is important prior to proceeding with repeat ablation.

2. Number of postablative arrhythmias: whether a patient is presenting with 1 consistent atrial tachycardia or flutter or multiple is of additional importance because it may have an impact on the likelihood of ablation success. In cases of a single arrhythmia, a targeted approach to arrhythmia induction, matching to the clinically documented arrhythmia, and assuring successful elimination or blocking of the circuit are critical. In the case of multiple arrhythmias, this may have an impact on ablation success rates.

3. Drivers of arrhythmia: consideration of how the arrhythmia is triggered may facilitate follow-up ablation. Specifically, arrhythmias triggered solely by exercise or stress may be better ablated under mild or moderate sedation whereas those that occur spontaneously and independent of autonomic state may be targeted under any level of anesthesia.

APPROACH TO MAPPING AND ABLATION

A targeted approach to mapping and ablation is critical when considering postablation arrhythmias. **Fig. 1** suggests a systematic approach to setting up for a procedure. Cardiac MRI, in select centers with experience, may be useful in delineating atrial fibrosis and identifying gaps in prior lesion sets.[19] These preoperative images may be segmented and imported into mapping systems to facilitate anatomic mapping and correlation with voltage data. The optimal approach to radiologic imaging and whether delayed enhancement imaging has the resolution to identify minor gaps, however, are unclear.

In addition, review of the prior ablation may help facilitate understanding of the substrate being dealt with. For example, prior ablation of complex fractionated electrograms along with pulmonary vein isolation may lead to patchy scar and require careful attention to voltage mapping throughout the atria. In turn, pulmonary

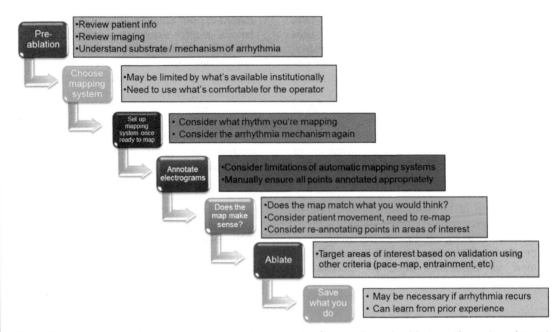

Fig. 1. Schematic approach to set up and approach to mapping for complex redo ablations. Shown is a schematic approach to decision making, setup, and approach for mapping and ablation. Critical aspects include consideration of the mechanism of the arrhythmia in question, the mapping system of choice to characterize the relevant substrate, and decisions during procedure on annotation and localization of relevant signals.

vein isolation in the absence of significant other atrial scar may lead to pulmonary vein reconnection or roof and/or mitral flutter being more likely. These issues are of critical importance when considering density of mapping needed and the potential complexity of the subsequent ablation.

Pulmonary Vein and Prior Ablation Set Assessment

The first and most critical consideration at the time of repeat ablation is assessment of the prior ablation lesion set, including for pulmonary vein reconnection. Most cases of arrhythmia recurrence after prior ablation are due to recurrent electrical conduction from previously isolated pulmonary veins rather than novel arrhythmogenic sites. The decision to assess and ablate the pulmonary veins prior to arrhythmia induction versus afterward may be operator dependent. Consolidating prior lines through which reconduction is seen, however, should be considered a cornerstone of repeat ablation. Another consideration is the use of adenosine to unmask dormant pulmonary vein conduction. Although demonstrated to potentially unmask latent conduction after index pulmonary vein isolation, trials have not consistently demonstrated benefit in adenosine infusion post–

pulmonary vein isolation.[20] Furthermore, the value at the time of redo procedures has not been demonstrated.

Voltage Mapping

Characterizing the atrial substrate at the time of repeat ablation is critical and may help inform likely arrhythmogenic regions, even in the absence of inducible arrhythmias. Voltage mapping may help identify areas of low voltage or scar and gaps in prior lines of block (including the pulmonary vein lesion set). In the absence of inducible arrhythmias but with recorded clinical arrhythmias, it may be reasonable to consider a substrate ablation approach in such situations. Optimal voltage cutoffs vary between studies and may be dependent on the region of the left or right atria being mapped.[21] Furthermore, the voltage cutoff may be dependent on whether mapping is done during atrial fibrillation, organized atrial arrhythmia, or sinus rhythm. In sinus rhythm, a voltage cutoff range of 0.2 mV to 0.45 mV may accurately demarcate scar region and identify areas of reconnection around the pulmonary veins.[22] A combination of mapping of the substrate with induction may further help facilitate identification of atypical, nonpulmonary vein triggers **(Fig. 2)**.

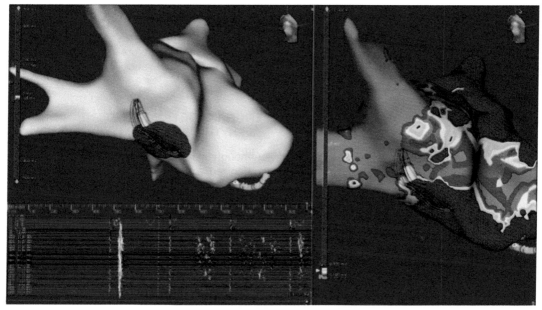

Fig. 2. Identification of trigger site for atrial fibrillation below site of prior ablation. Shown is an example of a patient at the time of redo ablation who had split potentials in a region just below the prior right pulmonary vein circumferential ablation lesion set. During coronary sinus pacing, as seen in the bottom left panel, there is disorganization in the signals on the multipolar catheter (seen in the right and top left images). This eventually degenerates the remainder of the atrium into atrial fibrillation.

Arrhythmia Induction and Clarification of Mechanism/Site of Origin

Arrhythmia induction at the time of repeat ablation is important to identify new sites of origin, especially if all prior lesion sets are intact (ie, pulmonary veins are chronically isolated and all other areas of ablation demonstrate persistent block). Induction consists of any combination of isoproterenol, atrial burst pacing, and atrial programmed stimulation from more than 1 site. Generally, inducible arrhythmias may be considered in the context of (1) how they correspond with the clinical arrhythmia, (2) whether arrhythmias are induced prior to vein reisolation/consolidation of prior lesion sets versus after, and (3) the presumed likelihood of induced arrhythmias being clinically relevant.

Correspondence of induced arrhythmia with clinical arrhythmia

One of the limitations of arrhythmia induction is the potential to induce arrhythmias that are not clinically relevant. In these cases, having prior electrocardiographic recordings of the clinical arrhythmia may be critical. Easy-to-induce arrhythmias may be considered clinical. Even if an induced arrhythmia does not match the clinically documented arrhythmia, it is possible that more than 1 arrhythmia can be present clinically, especially if not all clinical recurrences have been documented.

Induction prior to versus after ablation

One of the limitations of inducing after ablation is that extensive ablation to reisolate the pulmonary veins or consolidate prior lines may lead to edema and inflammation, resulting in nonspecific arrhythmias at study end. Prior studies have suggested that atrial arrhythmias induced with an aggressive postablation induction protocol may not predict long-term clinical recurrence.[23] Thus, having a targeted approach to induction, ablation, and reinduction is critical and likely needs to be contextualized to a given patient or procedure. For example, induction of a single arrhythmia, targeted mapping and ablation of that arrhythmia, and then attempt at reinduction to look for subsequent targetable arrhythmias may offer a systematic approach.

Likelihood of arrhythmia being clinically relevant

Recognizing whether an induced flutter is or is not clinically relevant can be extremely difficult. Generally, easy-to-induce arrhythmias may be more likely to be clinically relevant, albeit not universally. In the setting of extensive ablation, additional targeting of subsequent inducible arrhythmias may not be warranted to avoid loss of atrial contractility. Mappable, organized arrhythmias, however, likely should be mapped and ablated if feasible.

Mapping Induced Arrhythmias

Rapid recognition of the mechanism of a given arrhythmia may be facilitated through routine pacing maneuvers, as described elsewhere. Specifically, entrainment mapping from multiple sites may facilitate rapid localization of an induced flutter or organized atrial arrhythmia to a specific cardiac chamber. This may help in targeting mapping. If mapping was done prior to arrhythmia induction, targeted entrainment at sites that appear to be proarrhythmic based on abnormal voltage or narrow corridors of normal voltage amidst scar may facilitate targeted and rapid localization.[24] One approach to mapping when induction is done prior to transseptal may consist of entraining from the proximal coronary sinus catheter, the distal coronary sinus catheter, and a catheter placed in the high right atrium. This may facilitate localization to the annulus versus atrial body and left versus right atrium.

One critical consideration when proceeding with activation mapping is threshold settings for point acquisition, because low-voltage regions nevertheless may facilitate arrhythmia propagation, and bipolar voltage alone should not dictate whether an area is scar versus viable. Pacing in areas of presumed scar with lack of capture may more clearly reflect true scar than the bipolar voltage alone. Furthermore, setting an appropriate window of interest is critical at the time of activation mapping. High-density mapping may facilitate better appreciation of microreentrant circuits (ie, those ≤ 2 cm in diameter containing the entire tachycardia cycle length) where macroreentry may be identified with lower-density maps.

Activation and entrainment mapping are complementary to each other. After prior ablation, creation of scar may cause a focal tachycardia to appear macroreentrant due to conduction around a completely or through a near completely blocked ablation line. Thus, activation may mimic the activation sequence of macroreentry. In this case, activation mapping may not be sufficient. Alternatively, entrainment mapping during microreentry may cause an arrhythmia to appear focal unless pacing near the arrhythmia site of origin, in which case activation mapping may be complementary.

Thus, a deductive approach involving assessment of cycle-length stability, searching for macroreentry through a combination of entrainment and activation mapping, and searching for a focal source if macroreentry has been excluded may be useful in facilitating mapping. Cycle-length stability, however, should be considered in light of atrial activation sequence, because dual tachycardias are sometimes possible in which 2 paths for macroreentry may be coexisting with atrial activation altering down both paths.[25]

EPIDEMIOLOGY OF RECURRENT ARRHYTHMIAS

Although extensive prior ablation may lead to organized atrial arrhythmias pulmonary vein isolation alone also may be associated with the same. The extent of the index pulmonary vein lesion set may inform the likelihood of a subsequent atrial arrhythmia. It has been shown that segmental ostial vein isolation is associated with lower organized atrial arrhythmia recurrence than circumferential, wide-area pulmonary vein isolation.[26] In turn, however, broader areas of ablation may be more effective in preventing recurrent atrial fibrillation. Thus, a balanced approach is critical. The most common cause of organized arrhythmias after prior ablation include either reconnection across the prior pulmonary vein lesion set or creation of narrow zones of conduction in the roof or mitral isthmus. Particularly with extensive additional ablation or in the setting of a more extensive atrial myopathy with diffuse or patchy fibrosis, however, arrhythmias may arise from anywhere.

SPECIAL CONSIDERATIONS

Several special considerations with mapping and ablation of recurrent arrhythmias after prior ablation should be made:

1. High-density mapping: evolving catheter designs and mapping systems have allowed for high-density mapping wherein thousands of activation points may be obtained and automatically annotated. Using closely spaced bipolar electrodes, appreciation of local tissue activation and myocardial viability may allow for better recognition of small channels of activation through regions of low voltage or appreciation of small, microreentrant circuits. Whether high-density mapping offers benefits in terms of procedural success over traditional point-by-point mapping is unclear. Furthermore, although automated annotation algorithms have advanced over time with improved computational processing speeds, it remains a challenge as to how to best annotate complex, fractionated electrograms.[27,28]

2. Mapping fractionated potentials: older mapping systems would only allow annotation along a single aspect of a given acquired point. This creates limitations in activation mapping because signals characterized by multiple peaks over a broad time range may reflect proarrhythmic sites that may not otherwise be appreciated without specifically manually tagging them. Automated features in mapping systems may help identify these multicomponent signals and localize them. When considering multicomponent signals, however, it remains important to consider their location. For example, points along the atrial septum may be multicomponent due to delay between left and right atrial activation (**Fig. 3**).

3. Epicardial mapping: at least 1 study has suggested potential value in combined epicardial and endocardial mapping in patients with complex atrial arrhythmias.[29] It is well recognized that, particularly during atrial arrhythmias, endocardial and epicardial activation may be different. In addition, there is the potential for epicardial circuits not appreciated during endocardial mapping. Whether epicardial mapping at the time of redo ablation may facilitate improved arrhythmia-free outcomes, however, is as yet unclear and requires further study.

4. Apparent organization on 12-lead or in a single chamber: in cases of extensive prior ablation, it is possible to see apparent organization on a 12-lead, or even in 1 atrium, even if the other atrium is in a different rhythm and acting as a driver. This may be due, for example, to the extent of scarring in the other atrium driving the arrhythmia, leading to lack of contribution to voltage on a 12-lead. In addition, it is possible for the coronary sinus, the right atrium, or the left atrium to appear organized even though there is a fibrillatory driver elsewhere (**Fig. 4**).

5. Rotor ablation: although cases of recurrent arrhythmia after prior ablation can be complicated to target, particularly if all prior targeted structures and sites remain isolated and/or blocked, it is unclear if targeting rotors offers additional benefit.[30] Whether this is due to limitations in available techniques to map rotors, or whether ablating rotors actually is relevant to ablating atrial fibrillation, remains to be seen. The benefit of trying to identify and target rotors, however, is unclear.

6. Post-maze atrial arrhythmias: most of this discussion focuses on ablations after prior atrial fibrillation ablation. Recurrent atrial arrhythmias after maze, however, also are not uncommon. Ablation of post-maze atrial arrhythmias is feasible and highly successful, according to studies.[31] Approach to mapping and ablation takes a similar course to that of postablation arrhythmias, involving understanding what was done previously, appropriate substrate mapping, and targeted understanding of the arrhythmia mechanism.

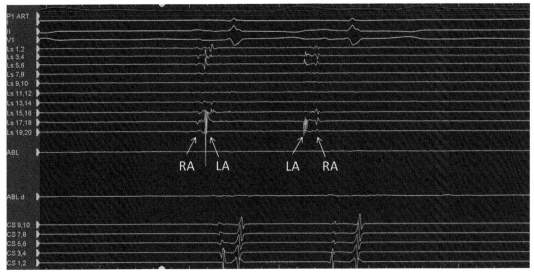

Fig. 3. Example of multicomponent signals. Shown is an example of multicomponent signals where the multipolar catheter (LS 1,2 through LS 19,20) is placed along the left atrial aspect of the interatrial septum. Labeled are the signals corresponding with the right atrium (RA) and left atrium (LA). Note reversal of signals with an atrial premature contraction.

A

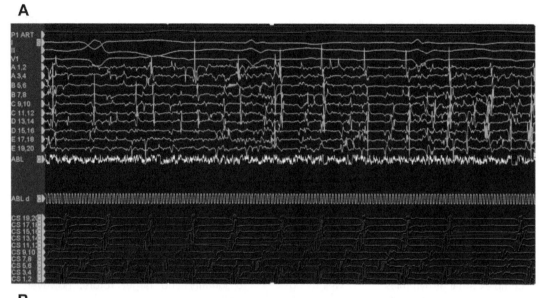

B

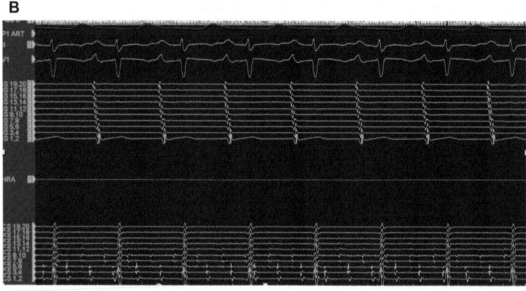

Fig. 4. Differential activation in sites after prior atrial fibrillation ablation during atrial arrhythmias. Differences in activation between different sites in the atrium are demonstrated, suggesting the overlying complexity in interpreting what may appear to be organized arrhythmias. (*A*) Demonstrates a coronary sinus catheter in blue (*bottom*) placed in the coronary sinus with the multipolar catheter (A 1,2 through E 19,20) placed at the coronary sinus ostium just against the right atrial side of the septum. Note that the coronary sinus catheter appears more organized than the site at the coronary sinus ostium, suggesting fibrillation rather than an organized arrhythmia. (*B*) Similarly shows a catheter in the coronary sinus (*bottom*) along with a multipolar catheter placed along the lateral right atrium (IS 19,20 through IS 1,2). Note the activation in the distal coronary sinus suggests a complex atrial arrhythmia but the 12-lead electrocardiogram suggests sinus rhythm corresponding with the activation pattern in the right atrium, suggesting dissociation between the 2 atria.

SUMMARY

Recurrent atrial arrhythmias after prior ablation are not uncommon. They may consist of recurrent atrial fibrillation or organized atrial arrhythmias, including focal atrial tachycardias or microreentrant or macroreentrant atrial flutters. Mapping and ablation of these may consist of a combination of activation and entrainment mapping and require close consideration of the atrial substrate as appreciated by noninvasive MRI or invasive voltage mapping. Novel technologies may help facilitate better understanding of arrhythmias, especially amidst complex substrate, but require further study to understand their impact on procedural outcomes.

REFERENCES

1. Calkins H, Hindricks G, Cappato R, et al. 2017 HRS/EHRA/ECAS/APHRS/SOLAECE expert consensus statement on catheter and surgical ablation of atrial fibrillation. Heart Rhythm 2017;14:e275–444.

2. Lellouche N, Jais P, Nault I, et al. Early recurrences after atrial fibrillation ablation: prognostic value and effect of early reablation. J Cardiovasc Electrophysiol 2008;19:599–605.

3. Andrade JG, Khairy P, Macle L, et al. Incidence and significance of early recurrences of atrial fibrillation after cryoballoon ablation: insights from the multicenter Sustained Treatment of Paroxysmal Atrial Fibrillation (STOP AF) trial. Circ Arrhythm Electrophysiol 2014;7:69–75.

4. Ballesteros G, Ravassa S, Bragard J, et al. Association of left atrium voltage amplitude and distribution with the risk of atrial fibrillation recurrence and evolution after pulmonary vein isolation: an ultrahigh-density mapping study. J Cardiovasc Electrophysiol 2019;30(8):1231–40.

5. Providencia R, Elliott P, Patel K, et al. Catheter ablation for atrial fibrillation in hypertrophic cardiomyopathy: a systematic review and meta-analysis. Heart 2016;102:1533–43.

6. Tan NY, Mohsin Y, Hodge DO, et al. Catheter ablation for atrial arrhythmias in patients with cardiac amyloidosis. J Cardiovasc Electrophysiol 2016;27:1167–73.

7. Ali RL, Hakim JB, Boyle PM, et al. Arrhythmogenic propensity of the fibrotic substrate after AF ablation: a longitudinal study using MRI-based atrial models. Cardiovasc Res 2019. [Epub ahead of print].

8. Sau A, Al-Aidarous S, Howard J, et al. Optimum lesion set and predictors of outcome in persistent atrial fibrillation ablation: a meta-regression analysis. Europace 2019. [Epub ahead of print].

9. Lee JM, Fynn SP. P wave morphology in guiding the ablation strategy of focal atrial tachycardias and atrial flutter. Curr Cardiol Rev 2015;11:103–10.

10. Leong-Si P, Roux JF, Zado E, et al. Antiarrhythmics after ablation of atrial fibrillation (5A study): six-month follow-up study. Circ Arrhythm Electrophysiol 2011;4:11–4.

11. Noseworthy PA, Van Houten HK, Sangaralingham LR, et al. Effect of antiarrhythmic drug initiation on readmission after catheter ablation for atrial fibrillation. JACC Clin Electrophysiol 2015;1:238–44.

12. Narui R, Matsuo S, Isogai R, et al. Impact of deep sedation on the electrophysiological behavior of pulmonary vein and non-PV firing during catheter ablation for atrial fibrillation. J Interv Card Electrophysiol 2017;49:51–7.

13. Chang TY, Lo LW, Te ALD, et al. The importance of extrapulmonary vein triggers and atypical atrial flutter in atrial fibrillation recurrence after cryoablation: insights from repeat ablation procedures. J Cardiovasc Electrophysiol 2019;30:16–24.

14. Santangeli P, Marchlinski FE. Techniques for the provocation, localization, and ablation of non-pulmonary vein triggers for atrial fibrillation. Heart Rhythm 2017;14:1087–96.

15. Romero J, Gianni C, Natale A, et al. What is the appropriate lesion set for ablation in patients with persistent atrial fibrillation? Curr Treat Options Cardiovasc Med 2017;19:35.

16. McGarry TJ, Narayan SM. The anatomical basis of pulmonary vein reconnection after ablation of atrial fibrillation: wounds that never felt a scar? J Am Coll Cardiol 2012;59(10):939–41.

17. Kallergis EM, Goudis CA, Vardas PE. Atrial fibrillation: a progressive atrial myopathy or a distinct disease? Int J Cardiol 2014;171:126–33.

18. Yang Y, Liu Q, Wu Z, et al. Stiff left atrial syndrome: a complication undergoing radiofrequency catheter ablation for atrial fibrillation. J Cardiovasc Electrophysiol 2016;27:884–9.

19. Jefairi NA, Camaioni C, Sridi S, et al. Relationship between atrial scar on cardiac magnetic resonance and pulmonary vein reconnection after catheter ablation for paroxysmal atrial fibrillation. J Cardiovasc Electrophysiol 2019;30:727–40.

20. Blandino A, Biondi-Zoccai G, Battaglia A, et al. Impact of targeting adenosine-induced transient venous reconnection in patients undergoing pulmonary vein isolation for atrial fibrillation: a meta-analysis of 3524 patients. J Cardiovasc Med (Hagerstown) 2017;18:478–89.

21. Lim HS, Yamashita S, Cochet H, et al. Delineating atrial scar by electroanatomic voltage mapping versus cardiac magnetic resonance imaging: where to draw the line? J Cardiovasc Electrophysiol 2014;25:1053–6.

22. Kapa S, Desjardins B, Callans DJ, et al. Contact electroanatomic mapping derived voltage criteria for characterizing left atrial scar in patients undergoing ablation for atrial fibrillation. J Cardiovasc Electrophysiol 2014;25:1044–52.

23. Santangeli P, Zado ES, Garcia FC, et al. Lack of prognostic value of atrial arrhythmia inducibility and change in inducibility status after catheter ablation of atrial fibrillation. Heart Rhythm 2018;15:660–5.

24. Blandino A, Bianchi F, Grossi R, et al. Left atrial substrate modification targeting low-voltage areas for catheter ablation of atrial fibrillation: a systematic review and meta-analysis. Pacing Clin Electrophysiol 2017;40:199–212.

25. Misiri J, Kim RJ, Kusumoto FM. Atrial flutter with alternating cycle lengths: mechanism and mapping. J Innov Card Rhythm Manag 2012;727–30.

26. Proietti R, Santangeli P, Di Biase L, et al. Comparative effectiveness of wide antral versus ostial pulmonary vein isolation: a systematic review and meta-analysis. Circ Arrhythm Electrophysiol 2014; 7:39–45.

27. Liang JJ, Elafros MA, Muser D, et al. Comparison of left atrial bipolar voltage and scar using multielectrode fast automated mapping versus point-to-point contact electroanatomic mapping in patients with atrial fibrillation undergoing repeat ablation. J Cardiovasc Electrophysiol 2017;28:280–8.

28. Schaeffer G, Akbulak RO, Jularic M, et al. High-density mapping and ablation of primary nonfocal left atrial tachycardia: characterizing a distinct arrhythmogenic substrate. JACC Clin Electrophysiol 2019; 5:417–26.

29. Jiang R, Buch E, Gima J, et al. Feasibility of percutaneous epicardial mapping and ablation for refractory atrial fibrillation: insights into substrate and lesion transmurality. Heart Rhythm 2019;16(8): 1151–9.

30. Parameswaran R, Voskoboinik A, Gorelik A, et al. Clinical impact of rotor ablation in atrial fibrillation: a systematic review. Europace 2018;20: 1099–106.

31. Kajiyama T, Kondo Y, Ueda M, et al. Catheter ablation of atrial tachyarrhythmias after a MAZE procedure: a single center experience. J Cardiol Cases 2018;19:89–92.

Mapping and Ablation of Rotational and Focal Drivers in Atrial Fibrillation

Junaid Zaman, MD, PhD[a,b], Tina Baykaner, MD[c],
Sanjiv M. Narayan, MD, PhD[d],*

KEYWORDS

- Atrial fibrillation • Mapping • Ablation • Driver • Focal source • Rotor • Phase mapping

KEY POINTS

- Rotational and focal sources are increasingly identified in persistent atrial fibrillation using a variety of mapping methods.
- Ablation at these sites has both short-term and long-term efficacy in treating atrial fibrillation in meta-analyses and subgroups of recent randomized clinical trials.
- Most of these sites are remote to the pulmonary veins, even in the right atrium, and this may explain a ceiling for success of pulmonary vein-based ablation for treatment of persistent atrial fibrillation.
- There are technical, logistical, and theoretic considerations for successful mapping of rotational and focal drivers, which are not part of traditional electrophysiology training.

Video content accompanies this article at http://www.cardiacep.theclinics.com.

INTRODUCTION

Drivers are increasingly studied ablation targets for atrial fibrillation (AF), and rotational or focal activation patterns are supported by most translational studies,[1–3] with steadily increasing evidence in patients.[4–10] However, results from ablation studies remain controversial. First, despite promising outcomes of AF driver ablation in several meta-analyses,[11–13] outcomes vary between centers and patients. Second, it is unclear how best to perform driver ablation. Recent data from the Randomized

Evaluation of Atrial Fibrillation Treatment With Focal Impulse and Rotor Modulation Guided Procedures (REAFFIRM) trial showed 77.7% freedom from atrial arrhythmias by driver ablation plus pulmonary vein isolation (PVI) in persistent AF, trending higher than PVI,[14] but success was lower when lines and fractionated electrograms were added, which rendered the trial neutral overall. Because prior strategies beyond PVI have all trended to lower results,[15] these data provide a potential signal that driver ablation could improve persistent

Disclosure: Dr S. Narayan reports funding by NIH (R01 HL83359, K24 HL103800); intellectual property owned by the University of California Regents and Stanford University; consulting income from Abbott, the American College of Cardiology, Beyond Limits.ai, TDK Inc, and UpToDate. Dr T. Baykaner reports funding by American Heart Association. Dr Zaman reports funding from the British Heart Foundation and UK-US Fulbright Commission.

[a] Stanford University, 780 Welch Road, Suite CJ250F, Stanford, CA 94305, USA; [b] Imperial College London, London, UK; [c] Department of Medicine/Cardiovascular Medicine, Stanford University, 780 Welch Road, Suite CJ250F, Stanford, CA 94305, USA; [d] Department of Medicine/Cardiovascular Medicine and Cardiovascular Institute, Stanford University, 780 Welch Road, Suite CJ250F, MC 5773, Stanford, CA 94305, USA
* Corresponding author.
E-mail address: Sanjiv1@stanford.edu

Card Electrophysiol Clin 11 (2019) 583–595
https://doi.org/10.1016/j.ccep.2019.08.010
1877-9182/19/© 2019 Elsevier Inc. All rights reserved.

AF ablation outcomes overall. Third, there is a lack of practical guidance on how to optimally map and ablate AF drivers, particularly to differentiate critical from secondary sites using different AF mapping methods. This article addresses each of these issues.

MECHANISTIC TARGETS FOR THERAPY

There is now considerable evidence that localized rotational or focal drivers sustain fibrillation using optical mapping in isolated hearts from multiple species including human AF. Optical mapping (**Fig. 1**) uses video imaging of voltage-sensitive dye imaging, coupled with activation, phase, or other analysis approaches to map AF at high spatial and temporal resolution. **Fig. 1A** shows rapid irregular action potentials at 1 point mapped optically. **Fig. 1B** plots such action potentials across the cardiac surface in fibrillation. Each color represents phases of cardiac activation (from depolarization to repolarization), in which rotations are represented as a full color spectrum from red to blue. Points in the atrium where activation and repolarization meet (see **Fig. 1C**), (ie, an entire cycle) have undefined phase and are termed phase

singularities (PSs), which may represent rotor cores in fibrillating myocardium. AF rotational circuits are not fixed like macroreentry around an obstacle, but precess in small regions (see **Fig. 1C**). This property also distinguishes them from fleeting rotational activity in multiwavelet (leading circle) reentry. Fibrillation may thus terminate when the rotor collides with a boundary,[3] does not have enough room to spin, or by eliminating drivers such that fibrillatory waves are no longer replenished and progressively extinguish.

Optical mapping of AF in human hearts shows endocardial microreentrant circuits that may be focal on the epicardium,[16] and hence reconcile the apparent paradox between surgical and clinical mapping studies.[1–3] Intriguingly, these optically mapped drivers were correctly detected as rotational circuits by concurrent clinical baskets and mapping algorithms (focal impulse and rotor mapping [FIRM]),[17] validating these clinical tools. In these unique translational human studies, rotational circuits localized to regions of microfibrosis, which may or may not represent those sites identified by clinical atrial MRI.

Clinically, the terms rotational activity, rotational driver, or even reentry are equally effective to

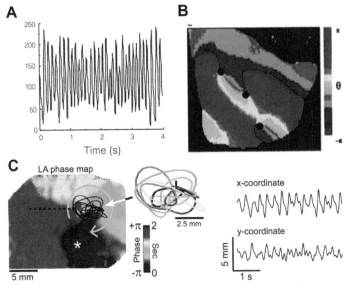

Fig. 1. Optical mapping of fibrillatory conduction from an AF source. (*A*) High-resolution optical action potentials obtained from explanted fibrillating tissue. (*B*) Snapshot of phase movie of a fibrillating rabbit ventricle, showing rotors as red to blue phase angles, and phase singularities (PSs) as dark black dots where all phases (colors) converge. (*C*) Rotor meandering and fractionation during AF in isolated sheep heart. On the left, a left atrial phase snapshot shows reentry in the left atrium (LA) free wall. The inset shows the time-space trajectory of the tip (PS), whereas the x and y coordinate signals are shown on the right. (*Adapted from* Gray R, Pertsov A, Jalife J. Spatial and temporal organization during cardiac fibrillation. Nature [Internet]. 1998 [cited 2013 Mar 13];392(May):75–8. Available from: http://www.nature.com/nature/journal/v392/n6671/abs/392075a0.html; and Zlochiver S, Yamazaki M, Kalifa J, Berenfeld O. Rotor meandering contributes to irregularity in electrograms during atrial fibrillation. Heart Rhythm [Internet]. 2008 Jun [cited 2013 May 14];5(6):846–54. Available from: http://www.pubmedcentral.nih.gov/articlerender.fcgi?artid=3079377&tool=pmcentrez&rendertype=abstract; with permission.)

describe mapped phenomena, and cannot be easily separated by the resolution of clinical tools. Classically, unlike anatomic reentry, entrainment is not possible because of complex or absent excitable gaps.[3]

COMPARING DIFFERENT ATRIAL FIBRILLATION MAPPING METHODS

Few studies have compared methods in the same patient data. The authors assembled an international registry to compare mapping methods in patients in whom ablation terminated persistent AF (NCT02997254), for which we have made data available online (http://narayanlab.stanford.edu). **Fig. 2** shows termination of persistent AF to sinus rhythm AF in a 65-year-old man. AF maps using traditional methods showed only partial and transient rotations (shown), which do not explain the site of termination. A freely available phase mapping approach[18] showed consistent rotations at this site, and were corroborated by FIRM maps, which show gray-scale activation maps and PSs (in red). Thus, sites of AF termination by ablation

may show rotational AF drivers by phase and activation plus phase (FIRM), which can be missed by traditional activation mapping of AF.[19]

Although termination of persistent AF by ablation is not equivalent to elimination, it is rare to terminate persistent AF by limited ablation of atrial tissue before PVI. Moreover, termination provides one of the few accepted acute end points for ablation. Long-term outcomes are clearly the ultimate goal but may not be ideal for assessing the accuracy of AF mapping, because they include long-term confounding issues unrelated to mapping, such as the effects of additional lesion sets, including PVI, lesion recovery, or disease progression. Thus, the approach of comparing maps and acute ablation response eliminates inappropriate comparisons of patient populations, and may continue to be a useful strategy to compare mapping method/algorithm moving forwards.

AF drivers have now been identified by multiple mapping systems, with many similarities.[7,20] The authors recently summarized these similarities in meta-analyses of mapping.[11,12] **Table 1** summaries some of these details. Studies of FIRM

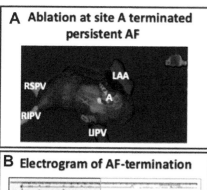
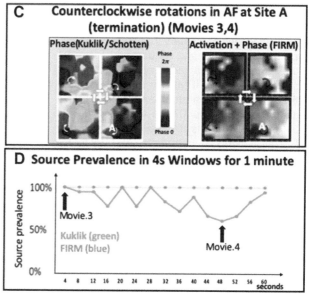
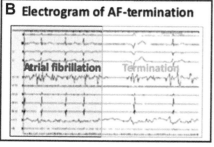

Fig. 2. At atrial fibrillation (AF) termination site, rotational activity without competing organized sites. In a 78-year-old man with persistent AF, (*A*) atrial shell on which ablation at site A, (*B*) terminated persistent AF. C, Clockwise rotation at site A by two independent mapping methods, including phase based method and clinical FIRM method. No rotations are seen at control site C. D, Prevalence of rotations at site A for successive 4-s windows over 1 minute of AF by both methods. At arrowed time points, Movie III in the original reference shows continuous rotations at site A by both methods; Movie IV in the original reference shows interrupted rotations by method 1 but continuous rotations by method 2. FIRM indicates focal impulse and rotor modulation; LAA, left atrial appendage; LIPV, left inferior pulmonary vein; RIPV, right inferior pulmonary vein; and RSPV, right superior pulmonary vein. (*From* Kowalewski CAB, Shenasa F, Rodrigo M, Clopton P, Meckler G, Alhusseini MI, et al. Interaction of Localized Drivers and Disorganized Activation in Persistent Atrial Fibrillation. Circ Arrhythmia Electrophysiol. 2018; 11(6):e005846; with permission.")

typically show 2 to 4 biatrial AF drivers, electrocardiographic imaging[5] showed 3 to 5, and other techniques, such as that by Lin and colleagues,[21] showed 2 to 3. When biatrial mapping is performed, about two-thirds of AF drivers lie in left atrium and one-third in right atrium, as also reported by other mapping modalities. This distribution may explain ablation outcomes, in which lesion sets may coincidentally hit AF drivers.[22]

Further comparative mapping studies are needed for new techniques, particularly those that compare methods in the same patient datasets, ideally compared with a reference such as optical mapping, as has been conducted for some methods.[17]

CLINICAL OUTCOMES OF FOCAL IMPULSE AND ROTOR MAPPING–GUIDED ABLATION

Multiple studies now exist on the outcomes from AF driver ablation. As with any new approach, initial reports were promising and some subsequent reports were disappointing. In recent meta-analyses, adjunctive driver-guided ablation was associated with higher rates of acute AF termination, lower recurrence of any atrial arrhythmia, and comparable complication incidence.[11]

Multicenter randomized data of AF driver ablation were recently presented. The REAFFIRM trial enrolled 375 patients and randomized them 1:1 to the intention-to-treat arms of PVI versus PVI plus rotor ablation (FIRM). By intention-to-treat analysis, freedom from atrial arrhythmias after a single procedure was 67.5% in the PVI and 69.3% in the FIRM arms at 1 year. However, nearly half of all patients in both limbs had additional ablation not prescribed by protocol. Examining on-treatment subgroups,[14] FIRM plus PVI (77.7%) achieved higher success than PVI (65.5%) with a trend ($P = .09$) because PVI success was higher than anticipated and the trial was not powered for these subgroups. Nonprescribed groups were PVI plus complex fractionated and linear ablation (69.6%), and all strategies combined with the lowest success (57.7%). Notably, the FIRM plus PVI result in REAFFIRM was similar to early studies (82.4% success in CONFIRM [Conventional Ablation for Atrial Fibrillation with or Without Focal Impulse and Rotor Modulation][4]). These results seem to reiterate the signal for lower success by ablation of complex fractionated atrial electrograms or lines observed in STAR-AFII (Substrate and Trigger Ablation for Reduction of Atrial Fibrillation Trial - Star AF II Study) and other recent randomized trials. The final publication of REAFFIRM is awaited and may address some unanswered questions, including ablation times in each limb, and what additional ablation was performed above the intention-to-treat strategies.

In FIRM studies from multiple groups, AF sources arise in diverse locations, overall with 25% to 40% near pulmonary veins, 25% to 40% elsewhere in the left atrium, and 25% to 40% in right atrium (**Fig. 3**, **Table 2**).[23] Body surface mapping and electrocardiogram (ECG) imaging show similar AF driver distributions but in larger regions,[5] which may represent greater so-called meander in projecting from the heart to the torso.[24] In multiple studies, right atrial drivers are mostly in the free wall, posterolateral to the right atrial appendage, and rarely near the superior vena cava (SVC) or cavotricuspid isthmus (see **Fig. 3**). AF drivers are present in higher numbers and more widely distributed in patients with persistent than paroxysmal AF.[25]

The emergence of randomized data of driver ablation with a favorable safety and procedure time profile, showing a trend to improve results from PVI, differs from all other additive strategies, which trended to worsen PVI.[15] This signal potentially improving outcomes from persistent AF ablation should prompt investigation into the most suitable patients in whom rotor mapping and ablation is performed. To address some of the variety in this technique, this article presents a practical guide for using FIRM mapping.

HOW TO CREATE BASKET-DERIVED DRIVER MAPS (FOCAL IMPULSE AND ROTOR MAPPING)

The general considerations for FIRM mapping and ablation are summarized in **Table 2**. The procedure requires skills that include assessing adequate basket coverage of the atrium, interpretation of complex AF maps, and appropriate ablation guidance. The authors estimate that approximately 20 cases are adequate for an operator to achieve proficiency.

The basket catheter should be sized to left atrial dimensions, then deployed sequentially in right then left atria via standard sheaths. New baskets cover greater than 80% of the atria (**Fig. 4**) and may improve on prior designs.[26] Suboptimal basket deployment (noncontact) may cause AF sources to be missed. Importantly, comprehensive atrial coverage may not be possible with a single basket position, and so repeat maps after repositioning may reveal all AF sources (**Fig. 5**). Video 1 shows preparation of the compliant basket, whose splines have rectangular cross section designed to not separate or spread significantly despite radial

Table 1
Summary of atrial fibrillation driver mapping and ablation strategies

Mapping Technique	AF Type Mapped	Number of Ablation Targets	Atrial Location (%)	Source Characterization (%)	Acute Termination (%)	Freedom From AF at 12 mo, With PVI (%)
FIRM[4,23,39]	Paroxysmal, persistent, and long-standing persistent	3–5	LA 70, RA 30, PV 24	Stable rotations 76, Focal sources 24[4]	56 (60 to sinus)[4], RA in 22[39]	Meta-analysis: 72.5[12], Persistent AF RCT: 77.7 (FIRM + PVI subgroup)[14]
Endocardial phase[19]	Paroxysmal, persistent, and long-standing persistent	3–5	LA 66, RA 34, PV 40	Stable rotations 100	100 (83 to sinus)	Similar to FIRM
Body surface, ECGI[5,40,41]	Persistent and long-standing persistent	3–6	LA 70, RA 30, LPV/LAA 82[5], LA 53, RA 27, Septum 20[40]	Reentries 80, Focal breakthrough 20[5]	80 (66 to AT)[5], 64 (79 to AT) (PVs 37, LA 35, RA in 28)[40]	85[5], 78[40]
CartoFinder[6,42–44]	Persistent and long-standing persistent	1–3	LA 63, RA 27, Non-PV 79[8]	Rotational activity 70, Focal activations 30[42], Focal activations 100[44]	63 (58 to AT)[42], 15 (all sinus)[8]	71[44], 70[8]
Spatiotemporal dispersion[10]	Persistent AF	4–6	LA 80, RA 20, PV/LAA 80	Regions of microreentry	95 (85 to AT)	85 without PVI (1.4 procedures, at 18 mo)
Dominant frequency[45]	Paroxysmal and persistent	3–4	LA 80, RA 20, PV>70	High-frequency sites	80–90 in HFSA arm	70 persistent
Charge/dipole density[7,46]	Persistent AF	2–3	RA not mapped, LA anterior 70	Localized irregular activity, Localized rotational activity, Focal activity	50–60	73[46]
Electrographic flow mapping[47,48]	Persistent AF	4–6	LA 70, RA 30, PV 40	Rotational 51, Focal 49	100, RA in 10	Pending
STAR[9]	Persistent AF	2–3 (after PVI)	LA 95, RA 5	Early sites of activation	29 (75 to AT)	80 (AT/AF at 18 mo)

Abbreviations: AT, atrial tachycardia; ECGI, electrocardiographic imaging; HFSA, high-frequency source ablation; LA, left atrium; LAA, left atrial appendage; LPV, left pulmonary vein; PV, pulmonary vein; RA, right atrium; RCT, randomized controlled trial; STAR, stochastic trajectory analysis of ranked signals.

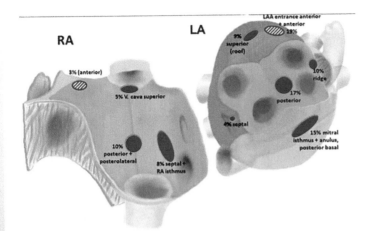

Fig. 3. Location of focal sources and rotors in patients using FIRM mapping. LAA, left atrial appendage; V. cava, vena cava. (*From* Spitzer SG, Károlyi L, Rämmler C, Scharfe F, Weinmann T, Zieschank M, et al. Treatment of Recurrent Non-Paroxysmal Atrial Fibrillation Using Focal Impulse and Rotor Mapping (FIRM) -Guided Rotor Ablation: Early Recurrence and Long-Term Outcomes Short title: FIRM ablation outcomes for recurrent non-paroxysmal AF. J Cardiovasc Electrophysiol. 2017;1–30; with permission.)

Table 2
Considerations for successful focal impulse and rotor mapping–guided ablation

General	• Basket coverage (multiple positions ideally used) and careful map interpretation are the cornerstones of AF driver ablation • Rotational and focal driver regions fluctuate but remain in spatially stable regions that are ablation targets • Sources lie in 2–3 cm^2 areas (1.5 × 1.5 cm) • FIRM sites lie between; that is, are typically bounded by physical electrodes • Given the size of each ablation lesion (>7 mm), the driver should be bracketed between electrodes rather than a precise core coordinate defined
Right Atrial Sources	• Observed in one-third of patients, paroxysmal as well as persistent AF (see **Fig. 3**) • Typically fewer than in LA • No stereotypical locations, but more likely in the free wall (where phrenic capture should be tested), septum, and posterior wall • Rarely at the superior vena cava or cavotricuspid isthmus
Left Atrial Sources	• Observed in nearly all patients • Typically multiple (average of 2–3), with higher numbers in patients with more advanced disease (persistent long-standing AF) • No stereotypical location, but 40%–50% at sites covered by a typical wide-area PV antral ablation

pressure. The basket is then collapsed for insertion into the femoral vein.

Right atrial contact is more forgiving of basket size. For the left atrium, a more anterior transseptal puncture orients the basket posteriorly, which is ideal, whereas a posterior puncture encourages partial prolapse across the mitral annulus, which is suboptimal. Basket size is selected by measuring distance from the interatrial septum to the Coumadin ridge via catheter spacing on fluoroscopy, intracardiac echocardiography, or preprocedural imaging to avoid the need to upsize or downsize.

Fig. 4 outlines deployment techniques for the basket catheter. In the right atrium the basket catheter is unsheathed in the SVC and slowly retracted into the right atrial body. Slight clockwise or counterclockwise torque is applied for optimal deployment. Particular care is required if a right atrial pacing lead is present, rotating the basket so that splines span the lead rather than displace it[27] and typically advancing from the inferior vena cava rather than pulling down from the SVC. Video 2 shows rapid creation of a right atrial geometry by insertion into the SVC, pulling down to the right atrium, then to the inferior vena cava. This process takes less than a minute, created several hundred geometric points with voltage data, and the basket is then used to map AF in 2 to 3 right atrial positions.

In left atrium, the basket is unsheathed in the left superior pulmonary vein and slowly retracted into the atrial body. Slight clockwise or counterclockwise torque may help achieve optimal basket deployment, maximizing endocardial contact with the fewest splines over the mitral valve orifice. Alternatively, the basket catheter can be carefully reflected off the carina of the left pulmonary veins. Video 3 shows rapid creation of left atrial geometry by insertion to the left superior

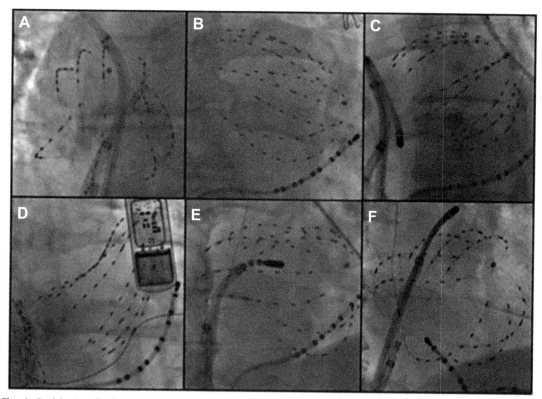

Fig. 4. Positioning basket catheters. (*A*) In right atrium, the sheath and catheter are advanced to the SVC, where retracting the sheath causes the basket to self-expand. Slight torque may be required to maximize expansion and apposition. Optimally only 0-1 splines should traverse the tricuspid valve orifice. (*B*) In left atrium, the sheath and catheter are advanced into the left superior pulmonary vein and the sheath is retracted. Slight manipulation may be needed to expand the basket outside of the vein. Again, only 0-1 spline should traverse the mitral valve orifice. (*C*) An undersized basket catheter assumes its natural spherical shape without any deformation, suggesting limited endocardial contact. Intracardiac echocardiography is often helpful in assessing endocardial contact. (*D*) An oversized basket catheter is most commonly recognized by an inability to expand the basket secondary to distal electrode restriction in a pulmonary vein antrum. Further basket withdrawal is limited by the proximal electrodes encountering the transseptal access site. (*E*) Withdrawal of basket out of the left upper pulmonary vein orifice results in slight spline prolapse into the left ventricle, although more than 56 electrodes are in contact with the left atrial walls. (*F*) Regional oversampling using the basket catheter. Here, the basket is manipulated to ensure higher sampling density at the LA roof, where a rotor was observed, at the cost of lower density sampling in the posterior and anterior walls, where rotors were previously not seen. If no AF sources are identified, repositioning to systematically sample regions of the atria is suggested. (*From* Narayan SM, Krummen DE, Rappel W-J. Clinical mapping approach to diagnose electrical rotors and focal impulse sources for human atrial fibrillation. J Cardiovasc Electrophysiol [Internet]. 2012 May [cited 2012 Aug 6];23(5):447–54. Available from: http://www.ncbi.nlm.nih.gov/pubmed/22537106; with permission.)

pulmonary vein, the posterior wall, the right pulmonary veins, then the anterior left atrium. This process takes less than a minute, created many hundred geometric points with voltage data, and the basket is then used to map AF in 2 to 3 left atrial positions.

Once the basket catheter is in place, AF electrograms are recorded in several 1-minute epochs, and exported for near-real-time analysis. Localization signals from electroanatomic mapping systems are best switched off while recording.

Signals are typically recorded in an unfiltered (0.05–250 Hz or 0.05–500 Hz) unipolar configuration, referenced to the Wilson central terminal, a body patch, or a catheter in the SVC. This method also serves to maximize the functional resolution of the basket by preserving spatial relations between 64 unipoles rather than 32 pairs of bipoles, and use of direction-sensitive bipolar data may hamper detection of rotational activity.

Computational analysis uses described algorithms[28] based on tissue physiology

Suboptimal

A Basket - poor coverage

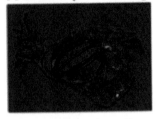

C Poor Basket Position

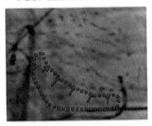

E Suboptimal Ablation

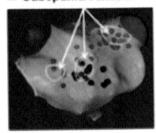

Optimal

B Multi-Basket Positions

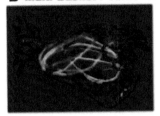

D Good Basket Position

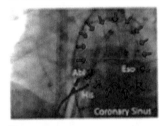

F Dense Source Ablation

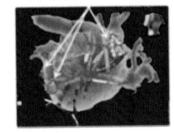

Fig. 5. Pearls and Pitfalls in AF Basket Placement. (*A*) Suboptimal basket position in left atrium. (*B*) Multi-Position Basket Mapping, the method of choice in large atria. (*C*) Poor Basket position, with inferior border shown (*arrows*) and missing much of posterior and inferior left atrium (dashed area).[49] (*D*) Good basket position outlined by arrows, covers atrium well; (*E*) Sparse lesions over source area in a disappointing report;[50] (*F*) Dense source area lesions in a successful series. Abl, ablation; Eso, esophagus. ([5C] From Narayan SM, Krummen DE, Rappel WJ. Clinical mapping approach to diagnose electrical rotors and focal impulse sources for human atrial fibrillation. J Cardiovasc Electrophysiol. 2012; 23(5): 447–54; with permission. [5D] From Miller JM, Kalra V, Das MK, et al. Clinical Benefit of Ablating Localized Sources for Human Atrial Fibrillation. J Am Coll Cardiol. 2017; 69(10): 1247–56; with permission. [5E] From Gianni C, Mohanty S, Di Biase L, et al. Acute and early outcomes of FIRM-guided rotors-only ablation in patients with non-paroxysmal atrial fibrillation. Heart Rhythm. 2016; 13(4): 830–835; with permission. [5F] From Sommer P, Kircher S, Rolf S, et al. Successful Repeat Catheter Ablation of Recurrent Longstanding Persistent Atrial Fibrillation with Rotor Elimination as the Procedural Endpoint: A Case Series. J Cardiovasc Electrophysiol 27. 2015;27(3):274–80. 27; with permission.)

(repolarization and conduction dynamics) in patients with persistent and paroxysmal AF[29–33] to create a propagation movie of the arrhythmia (AF). Three-dimensional activation on the basket catheter is translated to 2 dimensions to show a FIRM movie. **Fig. 6** A and B show 3 successive frames of a FIRM movie of AF spanning 100 to 160 milliseconds, showing a spiral wave and focal impulse, respectively. During a procedure, ~25 consecutive cycles (4 seconds) are typically viewed and analyzed per epoch. **Fig. 7** shows isochronal snapshots that summarize these movies. Rotational drivers (spiral waves) or focal sources are diagnosed using criteria in **Table 3**, and targeted only if they remain in stable regions for 1 minute or more, with precession that has been quantified in less than 2-cm² regions.[34] This criterion eliminates transient, partial, or migratory rotations.

HOW TO ABLATE FOCAL IMPULSE AND ROTOR MAPPING–IDENTIFIED ATRIAL FIBRILLATION DRIVERS

The basic approach to ablating AF drivers is to eliminate viable tissue in the region of precession. If right and left atria are mapped in that sequence, then ablation typically follows that sequence, but this order can be varied.

The rotational core or focal impulse origin of each driver is tagged relative to its closest electrode on the movie and on the multipolar catheter. **Figs. 2** and **5** show how drivers identified on AF maps are translated to physical electrode projections on electroanatomic shells. This process is straightforward in principle, but should avoid errors of projecting basket electrodes to the wrong regions of the shell. The authors ensure that the shell is viewed with the basket

Time = 1 cycle

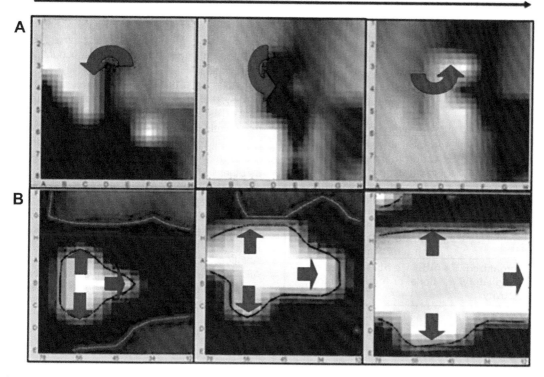

Fig. 6. AF sources on FIRM movies. Three successive FIRM movie snapshots showing (*A*) a counterclockwise AF rotor centered at electrode D3 to D4. (*B*) A focal impulse source for AF originating near electrode B5 to B6. Each AF source precessed within its spatially reproducible region for tens of minutes, until eliminated by brief FIRM targeted ablation.

spline en face, to avoid parallax errors, which would lead to the wrong regions marked on the shell. The ablation target area is an area of 1-cm to 2-cm diameter bounded by the electrodes that bracket it.

The ablation end point is elimination of the driver on a postablation map. Irrigated and nonirrigated radiofrequency and cryoablation energy have all

shown success in FIRM-guided ablation.[4,35] The typical approach using radiofrequency is to apply successive lesions, moving the catheter within the precession area. Local electrogram abatement and failure to capture with high-output pacing within the ablation target region can help ensure complete ablation of target area. If AF terminates during ablation, attempts are made to reinitiate

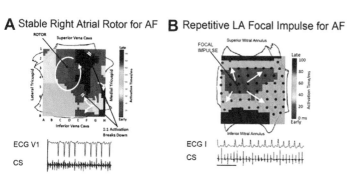

A Stable Right Atrial Rotor for AF   **B** Repetitive LA Focal Impulse for AF

Fig. 7. Snapshots illustrate FIRM-based AF movies. (*A*) Right atrial AF rotor lies at D3 to D4 (precesses between cycles), and was eliminated by ablation. Same patient as **Fig. 6**A. (*B*) Left atrial AF focal source lies at B56 (precesses between cycles), and was eliminated by ablation. Same patient as **Fig. 6**B. (*From* Narayan SM, Krummen DE, Rappel W-J. Clinical mapping approach to diagnose electrical rotors and focal impulse sources for human atrial fibrillation. J Cardiovasc Electrophysiol [Internet]. 2012 May [cited 2012 Aug 6];23(5):447–54. Available from: http://www.ncbi.nlm.nih.gov/pubmed/22537106; with permission.)

Table 3
Diagnostic criteria

Rotational AF Driver	• A rotational site that emanates waves to cause disorganized activity within the chamber • Driver may precess (meander) but should remain within a region of 1–2 cm² for ~ 1 min or more, with temporal fluctuations
Focal AF Driver	• A focal site with rapid activation that emanates waves to cause disorganized activation within the chamber • Driver may precess (meander) but should remain within a region of 1–2 cm² for ~ 1 min or more, with temporal fluctuations
Disorganized (Fibrillatory) Activity	• Absence of organized rotational or focal activation

AF for remapping. If AF does not terminate during ablation, repeat FIRM mapping sometimes identifies slight shifts of the driver. Additional AF drivers are sometimes clearer on a remap after competing sources are eliminated. **Table 4** summarizes how to approach common problems encountered in FIRM cases.

If AF driver ablation results in an atrial tachycardia, that mechanism is typically ablated as part of the procedure. Preliminary studies show that ablation of an AF driver may anchor activation to a localized microreentrant atrial tachycardia,[36] which may arise near the original driver, as well as other tachycardias.[37]

The safety profile of basket mapping and FIRM-guided ablation seems excellent,[38] with no documented cases of thromboembolism or perforation using basket catheters. This finding was supported by the safety profile in the REAFFIRM trial. Ablation safety seems similar to that of traditional AF ablation, and sensitive sites, such as near the esophagus or phrenic nerves, should be screened in routine fashion.

Table 4
Troubleshooting difficult cases

Basket Catheter Sizing and Positioning	• Select basket based on left atrial rather than right atrial size • Select basket based on measuring the distance from transseptal crossing to Coumadin ridge • Select a more anterior transseptal puncture, to advance the basket posteriorly into the LA • If in doubt, undersize rather than oversize the basket
Unable to Identify Focal Sources on a FIRM Map	• Assess for proper basket catheter size and position (See **Fig. 5**) • Maximize signal fidelity by catheter opposition; ensure adequate filtering and unipolar reference • Choose another time slice within the epoch, because AF drivers may fluctuate then reappear in the same location. Alternatively, collect another epoch • Play movie initially fast, to localize general region of rotation or focal activity, then slow movie down. For focal source, play movie in reverse to show activation collapse to an origin • Consider sources outside the mapping area • Evaluate regions of undersampling, adjust basket positioning, and resample • Choose an alternative spline to cut and open
Inability to Eliminate Rotor or Focal Source Despite FIRM Ablation	• Ensure adequate ablation at targeted sites by lack of capture with high-output pacing • Use additional ablation if needed, taking into account standard safety considerations; eg, near the esophagus or phrenic nerves • Repeat FIRM map. Sources may become clearer with elimination of other sources • Evaluate regions of undersampling, adjust basket positioning, and resample • Consider sources outside the mapping area

SUMMARY

There is mounting evidence that human AF is maintained by rotational and focal drivers, analogous to those long described in optical mapping of AF in animal models. Single-center studies and now multicenter randomized ablation trials show that driver ablation has the potential to improve outcomes for persistent AF, with a favorable safety profile and ablation time. Notably, additional ablation of complex electrograms and lines may reduce the success of AF driver ablation. Translational and clinical studies are needed to explain these clinical results, personalize mapping in individual patients, and reconcile technical differences between approaches. It is important for next-generation approaches to simplify the technique, including multipolar mapping and basket placement, AF map interpretation, and ablation guidance.

SUPPLEMENTARY DATA

Supplementary data related to this article can be found online at https://doi.org/10.1016/j.ccep.2019.08.010.

REFERENCES

1. Nattel S, Xiong F, Aguilar M. Demystifying rotors and their place in clinical translation of atrial fibrillation mechanisms. Nat Rev Cardiol 2017;14:509–20.

2. Nattel S, Dobrev D. Controversies about atrial fibrillation mechanisms: aiming for order in chaos and whether it matters. Circ Res 2017;120(9):1396–8. Available at: https://www.ahajournals.org/doi/10.1161/CIRCRESAHA.116.310489. Accessed June 9, 2019.

3. Pandit SV, Jalife J. Rotors and the dynamics of cardiac fibrillation. Circ Res 2013;112(5):849–62. Available at: http://circres.ahajournals.org/cgi/doi/10.1161/CIRCRESAHA.111.300158. Accessed March 1, 2013.

4. Narayan SM, Krummen DE, Shivkumar K, et al. Treatment of atrial fibrillation by the ablation of localized sources: CONFIRM (conventional ablation for atrial fibrillation with or without focal impulse and rotor modulation) trial. J Am Coll Cardiol 2012;60(7):628–36. Available at: http://linkinghub.elsevier.com/retrieve/pii/S0735109712021377. Accessed July 20, 2012.

5. Haissaguerre M, Hocini M, Denis A, et al. Driver domains in persistent atrial fibrillation. Circulation 2014;130(7):530–8. Available at: http://www.ncbi.nlm.nih.gov/pubmed/25028391. Accessed September 26, 2014.

6. Daoud EG, Zeidan Z, Hummel JD, et al. Identification of repetitive activation patterns using novel computational analysis of multielectrode recordings during atrial fibrillation and flutter in humans. JACC Clin Electrophysiol 2017;3(3):207–16. Available at: http://linkinghub.elsevier.com/retrieve/pii/S2405500X16302766. Accessed November 17, 2017.

7. Grace A, Willems S, Meyer C, et al. High-resolution noncontact charge-density mapping of endocardial activation. JCI Insight 2019;4(6) [pii:126422]. Available at: http://www.ncbi.nlm.nih.gov/pubmed/30895945. Accessed June 9, 2019.

8. Calvo D, Rubin J, Perez D, et al. Ablation of rotor domains effectively modulates dynamics of human long-standing persistent atrial fibrillation. Circ Arrhythm Electrophysiol 2017;10(12) [pii:e005740].

9. Honarbakhsh S, Hunter RJ, Ullah W, Keating E, Finlay M, Schilling RJ. Ablation in persistent atrial fibrillation using stochastic trajectory analysis of ranked signals (STAR) mapping method. JACC Clin Electrophysiol 2019;5(7):817–29. Available at: https://linkinghub.elsevier.com/retrieve/pii/S2405500X19302968. Accessed June 9, 2019.

10. Seitz J, Bars C, Théodore G, et al. AF ablation guided by spatiotemporal electrogram dispersion without pulmonary vein isolation: a wholly patient-tailored approach. J Am Coll Cardiol 2017;69(3):303–21. Available at: http://myaccess.library.utoronto.ca/login?url=http://search.ebscohost.com/login.aspx?direct=true&db=rzh&AN=120635135&site=ehost-live.

11. Lin CY, Lin YJ, Narayan SM, Baykaner T, Lo MT, Chung FP, et al. Comparison of phase mapping and electrogram-based driver mapping for catheter ablation in atrial fibrillation. Pacing Clin Electrophysiol 2019;42(2):216–23. Available at: https://onlinelibrary.wiley.com/doi/abs/10.1111/pace.13573. Accessed June 9, 2019.

12. Baykaner T, Rogers AJ, Meckler GL, et al. Clinical implications of ablation of drivers for atrial fibrillation. Circ Arrhythm Electrophysiol 2018;11(5). Available at: https://www.ahajournals.org/doi/10.1161/CIRCEP.117.006119. Accessed February 12, 2019.

13. Ramirez FD, Birnie DH, Nair GM, et al. Efficacy and safety of driver-guided catheter ablation for atrial fibrillation: a systematic review and meta-analysis. J Cardiovasc Electrophysiol 2017;1–8. Available at: http://doi.wiley.com/10.1111/jce.13313.

14. Brachmann J, Hummel JD, Wilber DJ, et al. S-LBCT01-02. Prospective randomized comparison of rotor ablation vs conventional ablation for treatment of persistent atrial fibrillation - The REAFFIRM trial. Heart Rhythm 2019;16(6):963–5. Available at: https://www.abstractsonline.com/pp8/#!/5753/presentation/31210. Accessed June 9, 2019.

15. Clarnette JA, Brooks AG, Mahajan R, et al. Outcomes of persistent and long-standing persistent

atrial fibrillation ablation: a systematic review and meta-analysis. Europace 2018;20(FI_3):f366–76. Available at: https://academic.oup.com/europace/article/20/FI_3/f366/4753706. Accessed June 9, 2019.

16. Hansen BJ, Zhao J, Csepe Ta, Moore BT, Li N, Jayne La, et al. Atrial fibrillation driven by micro-anatomic intramural re-entry revealed by simultaneous sub-epicardial and sub-endocardial optical mapping in explanted human hearts. Eur Heart J 2015;36(35):2390–401. Available at: http://eurheartj.oxfordjournals.org/cgi/doi/10.1093/eurheartj/ehv233.

17. Hansen BJ, Zhao J, Li N, Zolotarev A, Zakharkin S, Wang Y, et al. Human atrial fibrillation drivers resolved with integrated functional and structural imaging to benefit clinical mapping. JACC Clin Electrophysiol 2018;4(12):1501–15. Available at: https://linkinghub.elsevier.com/retrieve/pii/S2405500X1830793X. Accessed June 9, 2019.

18. Kuklik P, Zeemering S, Maesen B, et al. Reconstruction of instantaneous phase of unipolar atrial contact electrogram using a concept of sinusoidal recomposition and hilbert transform. IEEE Trans Biomed Eng 2015;62(1):296–302.

19. Alhusseini M, Vidmar D, Meckler GL, et al. Two independent mapping techniques identify rotational activity patterns at sites of local termination during persistent atrial fibrillation. J Cardiovasc Electrophysiol 2017;28(6):615–22.

20. Zaman JAB, Rogers AJ, Narayan SM. Rotational drivers in atrial fibrillation. Circ Arrhythm Electrophysiol 2017;10(12):e006022. Available at: http://www.ncbi.nlm.nih.gov/pubmed/29254949. Accessed December 21, 2017.

21. Lin Y-J, Lo M-T, Chang S-L, et al. Benefits of atrial substrate modification guided by electrogram similarity and phase mapping techniques to eliminate rotors and focal sources versus conventional defragmentation in persistent atrial fibrillation. JACC Clin Electrophysiol 2016;2(6):667–78. Available at: http://linkinghub.elsevier.com/retrieve/pii/S2405500X16302833.

22. Narayan SM, Krummen DE, Clopton P, et al. Direct or coincidental elimination of stable rotors or focal sources may explain successful atrial fibrillation ablation: on-treatment analysis of the CONFIRM (CONventional ablation for AF with or without Focal Impulse and Rotor Modulation) Trial. J Am Coll Cardiol 2013;62(2):138–47. Available at: http://www.ncbi.nlm.nih.gov/pubmed/23563126. Accessed June 1, 2013.

23. Spitzer SG, Károlyi L, Rämmler C, et al. Treatment of recurrent non-paroxysmal atrial fibrillation using focal impulse and rotor mapping (FIRM) -guided rotor ablation: early recurrence and long-term outcomes short title: FIRM ablation outcomes for recurrent non-paroxysmal AF. J Cardiovasc Electrophysiol 2017;28(1):31–8.

24. Rodrigo M, Guillem MS, Climent AM, et al. Body surface localization of left and right atrial high-frequency rotors in atrial fibrillation patients: A clinical-computational study. Heart Rhythm 2014;11:1584–91. Available at: http://www.ncbi.nlm.nih.gov/pubmed/24846374. Accessed July 15, 2014.

25. Krummen DE, Bayer JD, Ho J, Ho G, Smetak MR, Clopton P, et al. Mechanisms for human atrial fibrillation initiation: clinical and computational studies of repolarization restitution and activation latency. Circ Arrhythm Electrophysiol 2012;5(6):1149–59. Available at: http://www.ncbi.nlm.nih.gov/pubmed/23027797. Accessed November 12, 2012.

26. Honarbakhsh S, Schilling RJ, Providência R, et al. Panoramic atrial mapping with basket catheters: a quantitative analysis to optimize practice, patient selection, and catheter choice. J Cardiovasc Electrophysiol 2017;(12):1423–32. Available at: http://www.ncbi.nlm.nih.gov/pubmed/28862787. Accessed November 19, 2017.

27. Narayan SM, Krummen DE, Rappel W-J. Clinical mapping approach to diagnose electrical rotors and focal impulse sources for human atrial fibrillation. J Cardiovasc Electrophysiol 2012;23(5):447–54. Available at: http://www.ncbi.nlm.nih.gov/pubmed/22537106. Accessed August 6, 2012.

28. Narayan SM, Krummen DE, Enyeart MW, et al. Computational mapping identifies localized mechanisms for ablation of atrial fibrillation. PLoS One 2012;7(9):e46034. Available at: http://www.pubmedcentral.nih.gov/articlerender.fcgi?artid=3458823&tool=pmcentrez&rendertype=abstract. Accessed January 31, 2013.

29. Narayan SM, Bode F, Karasik P, et al. Alternans of atrial action potentials during atrial flutter as a precursor to atrial fibrillation. Circulation 2002;106(15):1968–73. Available at: http://circ.ahajournals.org/cgi/doi/10.1161/01.CIR.0000037062.35762.B4. Accessed March 11, 2013.

30. Narayan SM, Franz MR, Clopton P, et al. Repolarization alternans reveals vulnerability to human atrial fibrillation. Circulation 2011;123(25):2922–30. Available at: http://www.pubmedcentral.nih.gov/articlerender.fcgi?artid=3135656&tool=pmcentrez&rendertype=abstract. Accessed August 6, 2012.

31. Lalani GG, Schricker A, Gibson M, et al. Atrial conduction slows immediately before the onset of human atrial fibrillation: a bi-atrial contact mapping study of transitions to atrial fibrillation. J Am Coll Cardiol 2012;59(6):595–606. Available at: http://www.pubmedcentral.nih.gov/articlerender.fcgi?artid=3390156&tool=pmcentrez&rendertype=abstract. Accessed August 6, 2012.

32. Narayan SM, Krummen DE, Kahn AM, et al. Evaluating fluctuations in human atrial fibrillatory cycle length using monophasic action potentials. Pacing Clin Electrophysiol 2006;29(11):1209–18. Available

at: http://www.ncbi.nlm.nih.gov/pubmed/17100673. Accessed October 11, 2015.

33. Narayan SM, Kazi D, Krummen DE, et al. Repolarization and activation restitution near human pulmonary veins and atrial fibrillation initiation: a mechanism for the initiation of atrial fibrillation by premature beats. J Am Coll Cardiol 2008;52(15):1222–30. Available at: http://www.pubmedcentral.nih.gov/articlerender.fcgi?artid=2604131&tool=pmcentrez&rendertype=abstract. Accessed July 14, 2012.

34. Narayan SM, Shivkumar K, Krummen DE, et al. Panoramic electrophysiological mapping but not electrogram morphology identifies stable sources for human atrial fibrillation: stable atrial fibrillation rotors and focal sources relate poorly to fractionated electrograms. Circ Arrhythm Electrophysiol 2013;6(1):58–67. Available at: http://www.ncbi.nlm.nih.gov/pubmed/23392583. Accessed February 28, 2013.

35. Miller JM, Kowal RC, Swarup V, et al. Initial Independent outcomes from focal impulse and rotor modulation ablation for atrial fibrillation: multicenter FIRM registry. J Cardiovasc Electrophysiol 2014;25:921–9. Available at: http://www.ncbi.nlm.nih.gov/pubmed/24948520. Accessed June 23, 2014.

36. Baykaner T, Zografos TA, Zaman JAB, et al. Spatial relationship of organized rotational and focal sources in human atrial fibrillation to autonomic ganglionated plexi. Int J Cardiol 2017;240:234–9.

37. Rappel W-J, Zaman JAB, Narayan SM. Mechanisms for the termination of atrial fibrillation by localized ablation: computational and clinical studies. Circ Arrhythm Electrophysiol 2015;8(6):1325–33.

38. Krummen DE, Baykaner T, Schricker AA, et al. Multicentre safety of adding Focal Impulse and Rotor Modulation (FIRM) to conventional ablation for atrial fibrillation. Europace 2017;19(5):769–74. Available at: http://www.ncbi.nlm.nih.gov/pubmed/28339546. Accessed June 9, 2019.

39. Miller JM, Kalra V, Das MK, et al. Clinical benefit of ablating localized sources for human atrial fibrillation. J Am Coll Cardiol 2017;69(10):1247–56. Available at: http://linkinghub.elsevier.com/retrieve/pii/S0735109717301213.

40. Knecht S, Sohal M, Deisenhofer I, et al. Multicentre evaluation of non-invasive biatrial mapping for persistent atrial fibrillation ablation: The AFACART study. Europace 2017;19(8):1302–9. Available at: http://www.ncbi.nlm.nih.gov/pubmed/28204452. Accessed December 13, 2017.

41. Rodrigo M, Climent AM, Liberos A, et al. Technical considerations on phase mapping for identification of atrial reentrant activity in direct- and inverse-computed electrograms. Circ Arrhythm Electrophysiol 2017;10(9):e005008. Available at: http://www.ncbi.nlm.nih.gov/pubmed/28887361. Accessed November 17, 2017.

42. Honarbakhsh S, Schilling RJ, Dhillon G, et al. A novel mapping system for panoramic mapping of the left atrium. JACC Clin Electrophysiol 2018;4(1):124–34. Available at: https://linkinghub.elsevier.com/retrieve/pii/S2405500X17309490. Accessed June 10, 2019.

43. Honarbakhsh S, Schilling RJ, Dhillon G, et al. A novel mapping system for panoramic mapping of the left atrium. JACC Clin Electrophysiol 2017;546:124–34. Available at: http://linkinghub.elsevier.com/retrieve/pii/S2405500X17309490. Accessed December 13, 2017.

44. Honarbakhsh S, Schilling RJ, Providencia R, et al. Automated detection of repetitive focal activations in persistent atrial fibrillation: validation of a novel detection algorithm and application through panoramic and sequential mapping. J Cardiovasc Electrophysiol 2019;30(1):58–66. Available at: http://www.ncbi.nlm.nih.gov/pubmed/30255666. Accessed June 9, 2019.

45. Atienza F, Almendral J, Ormaetxe JM, et al. Comparison of radiofrequency catheter ablation of drivers and circumferential pulmonary vein isolation in atrial fibrillation. J Am Coll Cardiol 2014;64(23):2455–67. Available at: http://www.sciencedirect.com/science/article/pii/S073510971406584X. Accessed December 10, 2014.

46. Verma A. Utilizing novel dipole density capabilities to objectively visualize the etiology of rhythms in atrial fibrillation - UNCOVER-AF. Available at: https://clinicaltrials.gov/ct2/show/NCT02825992. Accessed June 10, 2019.

47. Swerdlow M, Tamboli M, Alhusseini MI, et al. Comparing phase and electrographic flow mapping for persistent atrial fibrillation. Pacing Clin Electrophysiol 2019;42(5):499–507. Available at: http://www.ncbi.nlm.nih.gov/pubmed/30882924. Accessed June 9, 2019.

48. Bellmann B, Lin T, Ruppersberg P, et al. Identification of active atrial fibrillation sources and their discrimination from passive rotors using electrographical flow mapping. Clin Res Cardiol 2018;107(11):1021–32. Available at: http://www.ncbi.nlm.nih.gov/pubmed/29744616. Accessed June 9, 2019.

49. Buch E, Benharash P, Frank P, et al. Quantitative analysis of localized sources identified by focal impulse and roter modulation mapping in atrial fibrillation. Circ Arrhythm Electrophysiol 2015;554–62. Available at: http://circep.ahajournals.org/cgi/doi/10.1161/CIRCEP.115.002721.

50. Gianni C, Mohanty S, Di Biase L, et al. Acute and early outcomes of FIRM-guided rotors-only ablation in patients with non-paroxysmal atrial fibrillation. Heart Rhythm 2015;13(4):830–5. Available at: http://www.ncbi.nlm.nih.gov/pubmed/26706193. Accessed January 10, 2016.

Mapping and Ablation of Ventricular Outflow Tract Arrhythmias

Magdi M. Saba, MD*, Anthony Li, MD

KEYWORDS

- Catheter ablation • Ventricular outflow tracts • Ventricular ectopy • Ventricular tachycardia
- 3d mapping

KEY POINTS

- Knowledge of intracardiac anatomy and the attitudinal orientation of the outflow tracts relative to each other is critical to mapping.
- Electrocardiographic algorithms to predict the origin of outflow tract arrhythmias can be useful in preprocedure planning but may also mislead.
- Pace-mapping has an inferior spacial resolution to activation mapping in the outflow tracts.
- Automated mapping systems should not replace careful interrogation of the local electrogram.

INTRODUCTION

This review focuses on outflow tract ventricular arrhythmias in the absence of structural heart disease.

Ventricular outflow tract arrhythmias represent a distinct form of arrhythmia. These are typically benign in nature and not associated with heart disease. However, a subset of patients may harbor subtle abnormalities of the outflow tract or elsewhere in the ventricles, and clinical management will be dictated not only by the burden of ectopy, but also by the presence or absence of coexisting structural heart disease. There are rare examples of outflow tract ectopy associated with polymorphic ventricular tachycardia or ventricular fibrillation.[1] By and large, in the absence of structural heart disease, outflow tract ectopy is not associated with sudden cardiac death.[2] The goals of management are the control of symptoms and the preservation of cardiac structure and function. In symptomatic patients, ablation is offered where significant symptoms persist despite attempts at suppressive medical therapy, or in those who cannot tolerate or decline medical therapy. In the absence of symptoms, ablation is considered in cases with a moderate to high burden (typically more than 15,000 in 24 hours), particularly in whom there is evidence of left ventricular dysfunction in the form of dilatation or depressed systolic function.[3]

MECHANISMS

Cyclic adenosine monophosphate–mediated triggered activity has been described as a mechanism of outflow tract ectopy. However, it is not well understood why right ventricular outflow tract (RVOT) ventricular ectopy (VE) is more commonly seen in women and left ventricular outflow tract (LVOT) VE more commonly in men.[4] Outflow tract site of origin and behavior are likely to be important factors associated with effects on left ventricular function.[5]

Financial Disclosures: None.
Cardiology Clinical Academic Group, St. George's University of London, Cranmer Terrace, London SW17 0QT, UK
* Corresponding author. St. George's University of London, Cranmer Terrace, London SW17 0QT, UK
E-mail address: msaba@sgul.ac.uk

Card Electrophysiol Clin 11 (2019) 597–607
https://doi.org/10.1016/j.ccep.2019.08.003
1877-9182/19/© 2019 Elsevier Inc. All rights reserved.

cardiacEP.theclinics.com

Management involves attempts at suppression with medical therapy in the first instance. Beta-blockers, and less commonly calcium channel blockers, are used as first-line therapy.[6] The efficacy of suppressive therapy is approximately 50% to 60% and side effects are not infrequent.[7] Ablation therefore offers the possibility of definitive control of the arrhythmia without requiring long-term medical therapy.[8]

PREPROCEDURE WORKUP

Echocardiography and cardiac MRI are used to rule out structural heart disease, the absence of which portends a good prognosis. Subtle abnormalities of the RVOT have been noted in patients with RVOT ectopy, although the clinical significance is unclear.[9] In this study, the location of subtle structural abnormalities in the RVOT by cardiac MRI colocated in 6 of 8 cases with the site origin of the clinical ventricular arrhythmias. In cases with more than one VE morphology, imaging is crucial to uncover possible underlying subtle pathology.

DIFFERENTIATING RIGHT FROM LEFT VENTRICULAR OUTFLOW TRACT ARRHYTHMIA

Differentiating right from left ventricular outflow tract arrhythmias is important both for decision-making and practical reasons. The challenges and risks associated with LVOT mapping are more serious than those associated with RVOT mapping and ablation. This should be discussed with the patient beforehand, considering the symptoms, burden of ectopy, response to suppressive medical therapy, and the likely origin of the arrhythmia. Many surface electrocardiogram (ECG) algorithms have been developed to try to differentiate the origins of VEs. However, beyond morphology, VE behavior, such as coupling interval variation and clinical features, also may be helpful.[4,10]

The 12-Lead Electrocardiogram

Based on the 12-lead ECG morphology of the ectopic beat, several algorithms have been developed to differentiate a left from right origin.[11,12] Additional ECG leads have also been shown to improve outflow tract localization.[13] Although right bundle branch block (RBBB) morphology of the ectopic beat indicates a left-sided origin, a left bundle branch block (LBBB) morphology only tends to favor an RVOT origin. The earlier the transition of the ectopic beat to a positive QRS in the precordial leads, the more likely it is to arise from the LVOT. It is the group of outflow tract arrhythmias with an LBBB morphology and positive transition by lead V3 that poses the problem. The transitional zone index is a concept recognizing that the heart is situated differently in different patients.[14] If the transition of the ectopic beat to a positive QRS in the precordial leads occurs before that of the intrinsically conducted beat, an LVOT origin is more likely. A later transition yields a positive index, favoring an RVOT origin. The width of the initial r wave in V1/V2 in LBBB VE is important. The wider the r wave in V1/V2, the more likely the origin is left-sided.[15]

Specific Morphologies Commonly Associated with Specific Sites of Origin

Left bundle branch block morphology with transition by V3

Early notching on the down-slope of the S wave or a "W" pattern in V1/V2 tends to indicate a right/left aortic sinus junction origin, and special attention should be paid to mapping that site with adequate catheter position and contact.[15]

Atypical right bundle branch block

A qR pattern in V1 indicates an origin below the aortic valve, typically at the segment of myocardium immediately anterior to the fibrous aortomitral continuity.[16]

RBBB pattern with a sharp, but diminutive q and prominent initial R wave and a smaller r' also indicates an origin below the aortic valve, at the left anterior fascicle.[17]

However, because of anatomic variations in the position of the outflow tracts relative to the surface ECG electrodes, ECG algorithms can be misleading. Therefore, it is our practice to start the mapping process by positioning a multipolar catheter at the great cardiac vein/anterior interventricular vein (GCV/AIV) junction, and the mapping/ablation catheter in the RVOT (**Fig. 1**).

The left ventricular (LV) summit is the epicardial segment of LVOT myocardium bounded by the bifurcation of the left main coronary artery superiorly and an imaginary line between the first septal perforator of the left anterior descending artery and the circumflex artery inferiorly. It is divided into basal and apical segments by the anterior interventricular vein as it courses across this segment of myocardium, which in itself can vary widely. Ectopy arising from this site, distant from the aortic sinus of Valsalva, is characterized by a wider initial r wave relative to the total QRS duration.[18] This ectopy typically arises from muscular components within close proximity to the venous drainage system. Thus, mapping epicardially via

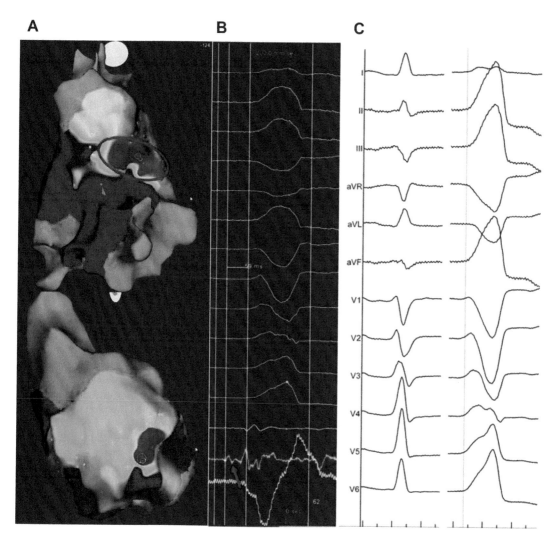

Fig. 1. 35-year-old woman with 35% burden VE. Normal cardiac MRI. (*A*) Top: Posterior-anterior view of LAT map showing broad area of earliest activation (*circled red*). Bottom: Left anterior oblique view of aortic sinuses showing a small area of early activation at the left coronary cusp/right coronary cusp junction. (*B*) Site of earliest activation showing prepotential (*red arrow*) 59 ms pre-QRS onset. Note unipolar activation occurs later. (*C*) Sinus rhythm and VE ECG: current algorithms differentiating left from right origin predicted an RVOT origin in this case.

the venous system, the distal great cardiac vein/ anterior interventricular vein, can yield a favorable target site for ablation. Given that the basal LV is often shrouded in fat, we find that the transpericardial approach is suboptimal. Both the quality of the electrograms (EGMs) and the ability to deliver effective ablative lesions are thus negatively impacted. However, ablation can be successful if the site of origin is within the "accessible" area of the summit, apical to the GCV and may be predicted by surface ECG configuration.[19]

The infero-septal process of the LV is a distinct origin of ectopy, accounting for 1.5% of ectopy

seen in high-volume centers. This ectopy is characterized by an atypical RBBB pattern, left superior axis morphology, with positive concordance and a small s wave in V5/V6. When met with this morphology, the infero-septal process should be mapped with retro-flexion of the mapping catheter below the aortic valve (in the infero-septal recess, or "Sibson vestibule") or via a transseptal approach using a deflectable sheath and directing the catheter to the most posterior, inferior-septal site below the aortic valve and the bundle of His.[20] This site is in close proximity to the compact Atrioventricular (AV) node and junctional rhythm can occur when delivering radiofrequency (RF) energy at this site. Careful monitoring of AV conduction is important during RF ablation at this site. Epicardial ablation of ectopy arising from this site can also be performed via the low septal right atrium.[21] However, as the AV nodal artery courses over the epicardial aspect of the infero-septal process, there is a risk of damage to this artery and consequent AV block.

PROCEDURAL CONSIDERATIONS

Because of the suppressive effect of sedation on the frequency of outflow tract ectopy, the use of benzodiazepine sedatives should be minimized or avoided altogether, if possible. This is particularly important with right-sided ectopy, which tends to show significantly more fluctuation in frequency compared with LVOT ectopy. We use the frequency spread on the Holter monitor to provide guidance on the likely effect of sedation in a particular patient.[22]

The problem of "no or minimal ectopy on the day" is a matter of significance. The use of stimulants, such as isoprenaline, to induce ectopy, is suboptimal. As these procedures are carried out under local anesthesia with little to no sedation, the patient will typically not tolerate several hours of this drug, with its associated tachycardia. Isoprenaline increases the speed of conduction and thus may alter the activation map by increasing the size of the area of earliest activation. This may lead to less precise activation maps and thus the delivery of unnecessary lesions.[23]

NEGOTIATING THE OUTFLOW TRACTS

When mapping the RVOT, it is advisable to advance the mapping catheter beyond the level of the pulmonic valve. This is important for 2 reasons. First, it is the safest method of RVOT mapping: rather than advancing the catheter repeatedly into the thin RVOT, which occasionally is significantly angulated leftward, with the possible existence of small outpouches. However, if after careful interrogation of the local signals a suitable site is not evident, then it may be necessary to gently retract and advance the catheter within the area of interest, as the catheter may find an additional site that, due to trabeculations and pouches, may not be immediately evident (**Fig. 2**). From above the pulmonary valve, gentle pull back, and counterclockwise rotation of the catheter from the pulmonary artery will allow it to safely fall into the highest, antero-septal region of the RVOT. This is the typical site of origin of RVOT VEs, followed by the posterior-septal and mid-RVOT and, least commonly, the free wall of the RVOT.[24] Second, the earliest activation may be above the pulmonic valve, requiring data acquisition from above the valve leaflets if this is not to be missed. The catheter tip may have to be flexed in tight curve or a reverse U fashion to best acquire EGMs from this site.[25]

Special care must be taken during LVOT mapping due to the proximity of the coronary artery ostia. In cases in which the plan includes LVOT mapping, we aim for full anticoagulation with a goal Activated clotting time of 350 to 450 seconds on gaining vascular access. Because of the high

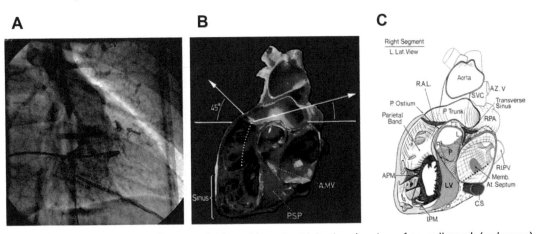

Fig. 2. (*A*) Right anterior oblique fluoroscopic view with contrast injection showing a free wall pouch (*red arrow*). (*B, C*) Coronal posterior-anterior dissection showing trabeculations and parietal band within the RVOT. AMV, anterior mitral valve; APM, anterior papillary muscle; AZV, azygous vein; CS, coronary sinus; IPM, inferior papillary muscle; PSP, posterior-superior process; RAL, right anterolateral leaflet of the pulmonary valve; RIPV, right inferior pulmonary vein; R, L, P, Right, Left, Posterior Aortic Leaflets; RPA, right pulmonary artery; SVC, superior vena cava. (*Courtesy* UCLA Cardiac Arrhythmia Center, Wallace A. McAlpine MD collection, reproduced with permission.)

variability of the relationship of the aortic root and the sinuses to the left ventricle from patient to patient, it is critical to be fully aware of the anatomy. As the procedure is usually carried out under local anesthesia with minimal to no sedation, transesophageal echocardiography is frequently not possible. Intracardiac echo is an option but can be costly and is not widely available.

Our practice is to obtain bilateral femoral arterial access, one to accommodate the mapping catheter and the other being a 4 to 5Fr sheath to allow aortic root angiography at the onset of LVOT mapping to serve as a road map for mapping, and subsequently immediately before ablation with the catheter tip on the site where energy is to be delivered to confirm a safe distance from the ostium of a coronary artery.

MAPPING

The goal of mapping is to localize the site of origin to the smallest possible area, to allow the abolition of the arrhythmia with the least amount of destructive energy. Activation mapping is the mainstay of mapping of outflow tract arrhythmias. Identifying the features of the local EGM at the site of origin of the ectopic beat is critical to the accurate targeting and judicious use of ablative energy in the outflow tract.

Bipolar EGMs preceding the QRS onset by at least 20 ms, typically 20 to 30 ms, are considered to be within close proximity to the site of origin and thus a good target for ablation.[26] The use of smaller-tip catheters, or mini-electrodes, may provide higher definition with the ability to discover very low amplitude local EGMs, but data on improved outcomes with such catheters compared with standard mapping catheters are lacking. During sinus rhythm, abnormal, low-amplitude, separately identifiable potentials may be discerned, typically following the far-field EGM, at the site of successful ablation in the aortic sinuses. During VE, a reversal of the activation sequence of these EGMs can be seen as isolated "prepotentials," preceding the QRS onset by more than 60 ms[15,27] (**Fig. 3**). However, care must be

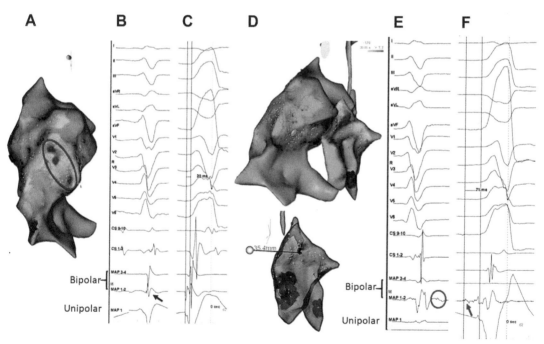

Fig. 3. 67-year-old man with symptomatic high burden VE and mild LV dysfunction. (*A*) Left lateral view of RVOT showing broad area of points with equally early activation on the septal aspect (*circled red*). (*B*) Sinus rhythm bipolar EGM from distal mapping electrode at early spot on RVOT septum (*black arrow*) showing bland EGM. (*C*) EGM during clinical VE showing activation 20 ms pre-QRS onset with negative unipolar signal. (*D*) Top: Steep left lateral view of the RVOT and aortic sinuses showing earliest site of activation and successful ablation site (*red*) at the right coronary cusp/left coronary cusp junction. Bottom panel shows the site of 96% pace-map match from the septal RVOT 35 mm from the site of successful ablation. (*E*) Sinus rhythm EGM at the site of successful ablation showing fractionated EGM with a late potential (*red circle*). (*F*) EGM during clinical VE demonstrating activation 71 ms pre-QRS onset with prepotential seen on bipolar EGM (red arrow). Unipolar EGM shows a small initial r and the steepest negative dV/dT later than the prepotential.

taken to avoid incorrectly annotating signals that are not due to local activation, such as artifactual signals created by aortic valve closure.[28] These may bear a fixed relationship to the true local EGM and thus masquerade as prepotentials during VE with a stable coupling interval. Discrete potentials, defined as sharp high-frequency potentials, often displaying multiple components, occurring during or after the local ventricular EGM in sinus rhythm or preceding the local ventricular EGM during VEs, have similarly been described at sites of successful ablation in RVOT[29] (**Fig. 4**).

The use of multi-electrode catheters during contact mapping may be counterproductive in cases of outflow tract activation mapping because of the irritable nature of that region and the high likelihood of catheter-induced ectopy leading to misleading data. During the acquisition of the activation map, it is critical to avoid mapping catheter-induced ectopy; currently available QRS-matching software cannot distinguish spontaneous from catheter-induced ectopy, which is more likely to occur the higher the number of contact points with the myocardium. In our experience, it is better to have a lower number of high-quality data points than a large amount of questionable data.

Local Electrogram Configuration

It is critical that the local bipolar EGM is scrutinized at the earliest sites. The EGM on the distal bipole should precede that on the proximal bipole and, ideally, a prominent negative deflection at the onset of the distal EGM and a prominent positive deflection at the onset of the proximal EGM should be carefully sought. Reversal of bipolar EGM polarity between the distal and proximal bipoles, when acquiring data from all contiguous electrodes, was shown to be present at 85% of successful ablation sites in patients with idiopathic

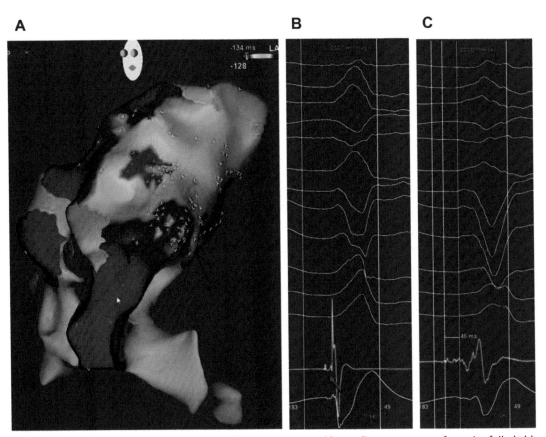

Fig. 4. 61-year-old woman with 30,000 VEs in 24 hours, no structural heart disease presents after prior failed ablation. (*A*) Left lateral view of RVOT showing a discrete area of early activation on the septum. (*B*) Earliest site of activation with a sharp Purkinje-like prepotential and corresponding location (*red arrow* denotes location of earliest activation shown in Panel B). (*C*) Shift in exit site after initial ablation. Note broader QRS and more notched limb leads. Local bipolar EGM with increased scale at this site showed fractionated low-amplitude activation 46 ms pre-QRS. Site of origin shifted to the free wall.

RVOT VE and absent at all unsuccessful sites.[30] In another study, the presence of negative concordance between the unipolar EGM and distal bipolar EGM complexes was shown to have a sensitivity and specificity of 94% and 95% in predicting the successful site of ablation in focal VEs.[31]

The local bipolar EGM at the site of earliest activation may appear normal by voltage criteria during sinus rhythm or may show signs of a subtle abnormality such as low voltage or fractionation circumscribed to a small area.[32] However, the local EGM during the ectopic beat at the site of earliest activation is typically of lower amplitude and of longer duration than in passive activation during sinus rhythm. Evidence of a local abnormality detectable in sinus rhythm based on local EGM complexity with corresponding good pace-map match has been shown to be useful in cases in which activation mapping is limited by infrequent clinical VEs on the day of the procedure.

Unipolar EGMs showing a QS pattern with a rapid downstroke and no initial r wave have been shown to be present at sites of successful activation. However, unipolar EGMs also have a wider field of view and therefore include significant far-field activation. Although the steepest part of the unipolar EGM has been shown to represent the true local activation at the recording electrode, its timing may not necessarily coincide with low-amplitude fractionated prepotentials seen in some cases in bipolar configuration (see **Fig. 3**). Furthermore, unipolar recordings are susceptible to noise such that the use of an indifferent electrode in the inferior vena cava as opposed to the Wilson central terminal may be needed. The spatial resolution of unipolar EGMs to localize the origin of VEs is suboptimal, with unipolar EGMs showing QS pattern greater than 1 cm from the site of origin.[33] Further, a QS intracavitary potential also can be seen where poor catheter contact is present, but usually can be distinguished by the lower dV/dT of the initial downstroke.

Three-Dimensional Mapping Features

A focal source of activation is expected where an area of earliest activation on a local activation timing (LAT) map is surrounded by progressively later activation isochrones, like ripples in a pond. The creation of these maps has been made less burdensome by the development of various automated annotation algorithms using morphology template matching. Beyond annotation of the earliest site, the appearance of the LAT can provide the operator with additional information. A broad area harboring sites of equally early

activation may suggest a breakthrough from a distant site of origin. In one study, an area of earliest activation greater than 1 cm^2 on the RVOT septum suggested an LVOT origin and a location greater than 1 cm below the pulmonary valve excluded an RVOT origin.[34] In another study, a broad area of the earliest 10-ms isochrone greater than 2.3 cm^2 on the RVOT septum gave a sensitivity and specificity of 83% and 92%, respectively, for predicting an LVOT origin.[35] Furthermore, a more ovoid shape of earliest activation with a longitudinal:perpendicular ratio less than 0.8 identified an LVOT origin with 68% sensitivity and 100% specificity[35] (see **Figs. 2** and **3**). However, these features may not be applicable when isoprenaline is used.[23]

Automated activation mapping, a feature of several 3-dimensional (3D) electroanatomic systems, may serve to speed up the process of activation mapping. When a VE meets a user-defined threshold for a match with a preacquired template, the local EGM is annotated automatically based on a combination of bipolar and unipolar (typically steepest negative dV/dT) EGM characteristics. Care should be taken when interpreting these maps, as automated mapping cannot easily discriminate features that the eye can discern. Problems can arise from incorrect automatic annotation of the local bipolar EGM based on current algorithms, as shown in **Fig. 3**. In this case, a prepotential 70-ms pre-QRS is not seen in the unipolar recording and was therefore annotated incorrectly by the automatic algorithm. In a recent study, validation of an automated annotation algorithm against manually annotated maps showed overall good correlation; however, earliest activation timing was consistently underestimated by the automated algorithm compared with manual annotation, particularly in the LVOT.[36] It is also critical to discern catheter-induced ectopy from spontaneous ectopy to avoid spurious data. The local bipolar EGM characteristics on the distal and proximal bipoles should be scrutinized for timing as well as features suggestive of spontaneous ectopy. The threshold for morphology matching when acquiring automated points should be set high, typically 90% to 95% match, to further reduce the likelihood of acquiring catheter-induced VEs.

Pace-Mapping

Pace-mapping is an inferior strategy to activation mapping in locating the site of origin of outflow tract VE due to a lower spatial resolution. In one study, the area of best pace-map match was shown to be larger than that of the earliest isochrone in an activation map (1.8 cm^2 vs 1.2 cm^2).[26] However, it is useful to regionalize the site of origin to allow more focused activation mapping in cases of low-burden ectopy on the day. It also may be a useful strategy when the area of best match colocates to an abnormal sinus rhythm EGM in the RVOT at the pulmonary valve transition zone.[32,37] It is advisable to perform pace-mapping at just over the threshold of tissue capture, and ideally at a similar coupling interval to the clinical VE, to minimize the volume of tissue captured and minimize the area of best match.[38] It also should be recognized that pace-mapping in the LVOT is more problematic. It is often the case that pacing fails to capture or requires high-amplitude stimulation in the aortic sinuses, due to the presence of isolated muscle bundles or preferential conduction pathways[39] (**Fig. 5**).

ACUTE RESPONSE TO ABLATION

It is our practice to routinely perform ablation with open irrigated catheters at 30 W, up to 40 W on occasion for up to 60 seconds per lesion in the RVOT and starting at 15 to 20 W in the aortic sinus region. The question of what an effective lesion is, is currently unclear. We use time to VE

suppression and, where present, the occurrence of ablation-induced automatic Ventricular tachycardia of similar morphology to the clinical beat as guides to effective lesions. Although indexes using force, time, and ablation power have been studied in the atrium, few data exist for the ventricle. In a recent retrospective study, higher ablation index values were associated with higher acute and 6-month success with an overall cutoff of 552 for the right ventricle, which gave a sensitivity and specificity of 80% and 70%, respectively, for long-term success.[40] This requires prospective evaluation.

DIFFICULT AND REDO CASES

Despite seemingly good initial data acquisition and ablation with good contact force and catheter stability, failure of VE elimination occasionally occurs. When mapping the anterior free wall of the RVOT, small movements of the catheter can locate a site that has been previously shielded by trabeculations or other structures, such as the parietal band (see **Fig. 2**). On the septum, it may be the case, as previously discussed, that the origin resides in the LVOT. Another possibility is that the exit of the VE has shifted to a different site,

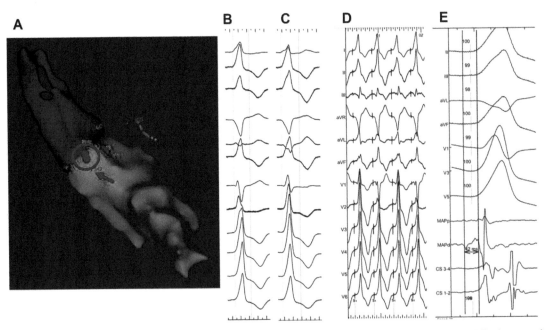

Fig. 5. 55-year-old man with high burden ectopy of 2 morphologies with prior myocarditis and mildly depressed LV function. (*A*) Anteroposterior view of aortic root showing successful ablation lesion set (*red circle*) that eliminated both clinical VEs. (*B, C*) 12-lead morphology of clinical VEs. (*D*) Pace-mapping in the LVOT below the level of the leaflets at constant pacing output showing QRS alternating between 2 morphologies similar in morphology to the clinical VEs, adjacent to the site of origin (*red arrow*, Panel A). (*E*) Site of earliest activation just below the aortic sinuses showing a prepotential 42 ms pre-QRS onset.

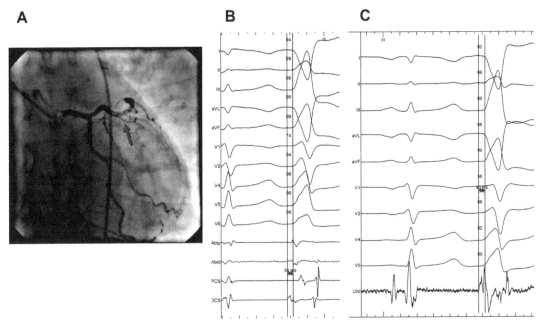

Fig. 6. 45-year-old woman with symptomatic 30% burden ectopy with normal cardiac MRI. (*A*) Right anterior oblique fluoroscopic view of angioplasty wire (*red arrow*) used to map the anterior interventricular vein showing close proximity to the Left Anterior Descending Artery. (*B*) EGMs 34 ms pre-QRS onset on the distal coronary sinus catheter positioned at the great cardiac vein-anterior interventricular vein junction (catheter not shown). (*C*) Unipolar mapping from angioplasty wire down the anterior interventricular vein showing earlier activation 40 ms pre-QRS onset.

and therefore the surface ECG should always be re-interrogated[41] (see **Fig. 4**).

For redo ablation cases, it is necessary to adopt an open mindset. Typically, redo cases will be more prolonged procedures, will require more careful mapping, and more ablation time. When dealing with redo cases, appraising and optimizing the local EGM is of critical importance, as signals can be of low amplitude in areas previously ablated. We routinely appraise the EGMs on both the 3D mapping system as well as the Electrophysiology recording system, which may aid in the recognition of these signals (see **Fig. 4**).

One study examined the reasons behind failed ablation in the RVOT. Among 38 patients subjected to a second procedure, the origin of the Ventricular arrhythmia was identified in 95% of the patients. In 28 (74%) of 38, the arrhythmia origin was not in the RVOT. The VA originated from intramural sites (n = 8, 21%), the pulmonary artery (n = 7, 18%), the aortic sinuses (n = 6, 16%), and the epicardium (n = 5, 13%). The VA was eliminated in 34 (89%) of 38 patients with repeat procedures.[42]

The LV summit is an area that is notoriously problematic. It is both difficult to access, and difficult to deliver energy to in terms of its relationship to the coronary arteries and sometimes deep intramural origin of the VA. A problematic procedure can be anticipated from the start when early signals from the Coronary Sinus catheter at the AIV-GCV junction are seen. Refinement in mapping can be achieved by means of a small multipolar catheter or by using an angioplasty wire down the AIV to record signals (**Fig. 6**). A deep intramural focus is suggested by signals that appear far-field/blunted with a timing and configuration that is unfavorable and pace-maps that are unable to fully match that of the clinical VE.[43] Ablation within the coronary venous system requires low power, typically 15 to 25 W, with high irrigation flow. Where conventional ablation is unsuccessful, alternative approaches, such as sequential or simultaneous unipolar ablation, can be attempted or, failing that, percutaneous or surgical epicardial access may be indicated. Similar to other reports, we have found percutaneous epicardial access is helpful in only a minority of cases in which the site of origin is apical to the course of the AIV.[19,44]

SUMMARY

Catheter ablation for outflow tract arrhythmias can be effective. However, because of the anatomic configuration of the outflow tracts, mapping and ablation can be challenging in some cases. With this in mind, one should not be married to either outflow tract during preprocedure planning and intraprocedural mapping. Although automated mapping has lessened the burden on the operator, it should not replace careful interrogation of the local EGM timing and configuration.

REFERENCES

1. Noda T, Shimizu W, Taguchi A, et al. Malignant entity of idiopathic ventricular fibrillation and polymorphic ventricular tachycardia initiated by premature extrasystoles originating from the right ventricular outflow tract. J Am Coll Cardiol 2005;46(7):1288–94.

2. Kennedy HL, Whitlock JA, Sprague MK, et al. Long-term follow-up of asymptomatic healthy subjects with frequent and complex ventricular ectopy. N Engl J Med 1985;312(4):193–7.

3. Al-Khatib SM, Stevenson WG, Ackerman MJ, et al. 2017 AHA/ACC/HRS guideline for management of patients with ventricular arrhythmias and the prevention of sudden cardiac death: executive summary. Heart Rhythm 2018;15(10):e190–252.

4. Penela D, De Riva M, Herczku C, et al. An easy-to-use, operator-independent, clinical model to predict the left vs. right ventricular outflow tract origin of ventricular arrhythmias. Europace 2015;17(7): 1122–8.

5. Bas HD, Baser K, Hoyt J, et al. Effect of circadian variability in frequency of premature ventricular complexes on left ventricular function. Heart Rhythm 2016;13(1):98–102.

6. Krittayaphong R, Bhuripanyo K, Punlee K, et al. Effect of atenolol on symptomatic ventricular arrhythmia without structural heart disease: a randomized placebo-controlled study. Am Heart J 2002;144(6):1–5.

7. Zhong L, Lee Y-H, Huang X-M, et al. Relative efficacy of catheter ablation vs antiarrhythmic drugs in treating premature ventricular contractions: a single-center retrospective study. Heart Rhythm 2014;11(2):187–93.

8. Ling Z, Liu Z, Su L, et al. Radiofrequency ablation versus antiarrhythmic medication for treatment of ventricular premature beats from the right ventricular outflow tract. Circ Arrhythm Electrophysiol 2014; 7(2):237–43.

9. Globits S, Kreiner G, Frank H, et al. Significance of morphological abnormalities detected by MRI in patients undergoing successful ablation of right ventricular outflow tract tachycardia. Circulation 1997; 96(8):2633–40.

10. Bradfield JS, Homsi M, Shivkumar K, et al. Coupling interval variability differentiates ventricular ectopic complexes arising in the aortic sinus of Valsalva and great cardiac vein from other sources: mechanistic and arrhythmic risk implications. J Am Coll Cardiol 2014;63(20):2151–8.

11. Betensky BP, Park RE, Marchlinski FE, et al. The V(2) transition ratio: a new electrocardiographic criterion for distinguishing left from right ventricular outflow tract tachycardia origin. J Am Coll Cardiol 2011; 57(22):2255–62.

12. Yoshida N, Yamada T, McElderry HT, et al. A novel electrocardiographic criterion for differentiating a left from right ventricular outflow tract tachycardia origin: the V2S/V3R index. J Cardiovasc Electrophysiol 2014;25(7):747–53.

13. Zhang F, Hamon D, Fang Z, et al. Value of a posterior electrocardiographic lead for localization of ventricular outflow tract arrhythmias. JACC Clin Electrophysiol 2017;3(7):678–86.

14. Yoshida N, Inden Y, Uchikawa T, et al. Novel transitional zone index allows more accurate differentiation between idiopathic right ventricular outflow tract and aortic sinus cusp ventricular arrhythmias. Heart Rhythm 2011;8(3):349–56.

15. Ouyang F, Fotuhi P, Ho SY, et al. Repetitive monomorphic ventricular tachycardia originating from the aortic sinus cusp: electrocardiographic characterization for guiding catheter ablation. J Am Coll Cardiol 2002;39(3):500–8.

16. Chen J, Hoff PI, Rossvoll O, et al. Ventricular arrhythmias originating from the aortomitral continuity: an uncommon variant of left ventricular outflow tract tachycardia. Europace 2012;14(3):388–95.

17. Nogami A, Naito S, Tada H, et al. Verapamil-sensitive left anterior fascicular ventricular tachycardia: results of radiofrequency ablation in six patients. J Cardiovasc Electrophysiol 1998;9(12): 1269–78.

18. Daniels DV, Lu Y-Y, Morton JB, et al. Idiopathic epicardial left ventricular tachycardia originating remote from the sinus of Valsalva: electrophysiological characteristics, catheter ablation, and identification from the 12-lead electrocardiogram. Circulation 2006;113(13):1659–66.

19. Santangeli P, Marchlinski FE, Zado ES, et al. Percutaneous epicardial ablation of ventricular arrhythmias arising from the left ventricular summit. Circ Arrhythm Electrophysiol 2015;8(2):337–43.

20. Li A, Zuberi Z, Bradfield JS, et al. Endocardial ablation of ventricular ectopic beats arising from the basal inferoseptal process of the left ventricle. Heart Rhythm 2018;15(9):1356–62.

21. Santangeli P, Hutchinson MD, Supple GE, et al. Right atrial approach for ablation of ventricular arrhythmias arising from the left posterior-superior process of the left ventricle. Circ Arrhythm Electrophysiol 2016;9(7):e004048.

22. Hamon D, Abehsira G, Gu K, et al. Circadian variability patterns predict and guide premature

ventricular contraction ablation procedural inducibility and outcomes. Heart Rhythm 2018;15(1): 99–106.

23. De Ponti R, Ho SY. Mapping of right ventricular outflow tract tachycardia/ectopies: activation mapping versus pace mapping. Heart Rhythm 2008; 5(3):345–7.

24. Joshi S, Wilber DJ. Ablation of idiopathic right ventricular outflow tract tachycardia: current perspectives. J Cardiovasc Electrophysiol 2005;16(s1): S52–8.

25. Liao Z, Zhan X, Wu S, et al. Idiopathic ventricular arrhythmias originating from the pulmonary sinus cusp. J Am Coll Cardiol 2015;66(23):2633–44.

26. Bogun F, Taj M, Ting M, et al. Spatial resolution of pace mapping of idiopathic ventricular tachycardia/ectopy originating in the right ventricular outflow tract. Heart Rhythm 2008;5(3):339–44.

27. Srivathsan KS, Bunch TJ, Asirvatham SJ, et al. Mechanisms and utility of discrete great arterial potentials in the ablation of outflow tract ventricular arrhythmias. Circ Arrhythm Electrophysiol 2008;1(1): 30–8.

28. Romero J, Ajijola O, Shivkumar K, et al. Characterization of aortic valve closure artifact during outflow tract mapping. Circ Arrhythm Electrophysiol 2017; 10(6). https://doi.org/10.1161/CIRCEP.116.004845.

29. Liu E, Xu G, Liu T, et al. Discrete potentials guided radiofrequency ablation for idiopathic outflow tract ventricular arrhythmias. Europace 2015;17(3): 453–60.

30. van Huls van Taxis CFB, Wijnmaalen AP, den Uijl DW, et al. Reversed polarity of bipolar electrograms for predicting a successful ablation site in focal idiopathic right ventricular outflow tract arrhythmias. Heart Rhythm 2011;8(5):665–71.

31. Sorgente A, Epicoco G, Ali H, et al. Negative concordance pattern in bipolar and unipolar recordings: an additional mapping criterion to localize the site of origin of focal ventricular arrhythmias. Heart Rhythm 2016;13(2):519–26.

32. Wang Z, Zhang H, Peng H, et al. Voltage combined with pace mapping is simple and effective for ablation of noninducible premature ventricular contractions originating from the right ventricular outflow tract. Clin Cardiol 2016;39(12):733–8.

33. Man KC, Daoud EG, Knight BP, et al. Accuracy of the unipolar electrogram for identification of the site of origin of ventricular activation. J Cardiovasc Electrophysiol 1997;8(9):974–9.

34. Acosta J, Penela D, Herczku C, et al. Impact of earliest activation site location in the septal right

ventricular outflow tract for identification of left vs right outflow tract origin of idiopathic ventricular arrhythmias. Heart Rhythm 2015;12(4):726–34.

35. Herczku C, Berruezo A, Andreu D, et al. Mapping data predictors of a left ventricular outflow tract origin of idiopathic ventricular tachycardia with V$_3$ transition and septal earliest activation. Circ Arrhythm Electrophysiol 2012;5(3):484–91.

36. Acosta J, Soto-Iglesias D, Fernández-Armenta J, et al. Clinical validation of automatic local activation time annotation during focal premature ventricular complex ablation procedures. Europace 2018; 20(FI2):f171–8.

37. Yamashina Y, Yagi T, Namekawa A, et al. Distribution of successful ablation sites of idiopathic right ventricular outflow tract tachycardia. Pacing Clin Electrophysiol 2009;32(6):727–33.

38. Goyal R, Harvey M, Daoud EG, et al. Effect of coupling interval and pacing cycle length on morphology of paced ventricular complexes: implications for pace mapping. Circulation 1996;94(11): 2843–9.

39. Yamada T, Murakami Y, Yoshida N, et al. Preferential conduction across the ventricular outflow septum in ventricular arrhythmias originating from the aortic sinus cusp. J Am Coll Cardiol 2007;50(9):884–91.

40. Casella M, Gasperetti A, Gianni C, et al. Ablation Index as a predictor of long-term efficacy in premature ventricular complex ablation: a regional target value analysis. Heart Rhythm 2019. https://doi.org/10.1016/j.hrthm.2019.01.005.

41. Shirai Y, Liang JJ, Garcia FC, et al. QRS morphology shift following catheter ablation of idiopathic outflow tract ventricular arrhythmias: prevalence, mapping features, and ablation outcomes. J Cardiovasc Electrophysiol 2018;29(12):1664–71.

42. Yokokawa M, Good E, Crawford T, et al. Reasons for failed ablation for idiopathic right ventricular outflow tract-like ventricular arrhythmias. Heart Rhythm 2013;10(8):1101–8.

43. Yokokawa M, Jung DY, Hero AO III, et al. Single- and dual-site pace mapping of idiopathic septal intramural ventricular arrhythmias. Heart Rhythm 2016; 13(1):72–7.

44. Yamada T, Doppalapudi H, Litovsky SH, et al. Challenging radiofrequency catheter ablation of idiopathic ventricular arrhythmias originating from the left ventricular summit near the left main coronary artery. Circ Arrhythm Electrophysiol 2016;9(10). https://doi.org/10.1161/CIRCEP.116.004202.

Mapping and Ablation of Fascicular Tachycardias (Reentrant and Nonreentrant)

Ahmed Karim Talib, MD, PhD[a,b,*], Mohammad Shenasa, MD, PhD, FHRS[c]

KEYWORDS

- Fascicular tachycardia • Verapamil-sensitive ventricular tachycardia • Catheter ablation
- Nonreentrant fascicular tachycardia • Upper septal ventricular tachycardia

KEY POINTS

- Fascicular ventricular tachycardia (FVT) is either reentrant or nonreentrant, and the left posterior fascicle is the most commonly involved fascicle in both types.
- Reentrant FVT has 3 distinct electrocardiographic characteristics: right bundle branch block (RBBB), left axis (common); RBBB, right axis (uncommon); and RBBB with identical axis to sinus rhythm (rare).
- Nonreentrant fascicular tachycardia (NRFT) is mainly seen in structural heart diseases involving the His-Purkinje system; however, NRFT constitutes approximately 3% of idiopathic ventricular tachycardia (VT).
- Reentrant FVT and NRFT cannot be distinguished by surface electrocardiogram; however, NRFT is verapamil resistant, nonentrainable, and does not show any diastolic potential during VT.
- Although the successful rate of reentrant FVT ablation is high, NRFT ablation outcome is less (83% success), mainly because of noninducibility and the presence of multiple exits.

FASCICULAR VENTRICULAR TACHYCARDIA
Classification

Fascicular ventricular tachycardia (FVT) can be seen in normal heart or in the setting of structural heart diseases, with idiopathic left FVT representing from 10% to 17% of idiopathic ventricular tachycardia (VT) cases referred for ablation.[1,2]

Box 1 shows FVT classification according to VT mechanism.

Monomorphic FVT can be reentrant or nonreentrant, and verapamil-sensitive left FVT is the second most common type of idiopathic VT after right ventricular outflow tract VT.

Reentrant Left Fascicular Ventricular Tachycardia

Idiopathic reentrant left fascicular ventricular tachycardia

Electrocardiogram features Idiopathic reentrant left FVT was first described as a narrow QRS-VT in 1972.[3] In 1979, Zipes and colleagues[4] identified the diagnostic characteristics of reentrant FVT: (1) induction with atrial pacing, (2) right bundle branch block (RBBB) and a left-axis configuration, and (3) absence of structural heart disease. In 1981, verapamil sensitivity of this tachycardia was described as the fourth identifying feature.[5]

[a] Cardiac Electrophysiology Division, Najaf Center for Cardiac Surgery and Trans-catheter Therapy, Najaf city, Iraq; [b] Cardiovascular Division, Faculty of Medicine, University of Tsukuba, Tsukuba, Japan; [c] Heart and Rhythm Medical Group, 105 North Bascom Avenue, Suite 204, San Jose, CA 95128, USA
* Corresponding author. Cardiac Electrophysiology Division, Najaf Center for Cardiac Surgery and Trans-catheter Therapy, P.O.Box:527, Najaf city, Iraq.
E-mail address: ahmed@asahikawa-med.ac.jp

Card Electrophysiol Clin 11 (2019) 609–623
https://doi.org/10.1016/j.ccep.2019.08.004
1877-9182/19/© 2019 Elsevier Inc. All rights reserved.

cardiacEP.theclinics.com

> **Box 1**
> **Fascicular ventricular tachycardia classification**
>
> A. Reentrant
>
>   1. Idiopathic verapamil-sensitive left FVT
>
>   i. Left posterior type and its variant
>
>   ii. Left anterior type and its variant
>
>   iii. Upper septal type
>
>   2. Structural FVT (eg, infarction and sarcoidosis)
>
>   3. Bundle branch reentry VT and interfascicular reentry
>
> B. Nonreentrant
>
>   i. Idiopathic (focal) FVT
>
>   ii. Structural (focal) FVT

Pathophysiology of idiopathic reentrant left fascicular ventricular tachycardia Because FVT is associated with exercise and digoxin toxicity and can be induced by burst and programmed stimulation, any arrhythmia mechanism can cause FVT; therefore, determination of VT mechanism has important clinical implications in the electrophysiology laboratory (discussed later).

There is growing evidence that the mechanism of verapamil-sensitive idiopathic left FVT is reentry involving a single left fascicle (posterior, anterior, or rarely upper septal) associated with a slower-conducting myocardial component, with anatomic distribution of FVT paralleling the topological extent of the respective fascicles. The induction, entrainment, and termination of VT by programmed stimulation provide evidence for a reentrant mechanism.

A close association of FVT with intracavitary structures, especially false tendon, was reported.[6,7]

Although surgical resection of left ventricular (LV) false tendon could eliminate idiopathic VT in 1 case report,[6] an arrhythmogenic role of false tendons in providing the anatomic basis for the macroreentrant circuit is still controversial. Thakur and colleagues[7] found that false tendons were seen in all patients with idiopathic left VT compared with only 5% of control subjects; however, when studied systematically, false tendons are equally prevalent among patients with and without FVT.[8]

Regardless of whether such intracavitary structures contribute to FVT or not, special attention is required to determine their presence, especially with widespread use of intracardiac echocardiography, because detecting the Purkinje networks in these small anatomic structures might be the key to successful ablation.

Reentrant fascicular ventricular tachycardia circuit The predominant mechanism of FVT is reentry with an area of slow conduction[9]; however, the reentry circuit was not completely defined. A seminal work by Nogami and colleagues[10] showed the VT circuit with the use of multipolar catheters positioned along the inferior LV septum.

During sinus rhythm, the conduction propagates antegradely (basal to apical) and rapidly down the left posterior fascicle (LPF) generating a presystolic potential (P2), which was recorded after the His-bundle potential and followed by ventricular activation (QRS complex). The anterograde conduction occurs over the LPF, as well as over the abnormal, slowly conducting Purkinje/adjacent ventricular tissue, with activation going from P2 to P1 (a diastolic potential) at the point of collision of retrograde and antegrade wave fronts; therefore, P1 is buried in the local ventricular activation (**Fig. 1**A).[10] During FVT, activation propagates anterogradely (basal to apical direction) over the abnormal Purkinje tissue, giving rise to P1, and the reentrant wave front then turns around in the lower third of the septum and activates the fast-conducting Purkinje fibers along the LPF, generating a retrograde P2. From the lower turnaround point, the wave front propagates anterogradely down the septum to exit the reentrant circuit and activate the posterior septal myocardium, and retrogradely over the LPF from apical to basal septum, forming the retrograde limb of the tachycardia.[10]

Hence 2 distinct potentials, P1 and P2, were recorded at the midseptum, where there is orthodromic activation of the diastolic potential P1 and retrograde activation of P2. The investigators suggested that P1 represented a critical pathway composed of specialized Purkinje tissue with decremental properties and verapamil sensitivity (**Fig. 1**B). Recently, Nogami and coworkers showed that LPF negatively participates in the VT circuit[11] and P2 of the LPF is a bystander in the VT circuit.[12] Nevertheless, the slowed conduction over P1 was not slow enough to explain the entire VT circuit and thus the entire circuit was poorly defined.[13] More recently, this concept was reinforced by Liu and colleagues,[14] who showed that the mechanism of LPF-VT is macroreentry involving the ventricular myocardium, a part of the LPF, a slow conduction zone, and in some cases a P1 fiber with a slow conduction zone located between the proximal portion of recorded P1 and ventricular myocardium. Despite considerable progress in defining LPF-VT circuit, the upper

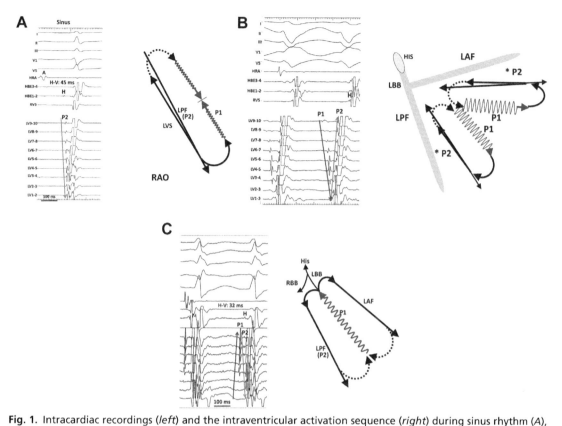

Fig. 1. Intracardiac recordings (*left*) and the intraventricular activation sequence (*right*) during sinus rhythm (*A*), LPF-VT/left anterior fascicle (LAF) VT(*B*), and USF-VT (*C*). (*A*) During sinus rhythm, the conduction propagates antegradely (basal to apical) and rapidly down the LPF generating a presystolic potential (P2), which was recorded after the His-bundle potential and followed by ventricular activation (QRS complex). The anterograde conduction occurs over the LPF, as well as over the abnormal, slowly conducting Purkinje/adjacent ventricular tissue, with activation going from P2 to P1 (a diastolic potential) at the point of collision of retrograde and antegrade wave fronts; therefore, P1 is buried in the local ventricular activation. (*B*) During LPF/LAF-VT, a diastolic potential (P1) and a presystolic Purkinje potential (P2) were recorded. Although P1 was recorded earlier from the proximal rather than the distal electrodes, P2 was recorded earlier from the distal rather than the proximal electrodes and His-bundle potential was recorded after the onset of the QRS complex (negative H-V interval) (*left*). Activation propagates anterogradely (basal to apical direction) over the abnormal Purkinje tissue, giving rise to P1. The reentrant wave front then turns around in the lower third of the septum and activates the fast-conducting Purkinje fibers along the LPF/LAF, generating a retrograde P2. From the lower turnaround point, the wave front propagates anterogradely down the septum to exit the reentrant circuit and activate the posterior (LPP-VT) or anterior (LAF-VT) septal myocardium, and retrogradely over the LPF/LAF from apical to basal septum, forming the retrograde limb of the tachycardia. Although the lower turnaround point is known (*solid line*), the upper turnaround point (*dashed line*) is still ill-defined (*B*). Recent evidence suggests that the retrograde limb consists of myocardial potential, but not of P2 (asterisk). (*C*) During upper septal idiopathic left fascicular VT, P1 was recorded earlier from the distal rather than from the proximal electrodes, whereas P2 was recorded earlier from the proximal rather than from the distal electrodes, similar to that during sinus rhythm. His-bundle potential preceded the onset of the QRS complex by 32 milliseconds, which was shorter than that during sinus rhythm in (*A*) (*left*). Left upper septal VT. P1 represents the activation potential of the specialized Purkinje tissue at LV upper septum. P2 represents the activation of the left anterior and posterior fascicles. Both left anterior and posterior fascicles are the antegrade limbs of the reentrant circuit in VT, which explains why this VT shows a narrow QRS configuration and inferior axis (*right*). H, His potential; LBB, left bundle branch; LVS, left ventricular septum; RAO, right anterior oblique; RBB, right bundle branch; V, ventricle.

turnaround point of LPF-VT is still undetermined, whereas a long H-V interval during LPF-VT may indicate that the lower turnaround point is located basally. Conversely a short H-V interval during LPF-VT indicates that the lower turnaround point is more apical far from the His bundle.[15] Ma and colleagues[16] showed that the more negative the H-V interval during LPF-VT, the further the breakthrough site in the LV is from the proximal His-Purkinje system.

However, complexity of both functional and anatomic aspects of the His-Purkinje system results in complex tachycardia circuits and difficulties in predicting its exact origin.[15]

The left anterior fascicle (LAF)-VT circuit is similar to LPF-VT, the difference being in the fascicle involved.[17] Namely, the diastolic potential (P2) is propagated antegradely over the midseptal area, similar to the common type of LPF-VT, then retrogradely propagates over the area near the LAF (see **Fig. 1**B). Some investigators suggested that both LPF and LAF-VT shared the midseptal area as an antegrade limb of the circuit because ablation of such area could successfully eliminate both LAF-VT and LPF-VT in the same patient.[17]

Upper-septal (USF)-VT is very rare. To show its circuit, the authors used an octapolar catheter at the LV midseptum where the activation sequence of P1 was from the distal to proximal septum, whereas the activation sequence of P2 was from the proximal to distal septum, similar to that during sinus rhythm.[18] We hypothesized that the USF-VT is an orthodromic, or fast-slow, variant of LPF-VT and LAF-VT, in which both LAF and LPF are the antegrade limbs of the reentrant circuit, whereas the retrograde activation occurs via the abnormal Purkinje fiber at the middle fascicular area. Although His and right bundle branch (RBB) are bystanders, they were activated just after the activation of LAF and LPF. This finding explains why this VT shows a narrow QRS configuration with a near-normal activation sequence and inferior axis. P1 represents the common retrograde limb of the circuit during the VT and can be a suitable ablation target (**Fig. 1**C).

The cause of USF-VT is unknown; however, the authors found that all patients had minor electrocardiogram (ECG) morphologic abnormalities, including Q waves in the inferior limb leads and/or S waves in limb leads I and/or aVL; these changes were caused by previous LPF-VT ablation session(s) in half of the cases these findings suggest that, whether iatrogenic or not, such morphologic abnormalities might provide a potential substrate for this type of VT.[18]

APPROACH TO REENTRANT FASCICULAR TACHYCARDIA
Electrocardiographic Recognition

After detailed history and examination with the necessary investigations to rule out structural heart disease; 3 main questions should be answered before planning ablation:

1. Confirm the diagnosis of VT by the usual diagnosis criteria, such as presence of capture and fusion beats and atrioventricular dissociation, in order to differentiate VT from supraventricular tachycardia (SVT), because SVT with aberrancy can easily be confused with FVT and sometimes it is very difficult to differentiate between 2 arrhythmias, particularly in patients with USF-VT. Failure of adenosine to terminate a tachycardia that responds well to verapamil may provide a clue that the tachycardia is probably FVT. This possibility is important to consider before planning the ablation strategy and the chamber to be mapped.

2. Differentiation from other types of VT. Nonreentrant FVT, papillary muscle VT, and mitral annular VT are the most important differential diagnoses. LPF-VT and LAF-VT mimic posteromedial and anterolateral papillary muscle VT, respectively. There are several criteria that can differential FVT from the other arrhythmias, such as QRS duration during VT, R(r')-pattern in V1 and V5, and R-wave concordance.[19,20] However, there is close overlap between these types because of the complexity of the Purkinje network that covers the papillary muscles, making ECG differentiation very difficult.[21]

3. Defining the fascicle involved. According to the fascicle involved in the reentry circuit, there are 3 main ECG types of verapamil-sensitive left FVT:

   A. LPF-VT is the most common form of idiopathic reentrant FVT. As described earlier,[4] LPF-VT is RBBB and a left-axis configuration (**Fig. 2**A). Based on QRS duration, R/S ratio in lead I and lead V6, Ma and colleagues[16] could predict LPF-VT exit with reasonable sensitivity and specificity. Namely, proximal exit of LPF-VT is characterized by QRS duration less than or equal to 120 milliseconds, R/S ratio in lead I greater than or equal to 1.0, and in lead V6 greater than or equal to 0.6, whereas QRS duration greater than or equal to 135 milliseconds and R/S less than or equal to 0.5 in lead I and less than or equal to 0.3 in V6 could predict a distal exit of LPF-VT. Recently the authors described a subtype of LPF-VT that shows RBBB configuration and superior right axis deviation or horizontal axis. This variant originates from Purkinje arborization around the posterior papillary muscle.[21]

   B. LAF-VT is uncommon form of reentrant FVT. It is characterized by RBBB morphology and right axis deviation (**Fig. 2**B).[17] A papillary-Purkinje subtype shows RBBB configuration and right axis deviation with a deep S wave in leads I, V5, and V6.[21]

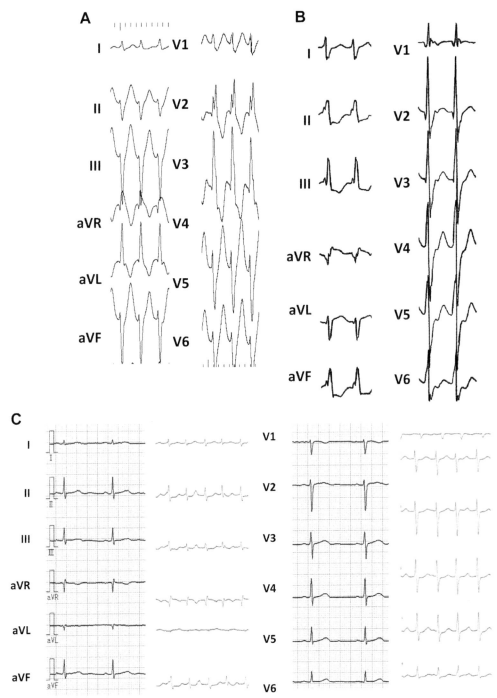

Fig. 2. Twelve-lead ECG of clinically documented LPF, LAF, and USF-VT. ECG of LPF-VT shows RBBB left-axis config-uration (*A*) and LAF-VT shows RBBB–right axis configuration (*B*) and 2 subtypes of USF-VT; namely, an identical precordial QRS configuration to that during sinus rhythm (*C*) and incomplete RBBB pattern (*D*).

C. USF-VT is a very rare reentrant type with incidence of 1% to a maximum of 6% among FVT in referral centers. USF-VT is characterized by QRS duration less than 120 milliseconds and right axis deviation or normal axis (identical to sinus axis) with identical precordial QRS configuration to that during sinus rhythm or right bundle block pattern (**Fig. 2**C, D).[22] The authors found that baseline sinus ECG always

D

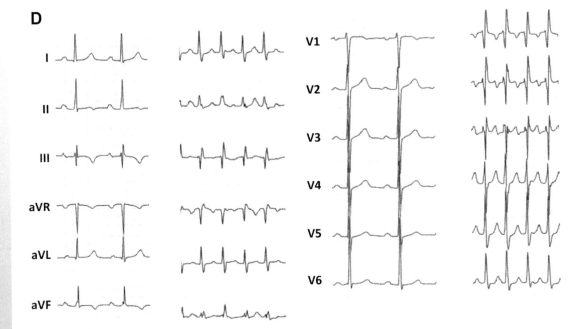

Fig. 2. (*continued*)

showed minor morphologic abnormalities, including Q-waves in the inferior limb leads and/or S-waves in limb leads I and/or aVL; these changes are caused by previous ablation sessions of LPF-VT in half of these patients.[22]

Mapping and Ablation

Catheter ablation is a highly effective long-term measure and is especially useful in patients in whom drug therapy is not successful, not tolerated, or not preferred.

Catheter setup

Under conscious sedation and using femoral approach, His, right ventricle (RV), and high right atrial catheters are typically used. Left ventricle mapping is better to be delayed after 2 important steps (1) confirm VT diagnosis and rule out SVT with aberrancy in the electrophysiology (EP) laboratory; (2) rule out other VTs, such as NRFT, papillary muscle VT, or mitral annular VT, by EP maneuvers before LV mapping because mapping the LV may cause mechanical bumping, rendering VT noninducible and resulting in difficult diagnosis.

Ablation can be performed conventionally under fluoroscopic guidance; however, a three-dimensional (3D) mapping system is useful to precisely tag the ablation points or line of interest, especially when the VT is noninducible. It is also useful to have intracardiac echocardiography to confirm false tendons, papillary muscles, or other intracavitary structures that may provide anatomic substrates of VT and guide ablation.

Induction

First burst atrial pacing is performed from the right atrium until the Wenckebach cycle is reached. Then programmed atrial pacing is used until the atrioventricular nodal effective refractory period is reached. If VT is noninducible, burst and programmed stimulation (up to double or triple stimuli) from the RV apex and RV outflow tract (RVOT) is performed. Pacing from the RVOT is particularly useful if RV apical pacing fails to induce FVT.

When sustained VT is still not inducible, then pharmacologic provocation is performed using atropine and isoproterenol. Both isoproterenol and atropine are effective in inducing FVT. Although isoproterenol enhances the inducibility of the VT by affecting the VT circuit, atropine does not affect the circuit itself. Atropine enhances the atrioventricular nodal conduction; therefore, it can increase the maximum stimulation rate to the Purkinje network during atrial stimulation[23] because one of the characteristic features of verapamil-sensitive left FVT is inducibility by atrial stimulation.[4] The authors usually use intravenous injection of atropine 0.5 to 1.0 mg if atrioventricular block occurs at a cycle length of longer than 300 milliseconds during atrial stimulation. Atropine has another benefit in the stability of mapping/ablation catheter. Unlike isoproterenol, atropine does not cause cardiac hyperkinetic contraction of the left ventricle.

After atropine injection, the same stimulation protocol (from RA, RV, RVOT) is repeated. If VT is still noninducible, the stimulation is repeated during isoproterenol infusion (0.5–2.0 Microgram (µg)/min).

During atrial pacing, repetitive ventricular response of fascicular origin may give a clue to the presence of FVT; this should be differentiated from aberrant conduction (**Fig. 3**A).

Entrainment

When tachycardia is induced, SVT with aberrancy should be ruled out. His bundle is usually activated after the onset of QRS complex in LPF-VT and LAF-VT, whereas His bundle is always activated before aberrant conduction beats (see **Fig. 3**A).

Once VT diagnosis is confirmed, demonstration of entrainment, resetting, and termination criteria from the atrium and/or ventricles is important to differentiate reentrant from nonreentrant VT. This differentiation is particularly important to exclude NRFT and papillary muscle VT. When performing overdrive pacing from the right atrium, ventricular capture should be confirmed before judging whether the tachycardia is entrainable or not because atrioventricular block during atrial overdrive pacing can be misleading. Entrainment can

also be performed locally at the area of interest to decide the ablation target (**Fig. 3**B).

Mapping and ablation

Inducible ventricular tachycardia Through a retrograde aortic approach, mapping is performed along the LV inferior septum (for LPF-VT), and along the anterolateral LV (for LAF-VT). During sinus rhythm, a 3D mapping system can be used to create LV geometry with voltage map and to delineate the His and fascicular system. The presystolic potential (so-called P2) is recorded after the His-bundle potential and before the onset of the QRS complex (see **Fig. 1**A). During VT, a diastolic potential (P1), a discrete, high-frequency potential that precedes the site of earliest ventricular activation by 15 to 42 milliseconds, is recorded at the posterior third of the LV septum. P1 and presystolic potential (P2) are activated in the reverse direction (see **Fig. 2**B). Although P1 propagates from the base to the apex, P2 is activated retrogradely. P1 is recorded within an area proximal to the earliest P2 recording site and is activated from the basal to apical septum toward the earliest P2 site.

There are 2 mains strategies to ablate FVT: (1) targeting any P1 in the circuit; (2) targeting the earliest P2.

Because P1 represents the critical diastolic potential, any P1 can be targeted for ablation. However, to avoid left bundle branch block and

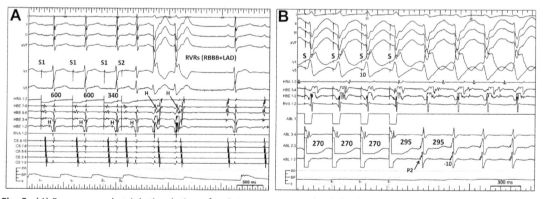

Fig. 3. (*A*) Programmed atrial stimulation after intravenous atropine injection. Programmed atrial stimulation after intravenous atropine injection induced wide QRS complexes with RBBB configuration and left-axis deviation, which is similar to the clinical VT. Negative H-V interval was observed during these complexes. H-V interval during FVT depends on the site of the upper turnaround. If the site of turnaround is high (or close to His bundle), H-V interval will be positive (but shorter than that during sinus rhythm) and vice versa (ie, if the lower turnaround site is more distal, the H-V interval will be negative). (*B*) Entrainment pacing at the VT termination site. At the VT termination site, fused presystolic P2 potential was recorded during VT and P2 preceded the onset of the QRS by 10 milliseconds; however, P1 potential was not recognized. Entrained QRS waves showed minimal fusion with 10-millisecond pacing delay. Postpacing interval (stimulus to returned P2) was 295 milliseconds, which was equal to the cycle length of VT. ABL, ablation catheter; BP, blood pressure; CS, coronary sinus; LAD, left axis deviation; HBE, his-bundle electrogram; HRA, high right atrium; RVA, right ventricular apex; RVR, repetitive ventricular response; 9-10, proximal bipole; 1-2, distal bipole.

atrioventricular block, P1 at the distal third of the septum is a suitable target for ablation.

It is reported that diastolic potential (P1) can be recorded in 64% to 75% of VT cases only.[1,10]

If P1 cannot be detected, the earliest P2 should be targeted. P2 represents the VT exit site. Some investigators suggested the H-V interval during VT can be used to anticipate the VT exit site (ie, more negative H-V interval during VT indicates that the VT exit site is more distal from the His recording site).[16]

A third ablation strategy has been recently reported by Zhang and colleagues.[24] They proposed fragmented antegrade Purkinje potential (FAP) as an arrhythmogenic substrate for LPF-VT. FAP is an abnormal wide, low-frequency potential noted before ventricular activation during sinus rhythm and LPF-VT. FAPs were usually clustered at the posterior septum and the middle segment of the LPF. Two or 3 radiofrequency (RF) energy applications at the area of FAP during sinus rhythm resulted in successful ablation with excellent midterm follow-up.

Ablation of FVT is typically performed during VT at the inferior septum in LPF-VT and midanterior in LAF-VT. When using irrigated system, the authors use a maximum power of 50 W. When using a nonirrigated catheter, ablation is undertaken in temperature-controlled mode at a maximal target temperature of 55°C and maximum power of 50 W.

Ideally, the P1-QRS interval is gradually prolonged during ablation until P1-P2 block results in VT termination.

One caveat to this approach is when VT is terminated by mechanical suppression of the VT circuit by the ablation catheter (ie, mechanical bump) or when the VT is terminated by premature ventricular contraction (PVC) caused by the ablation catheter.

USF-VT is a very rare type of FVT and shares the common characteristics of reentrant FVT, such as inducibility by ventricular and/or atrial stimulation, entrainment, and verapamil sensitivity (**Fig. 4**).[22] Because USF-VT is narrow with a similar axis to that during sinus rhythm and responds well to verapamil, USF-VT can be easily misdiagnosed as SVT.

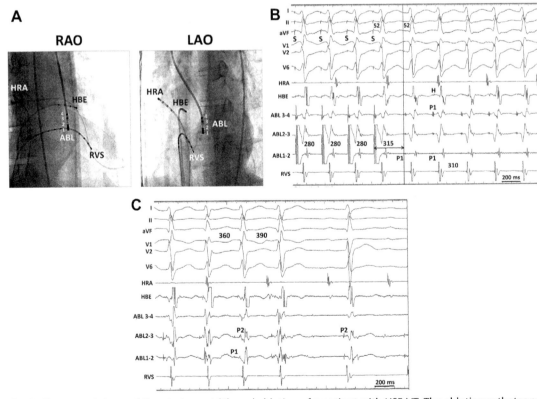

Fig. 4. Fluoroscopic image (A), entrainment (B), and ablation of a patient with USF-VT. The ablation catheter position at the upper-middle ventricular septum (A) where the diastolic P1 preceded the onset of the QRS interval by 52 milliseconds. Entrainment from this site resulted in concealed fusion and postpacing interval–VT cycle length difference of 5 milliseconds and an interval between the pacing stimulus and QRS onset of 52 milliseconds, equal to the P-QRS interval during VT (B). VT was slowed and terminated by RF energy application at this site within a few seconds (C) and VT became noninducible. LAO, left anterior oblique; RVS, right ventricular septum.

During USF-VT mapping, 2 characteristic features should be identified. First, the activation sequence of P1 is from the distal to proximal septum, whereas the activation sequence of P2 is from the proximal to distal septum, similar to that during sinus rhythm (see **Fig. 1**C); this explains why this VT shows a narrow QRS configuration with a near-normal activation sequence and inferior axis.

Second, retrograde activation of the His bundle occurs before the QRS onset, with an H-V interval significantly shorter during VT than during sinus rhythm.[22]

In USF-VT, the ablation site is at the left upper-middle ventricular septum, midway between the His-bundle recording site and the LV apex (see **Fig. 4**). Ablation at the most basal portion of the Left ventricular septum should not be performed to avoid left bundle/atrioventricular block. Electrophysiologically, the ablation site is characterized by the presence of the diastolic Purkinje potential (P1) during VT and the absence of both His-bundle and atrial potentials during sinus rhythm.

In USF-VT, ablation is performed during sinus rhythm in most cases. The authors use a low power output (ie, 10 W), which is increased gradually while carefully monitoring for the development of junctional rhythm or atrioventricular block.[22]

Noninducible ventricular tachycardia Noninducible VT, whether at baseline or after mapping, is a potential cause of unsuccessful procedures. Additional pharmacologic agents, such as class Ia antiarrhythmic drugs [24] or phenylephrine, can be used to induce VT.[25] Short-long-short sequence pacing can be useful.

If ventricular echo beats with similar morphology to those of FVT are observed, they can be mapped (see **Fig. 3**A); otherwise, anatomic linear ablation is performed. Ablation is performed by delivering RF energy ablation in a linear fashion approximately midway to two-thirds of the way toward the apex along the mid-septum to inferior septum and perpendicular to the plane of the septum.[26]

During anatomic ablation, FVT might become easily inducible. **Fig. 5** shows an example of linear

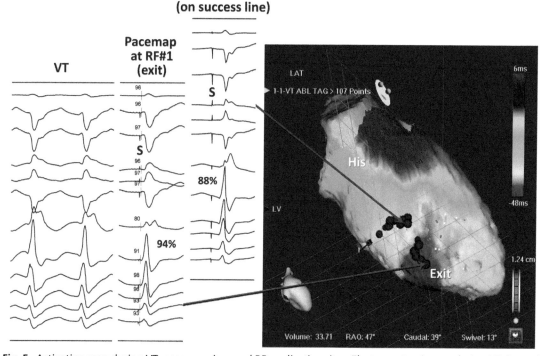

Fig. 5. Activation map during VT, pacemapping, and RF application sites. Electroanatomic map during VT showed a centrifugal pattern from the exit site, which was also determined by pacemapping. The second anatomic linear RF lesion (more proximal to the first RF [*line*]) was created and resulted in VT termination. Although a good pacemap (94% match) was observed at the VT exit site, RF application was ineffective. In contrast, the VT was terminated in a more basal site where less-perfect pacemap (88% matches) with a longer pacing latency, indicating a delay in capturing Purkinje fiber, was observed. LAT, local activation time.

ablation. A caveat to this approach is that pace-mapping at the successful ablation site is usually not effective, because selective pacing of P1 is difficult and there is an antidromic activation of the proximal P1 potential.[26]

Structural Reentrant Fascicular Ventricular Tachycardia

This type of VT occurs when the LV septum and subsequently the His-Purkinje system is diseased and involved in the reentry circuit; mainly caused by an ischemic process after myocardial infarction[27,28] and less commonly by an inflammatory process such as cardiac sarcoidosis.[29]

After myocardial infarction, FVT represents 5% to 11% of postinfarction VT cases.[27,28] The largest series of postinfarction FVT was reported by Bogun and colleagues,[28] who found that about 11% of postinfarction patients developed FVT; among them, 82% showed RBBB morphology with left-axis deviation, suggesting involvement of LPF in the reentry circuit, whereas only 1 patient (9%) had LAF-VT morphology (RBBB–right axis deviation). In cardiac sarcoidosis, both reentrant and nonreentrant FVT were observed, and reentrant FVT represents 10% of all sarcoid-related VT cases[29] with equal distribution between posterior FVT (RBBB, left-axis deviation) and anterior fascicular type (RBBB, right axis deviation). Note that QRS duration and VT cycle length of structural FVT are longer than those of the idiopathic fascicular type.[27,29]

Ablation End Point

Noninducibility despite a full stimulation protocol should be confirmed. Appearance of retrograde P1 during sinus rhythm after ablation might indicate myocardial-P1 block.[30,31]

Creation of left fascicular block as an ablation end point is debated. In contrast, the authors found that ablation-induced ECG changes might lead to USF-VT; however, this has not been systematically assessed.

Bundle Branch Reentry Ventricular Tachycardia and Interfascicular Reentry

This type of macroreentry typically occurs in diseased His-Purkinje systems where relative conduction delay provides the reentrant substrate. This form of tachycardia uses the right bundle (typically as the antegrade limb) and the left bundle branch/fascicles as the retrograde limb. Atypical bundle branch reentry uses the RBB as the retrograde limb. VT morphology shows left bundle branch block (LBBB) or RBBB pattern (LBBB pattern is the most common VT morphology), and it usually has normal or left-axis deviation.

Typical diagnostic findings are His recording preceding the QRS, H-V interval equal to or longer than that during sinus rhythm, and H-H changes driving V-V changes. It responds poorly to pharmacologic therapy and can be cured effectively with catheter ablation, mainly by targeting the right bundle. However, even after ablation, patients may remain at risk for total mortality and sudden cardiac death, and may require further therapies, including, but not limited to, cardiac resynchronization therapy or an implantable cardioverter-defibrillator.[31]

Nonreentrant fascicular tachycardia

This type of VT is usually induced by exercise, emotional stress, and fever, and it is classified as propranolol-sensitive VT. It is thought to be caused by abnormal automaticity in most cases.[32]

Focal nonreentrant fascicular tachycardia (NRFT) was reported in patients with structural heart diseases involving the Purkinje system, such as those associated with myocardial infarction.[33] In structurally normal heart, the authors recently found that 2.8% of idiopathic VT cases referred for ablation were caused by idiopathic NRFT.

Electrocardiographic Characteristics

The patients present with narrow QRS tachycardia (123 ± 12 milliseconds). Verapamil was ineffective for VT termination in all patients.

The VT showed 3 distinct QRS morphologies: (1) RBBB and superior axis configuration in 73% of the patients (LPF origin) (**Fig. 6**A); (2) RBBB and inferior axis configuration 20% (LAF origin) (**Fig. 6**B); and (3) LBBB and superior axis configuration in 7% (right Purkinje arborization) (**Fig. 6**C).

Mapping and Ablation

This type of FVT is difficult to induce. Because fascicular reentrant circuits are notoriously liable to be bumped during mapping, the VT stimulation protocol should be performed before introducing the mapping/ablation catheter into the ventricle, rendering noninducibility of NRFT unlikely to be bump related. Isoproterenol infusion and/or burst ventricular pacing is the most effective method of induction. Even if clinical VT is not inducible, PVC with an identical morphology to the clinical VT can be mapped. Clinical VT/PVC could not be induced in 20% of our series, and pacemap-guided ablation was performed.

It is difficult to differentiate between reentrant FVT and NRFT based on surface ECG alone.

There are 3 important electrophysiologic characteristics that favor the diagnosis of NRFT:

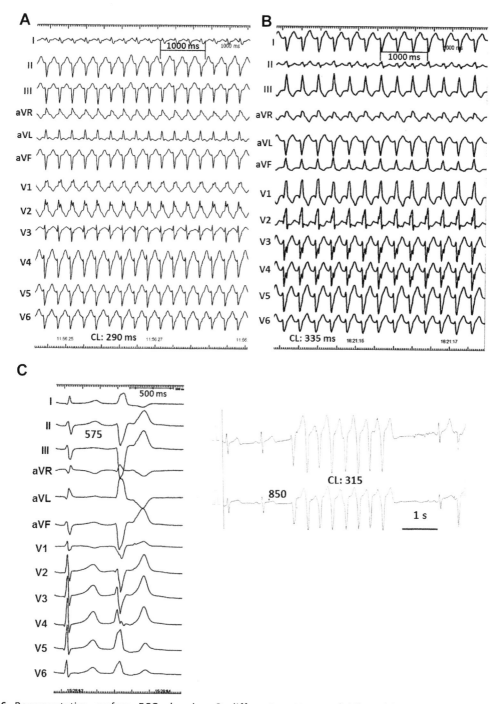

Fig. 6. Representative surface ECG showing 3 different patterns of idiopathic NRFT. (*A*) Pattern 1: RBBB configuration and superior axis. (*B*) Pattern 2: RBBB configuration and inferior axis. (*C*) Pattern 3: VT with a long coupling interval (850 milliseconds) was documented by Holter monitoring. During ablation, an identical PVC was induced. (*D*) Twelve-lead ECG showing absence of constant fusion during right ventricular apex overdrive pacing. Pacing cycle length was 310 milliseconds, whereas VT cycle length was 330 milliseconds. This finding proves that NRFT is a nonreentrant tachycardia. CL, cycle length; S, pacing stimulus.

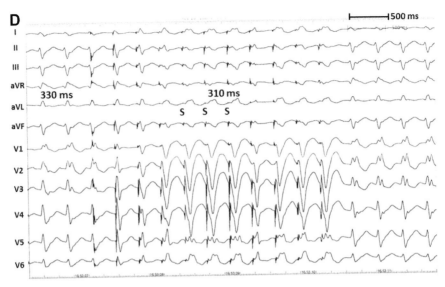

Fig. 6. (*continued*)

1. Verapamil resistance.
2. Absence of reentry criteria. When performing overdrive pacing from the right atrium, RV, and locally from the ablation catheter at the area of interest, VT could not be entrained by overdrive pacing. **Fig. 6**D shows absence of constant fusion during right ventricular apex overdrive pacing. This finding proves that NRFT is a nonreentrant tachycardia.

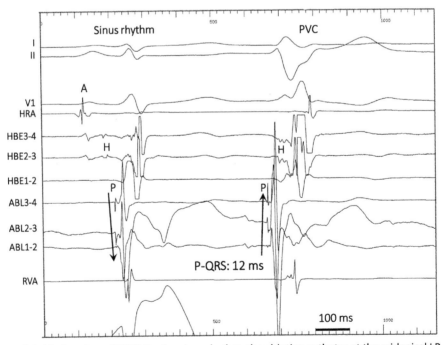

Fig. 7. Successful ablation sites of NRFT. During sinus rhythm, the ablation catheter at the midapical LPF showed a presystolic Purkinje potential, which was recorded after His potential and followed by ventricular activation. During PVC (PVC) of the same morphology of clinically documented VT (RBBB configuration and superior axis), the Purkinje potential preceded the QRS onset of the PVC by 12 milliseconds. The PVC/VT was eliminated by RF catheter ablation (RFCA) at the same site. Note that the Purkinje potential was activated antegradely (proximal to distal) during sinus rhythm, whereas/although during PVC, the Purkinje potentials were activated retrogradely (*arrows*).

3. VT mapping does not show any diastolic potential that suggests a reentrant circuit.

After mapping the left His-Purkinje System, the ablation target is the earliest presystolic Purkinje potential during VT/PVC (**Fig. 7**). One caveat is that targeting a Purkinje potential that is not the earliest one may only change the VT exit and may not eliminate the clinical arrhythmia.

NONREENTRANT FASCICULAR TACHYCARDIA ABLATION END POINT

The ablation end point was elimination of clinical arrhythmia and the newly induced ventricular arrhythmias after repeating the same induction protocol.

CHALLENGES IN NONREENTRANT FASCICULAR TACHYCARDIA ABLATION

Ablation of NRFT is hampered by a high recurrence rate (27%) compared with other forms of idiopathic VT, such as outflow tract VT. Our data suggest that the high recurrence rate is mainly caused by 3 factors: the nature of VT, mapping limitations, and potential risk of complications. If VT is noninducible, pacemapping would be a reasonable alternative option. The authors found that pacemapping at the successful ablation site cannot produce an excellent QRS match in most (93%) cases, because selective pacing of the Purkinje potential of interest is difficult, and local myocardial capture may result in different QRS morphologies. In addition, good pacemapping does not always indicate the site of origin. Pacing

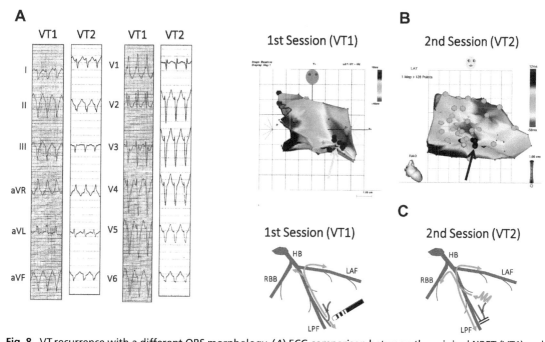

Fig. 8. VT recurrence with a different QRS morphology. (*A*) ECG comparison between the original NRFT (VT1) and another VT that recurred 2 months after the first session (VT2). The VT cycle length and morphology in limb leads were almost identical, whereas the precordial recording was different. VT2 showed an atypical RBBB configuration. (*B*) CARTO mapping of the first and second sessions. The red tags indicate the ablation sites, and the green tags represent presystolic Purkinje potential sites. During the first session, the ablation site (*blue arrow*) was determined by pacemapping because VT/PVC could not be induced. During the second session, PVC with the same morphology of VT2 could be mapped, and the earliest presystolic Purkinje potential was observed slightly proximal to the site of the midapical LPF lesion. PVC was eliminated by RF delivery to this lesion. The yellow tags indicate the sites of presystolic Purkinje potential during sinus rhythm. These findings suggest that both VTs had the same origin but ablation of the exit site, as determined by pacemapping, does not necessary eliminate the origin of NRFT but may change its exit to an adjacent Purkinje arborization or to the myocardium. (*C*) VT1 and VT2. The focal origin of VT1 and VT2 was the same and located at the distal site of Purkinje arborization near the LPF. RFCA at the first session created a conduction block in the Purkinje network and conduction from the origin to another Purkinje arborization via the septal muscle occurred. This finding explains why VT2 had a similar cycle length, slightly less superior axis, and less RBBB configuration. RFCA was successful at the proximal site of the Purkinje potential during PVC.

at the exit site from the Purkinje network to the ventricular myocardium may reproduce an identical QRS configuration. VT recurrence was observed in 4 patients, 3 of whom had noninducible VT at baseline, and pacemap-guided ablation was performed during the first ablation session. In our cohort, 2 cases developed a new VT of a different morphology, suggesting that ablating the exit site, as determined by pacemapping, did not necessarily eliminate the VT origin; instead, it may have only changed the VT exit to an adjacent Purkinje arborization or to the myocardium.

It is also possible that the Purkinje focus has several exit sites that produce different morphologies. Of note, after suppressing the original VT, a new VT of a different morphology was observed during the procedures in some patients (**Fig. 8**).

REFERENCES

1. Lin D, Hsia HH, Gerstenfeld EP, et al. Idiopathic fascicular left ventricular tachycardia: linear ablation lesion strategy for noninducible or nonsustained tachycardia. Heart Rhythm 2005;2:934–9.
2. Talib AK, Nogami A, Morishima I, et al. NonReentrant fascicular tachycardia: clinical and electrophysiological characteristics of a distinct type of idiopathic ventricular tachycardia. Circ Arrhythm Electrophysiol 2016;9(10) [pii:e004177].
3. Cohen HC, Gozo EG, Pick A. Ventricular tachycardia with narrow QRS complexes (left posterior fascicular tachycardia). Circulation 1972;45:1035–43.
4. Zipes DP, Foster PR, Troup PJ, et al. Atrial induction of ventricular tachycardia: reentry versus triggered automaticity. Am J Cardiol 1979;44:1–8.
5. Belhassen B, Rotmensch HH, Laniado S. Response of recurrent sustained ventricular tachycardia to verapamil. Br Heart J 1981;46:679–82.
6. Suwa M, Yoneda Y, Nagao H, et al. Surgical correction of idiopathic paroxysmal ventricular tachycardia possibly related to left ventricular false tendon. Am J Cardiol 1989;64:1217–20.
7. Thakur RK, Klein GJ, Sivaram CA, et al. Anatomic substrate for idiopathic left ventricular tachycardia. Circulation 1996;93:497–501.
8. Lin FC, Wen MS, Wang CC, et al. Left ventricular fibromuscular band is not a specific substrate for idiopathic left ventricular tachycardia. Circulation 1996;93:525–7.
9. Okumura K, Matsuyama K, Miyagi H, et al. Entrainment of idiopathic ventricular tachycardia of left ventricular origin with evidence for reentry with an area of slow conduction and effect of verapamil. Am J Cardiol 1988;62(10 pt 1):727–32.
10. Nogami A, Naito S, Tada H, et al. Demonstration of diastolic and presystolic Purkinje potentials as critical potentials in a macroreentry circuit of verapamil-sensitive idiopathic left ventricular tachycardia. J Am Coll Cardiol 2000;36:811–23.
11. Morishima I, Nogami A, Tsuboi H, et al. Negative participation of the left posterior fascicle in the reentry circuit of verapamil-sensitive idiopathic left ventricular tachycardia. J Cardiovasc Electrophysiol 2012;23:556–9.
12. Maeda S, Yokoyama Y, Nogami A, et al. First case of left posterior fascicle in a bystander circuit of idiopathic left ventricular tachycardia. Can J Cardiol 2014;30. 1460.e11–13.
13. Nogami A. What is the real identity of the mysterious potential P1, and what Is the most important segment of the fascicular ventricular tachycardia circuit? Circ Arrhythm Electrophysiol 2016;9 [pii:e004517].
14. Liu Q, Shehata M, Jiang R, et al. The Macro-reentrant loop in ventricular tachycardia from the left posterior fascicle: new implications for mapping and ablation. Circ Arrhythm Electrophysiol 2016;9: e004272.
15. Talib AK, Nogami A. Purkinje arrhythmia origin made easy. Circ Arrhythm Electrophysiol 2017;10 [pii: e005889].
16. Ma W, Lu F, Shehata M, et al. Catheter ablation of idiopathic left posterior fascicular ventricular tachycardia: predicting the site of origin via mapping and electrocardiography. Circ Arrhythm Electrophysiol 2017;10:e005240.
17. Ohe T, Shimomura K, Aihara N, et al. Idiopathic sustained left ventricular tachycardia: clinical and electrophysiologic characteristics. Circulation 1988;77: 560–8.
18. Kottkamp H, Hindricks G, Willems S, et al. Idiopathic left ventricular tachycardia: new insights into electrophysiological characteristics and radiofrequency catheter ablation. Pacing Clin Electrophysiol 1995; 18:1285–97.
19. Al'Aref SJ, Ip JE, Markowitz SM, et al. Differentiation of papillary muscle from fascicular and mitral annular ventricular arrhythmias in patients with and without structural heart disease. Circ Arrhythm Electrophysiol 2015;8:616–24.
20. Good E, Desjardins B, Jongnarangsin K, et al. Ventricular arrhythmias originating from a papillary muscle in patients without prior infarction: a comparison with fascicular arrhythmias. Heart Rhythm 2008;5:1530–7.
21. Komatsu Y, Nogami A, Kurosaki K, et al. Fascicular ventricular tachycardia originating from papillary muscles: Purkinje network involvement in the reentrant circuit. Circ Arrhythm Electrophysiol 2017;10: e004549.
22. Talib AK, Nogami A, Nishiuchi S, et al. Verapamil-sensitive upper septal idiopathic left ventricular tachycardia: prevalence, mechanism, and electrophysiological characteristics. JACC Clin Electrophysiol 2015;1:369–80.

23. Zhan XZ, Liang YH, Xue YM, et al. A new electro-physiologic observation in patients with idiopathic left ventricular tachycardia. Heart Rhythm 2016;13: 1460–7.

24. Nagai T, Suyama K, Shimizu W, et al. Pilsicainide-induced verapamil sensitive idiopathic left ventricular tachycardia. Pacing Clin Electrophysiol 2006; 29:549–52.

25. Gopi A, Nair SG, Shelke A, et al. A stepwise approach to the induction of idiopathic fascicular ventricular tachycardia. J Interv Card Electrophysiol 2015;44:17–22.

26. Talib AK, Nogami A. Anatomical ablation strategy for noninducible fascicular tachycardia. Card Electrophysiol Clin 2016;8:115–20.

27. Hayashi M, Kobayashi Y, Iwasaki Y, et al. Novel mechanism of postinfarction ventricular tachycardia originating in surviving left posterior Purkinje fibers. Heart Rhythm 2006;3:908–18.

28. Bogun F, Good E, Reich S, et al. Role of Purkinje fibers in post-infarction ventricular tachycardia. J Am Coll Cardiol 2006;48:2500–7.

29. Naruse Y, Sekiguchi Y, Nogami A, et al. Systematic treatment approach to ventricular tachycardia in cardiac sarcoidosis. Circ Arrhythm Electrophysiol 2014; 7:407–23.

30. Tada H, Nogami A, Naito S, et al. Retrograde Purkinje potential activation during sinus rhythm following catheter ablation of idiopathic left ventricular tachycardia. J Cardiovasc Electrophysiol 1998;9: 1218–24.

31. Nogami A. Purkinje-related arrhythmias part I: monomorphic ventricular tachycardias. Pacing Clin Electrophysiol 2011;34:624–50.

32. Gonzalez RP, Scheinman MM, Lesh MD, et al. Clinical and electrophysiologic spectrum of fascicular tachycardia. Am Heart J 1994;128: 147–56.

33. Lopera G, Stevenson WG, Soejima K, et al. Identification and ablation of three types of ventricular tachycardia involving the His-Purkinje system in patients with heart disease. J Cardiovasc Electrophysiol 2004;15:52–8.

Ablation of Neuroaxial in Patients with Ventricular Tachycardia

Yuhong Wang, MD[a], Lilei Yu, MD, PhD[a], Sunny S. Po, MD, PhD[b],*

KEYWORDS

- Autonomic nervous system • Ventricular tachycardia • Sympathetic activation
- Left cardiac sympathetic denervation • Renal sympathetic denervation

KEY POINTS

- Patients with ventricular tachycardia (VT) usually have autonomic imbalance with reduced vagal and increased sympathetic activities.
- Sympathetic activation contributes to VT, and sympathetic denervation has emerged as a novel therapy to treat VT.
- Animal and human studies show that left cardiac sympathetic denervation (LCSD) and renal sympathetic denervation (RDN) are important approaches of sympathetic denervation.

INTRODUCTION

Patients with ventricular tachycardia (VT) are at a high risk of developing ventricular fibrillation (VF) and sudden cardiac death (SCD). To treat VT, pharmacologic therapy remains the first-line therapy, but antiarrhythmic agents may not be effective or carry significant side effects. Catheter ablation is an effective treatment of drug-refractory VTs. In past decades, inhibition of the sympathetic nervous system to suppress VT has emerged as a novel therapy to treat VT resulting from various etiologies. The earliest clinical study on effective prevention of recurrent VT by left cardiac sympathetic denervation (LCSD) was reported by Estes and Izlar[1] in 1961 and later by Zipes and coworkers[2] in 1968. Krum and colleagues[3] first demonstrated the effectiveness of renal sympathetic denervation (RDN) in patients with resistant hypertension in 2009.

SYMPATHETIC ACTIVATION CONTRIBUTES TO VENTRICULAR TACHYCARDIA

The cardiac autonomic nervous system has two main components: the sympathetic nervous system and the parasympathetic nervous system. Sympathetic nervous system is cardiostimulatory, which increases the heart rate and blood pressure, whereas parasympathetic nervous system is cardioinhibitory. The balance between the sympathetic and parasympathetic nervous system is crucial for preventing cardiovascular diseases. It is well-known that autonomic imbalance, especially hyperactivity of the sympathetic nervous system, plays an important role in the genesis of VT; resetting balance by suppressing sympathetic neural activity has emerged as a potential therapy to treat VT.

Multiple lines of evidence revealed a strong correlation between sympathetic activation and ventricular arrhythmias as early as 1950s.[4–7] In 1975,

[a] Department of Cardiology, Renmin Hospital of Wuhan University, Cardiovascular Research Institute, Wuhan University, Hubei Key Laboratory of Cardiology, No. 9 ZhangZhiDong Street, Wuchang District, Wuhan, Hubei, China; [b] Department of Medicine, Heart Rhythm Institute, University of Oklahoma Health Sciences Center, Oklahoma City, OK, USA
* Corresponding author.
E-mail address: sunny-po@ouhsc.edu

Card Electrophysiol Clin 11 (2019) 625–634
https://doi.org/10.1016/j.ccep.2019.08.001
1877-9182/19/© 2019 Elsevier Inc. All rights reserved.

Kliks and colleagues[8] demonstrated that stellate stimulation, which increased cardiac sympathetic tone, reduced VF threshold an average of 42% compared with control subjects. Stellate ganglion stimulation plus coronary occlusion reduced the threshold by an average of 63% compared with control subjects, indicating the arrhythmogenic effect of sympathetic activation. Janse and colleagues[9] further demonstrated that left stellate ganglion (LSG) stimulation significantly increased the degree of instability of cardiac electrophysiology. Multiple preclinical studies also reported the arrhythmogenic effects of sympathetic nerve sprouting and hyperinnervation.[10–12] A 41-day subthreshold LSG stimulation induced sympathetic nerve sprouting and hyperinnervation, leading to a high risk of ventricular arrhythmia and SCD.[11] Moreover, it was observed that malignant ventricular arrhythmias were preceded within 10 to 15 seconds by increasing sympathetic nerve activity through recording the activity of LSG, indicating the key role of sympathetic activation in the initiation of ventricular tachyarrhythmias.[12] Recent studies also demonstrated that inflammation and leptin can increase the activity of LSG, contributing to the genesis of VT.[13,14]

Clinical study by Shusterman and colleagues[15] also showed that increasing sympathetic activity contributed to VT, assessed by heart rate variability. Cao and colleagues[16] found hyperinnervation of cardiac sympathetic nerve fibers in transplant recipients with a history of tachyarrhythmia, suggesting that hyperinnervation sympathetic nerves may contribute to the ventricular arrhythmia and SCD in patients with heart failure. Other studies also support the role of sympathetic nervous system in ventricular arrhythmias[10–12,16–19] in patients with structural heart diseases. In patients without structural heart diseases, similar observation was made by Hayashi and colleagues[20] in seven patients with VT from right ventricular outflow tract to demonstrated the key role of sympathovagal imbalance in the initiation of VT.[20]

ANATOMY OF THE CARDIAC AND RENAL SYMPATHETIC NERVOUS SYSTEM

The cardiac sympathetic nervous system is composed of preganglionic and postganglionic neurons and their axons (**Fig. 1**). The former is located within the brain; the latter is located outside the brain and includes the superior cervical ganglia (C1-C3), the stellate ganglia (C7-T2), and the thoracic ganglia (T2-T7). Many of the preganglionic sympathetic fibers synapse with the stellate ganglion, which is located between

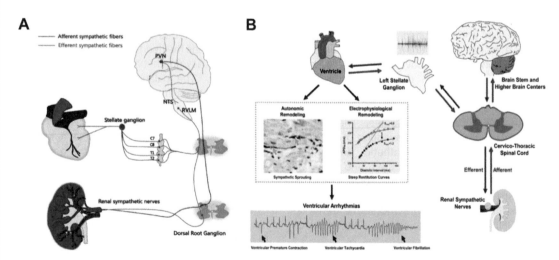

Fig. 1. Anatomic connection between cardiac and renal sympathetic nervous system (*A*) and the rationale of LCSD and RDN on ventricular arrhythmias (*B*). Systemic sympathetic nervous system includes two important members, cardiac and renal sympathetic nervous system, which connect each other via afferent and efferent sympathetic fibers. RDN can decrease the neural activity of the LSG by lowering central sympathetic outflow, whereas LCSD can directly decrease the cardiac sympathetic activity by removing the LSG. Decreased cardiac sympathetic nerve sprouting and electrophysiologic remodeling induced by RDN or LCSD can reduce the incidence of ventricular arrhythmias. NTS, nucleus tractus solitary; PVN, paraventricular nucleus of the hypothalamus; RVLM, rostral ventrolateral medulla. ([*B*] *Reprinted from* Clinical Research in Cardiology, Volume 104, Huang B, Scherlag BJ, Yu L, Lu Z, He B, Jiang H, Renal sympathetic denervation for treatment of ventricular arrhythmias: a review on current experimental and clinical findings, Pages No 535-543, Copyright (2019), with permission from Springer.)

the C6 and C7 vertebrae, and then travel to the myocardium of atria and ventricle.

In an attempt to alleviate the sympathetic activity of stellate ganglion to reduce the incidence of ventricular arrhythmia,[21] stellate ganglion block (SGB) was developed. This minimally invasive technique requires good understanding of the location of the LSG. Both the fluoroscopic-guided and ultrasound-guided SGB techniques are achieved by injection of local anesthetic into the stellate ganglion, lying anterior to the transverse process of the C6 or C7 vertebrae. It is just below the subclavian artery and close to the dome of pleura. The fluoroscopic-guided SGB can identify bony structure clearly, and the needle is inserted anterolateral to the longus colli muscle.

Renal sympathetic nerve (RSN) is another important component of systemic sympathetic nervous system, and most of the RSN are located in the adventitia of the renal artery.[22] Having efferent and afferent fibers, RSN is the bridge between the kidney and central nervous system. Afferent fibers carry information from kidneys to the dorsal ganglia (T6-L4) and eventually synapse with the autonomic control center in the brainstem. The efferent signal transmission from the autonomic control center passes through T10-L2 of the spinal cord. The complexity and diversity of RSN anatomic distribution have been reported, and the differences include the different number and size of fibers, the different density of fibers, and the different distance to arterial lumen in the proximal or distal part of the renal artery.[23] In a porcine model, Tellez and colleagues[24] divided each renal artery into three parts (proximal, mid, and distal part), and they assessed the number, size, and depth in the three parts, respectively. They found that the proximal part has the most number of nerves, and nerves of the distal part are located closer to the arterial lumen. However, the size of nerves are similar in the three parts. Sakakura and colleagues[25] (**Fig. 2**) studied the autonomic distribution of RSN in humans, and reported: (1) the number of RSN in proximal and middle parts are similar (39.6 ± 16.7 vs 39.9 ± 13.9 per section), whereas the distal part has fewer (33.6 ± 13.1 per section); (2) the depth of nerves is greatest in the proximal part, whereas it is least in the distal part; and (3) the predominant fibers are efferent, not afferent. Yu and colleagues[26] further demonstrated that only proximal RSN stimulation could increase the neural activity and function of cardiac sympathetic nervous system (eg, superior left ganglionated plexi and LSG), and decrease the inducibility of atrial fibrillation (AF).

The current RDN procedure is performed with a radiofrequency catheter. Using renal angiography or electroanatomic mapping makes the renal artery structure more visible; each renal artery receives six or eight ablations longitudinally and rotationally in hope of radiofrequency energy disrupting the renal nerve traffic. However, ablations are always anatomy-based without assurance that ablation lesions are applied to sites with rich RSN.

For this reason, the clinical end point (decreased blood pressure) was not achieved by the Simplicity III trial. Negative results from clinical trials prompted researchers to explore the possibility of selective RDN, which only ablates the sympathostimulatory fibers (hot spots). An approach to identifying these hot spots is to deliver high-frequency electrical stimulation to potential ablation targets. If stimulation leads to a significant increase in blood pressure, it suggests that there may be RSN at that site and radiofrequency ablation can be delivered there. However, it is not clear if this approach provides enough sensitivity and/or specificity of identifying the RSN innervation site. Further investigations are needed.

The interactions between cardiac and renal sympathetic nervous system have been reported.[26–29] Increasing the activity of RSN can activate the cardiac stellate ganglion; decreasing the activity of RSN leads to a reduced neural activity of cardiac stellate ganglion. The interplay between the two sympathetic systems led to the use of RSD to treat VT/VF. Huang and colleagues[30] showed that left RSN was able to increase the activity of cardiac sympathetic ganglion in canine model, providing the direct evidence of renal-cardiac sympathetic connection. Moreover, RSD could stabilize ventricular electrophysiologic properties and reduces the occurrence of VT.[27,28] Pokushalov and colleagues[31] accessed the effects of RSD in patients with AF and resistant hypertension. They found that pulmonary vein isolation plus RSD could significantly reduce blood pressure and AF recurrences compared with the only pulmonary vein isolation. The same team conducted a further clinical study, which demonstrated that RSD was more suitable for patients with persistent AF and/or severe resistant hypertension, rather than moderate hypertension.[32]

THE EFFECTS OF LEFT CARDIAC SYMPATHETIC DENERVATION TO TREAT VENTRICULAR TACHYARRHYTHMIAS

LCSD was the first approach of sympathetic denervation to treat life-threatening ventricular

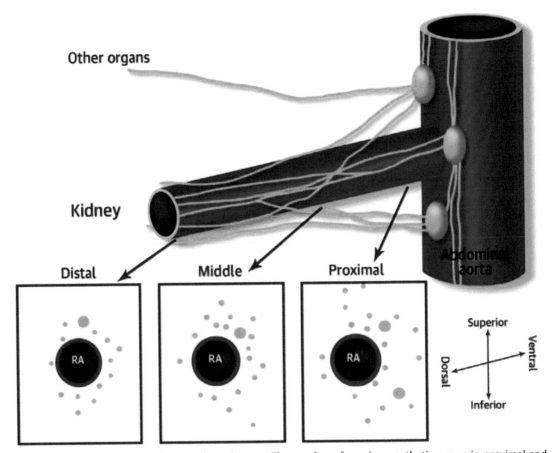

Fig. 2. The nerve location and density of renal artery. The number of renal sympathetic nerves in proximal and middle parts are similar, whereas the distal part has the smaller number. The depth of nerves is greatest in proximal part, and is least in distal part. RA, renal artery. (*Reprinted from* Journal of the American College of Cardiology, Volume 64, Sakakura K, Ladich E, Cheng Q, Otsuka F, Yahagi K, Fowler DR, Kolodgie FD, Virmani R and Joner M, Anatomic Assessment of Sympathetic Peri-Arterial Renal Nerves in Man, Pages No 635-643, Copyright (2019), with permission from Elsevier.)

arrhythmias.[33] LCSD is capable of rebalancing the sympathovagal activities by inhibiting sympathetic activation directly and enhancing parasympathetic activation indirectly in patients with VT.

LCSD was once used to treat patients with angina until the advent of β-blockers.[34] In the 1960s, the first human studies that reported the effective prevention of recurrent VT by LCSD were performed by Estes and Izlar[1] and Zipes and coworkers.[2] However, Yanowitz and colleagues[35] showed LCSD had no significant effects on QT intervals, thus the effectivity of LCSD was again controversial. In 1971, Moss and McDonald[36] demonstrated that LCSD could be a treatment of patients with long QT syndrome (LQTS) not taking β-blockers. Moreover, it was been suggested that one major trigger for LQTS may be the activity of LSG.[37,38] Stimulating the LSG was shown to induce the prolongation of QT intervals

and the macroscopic T-wave alternans,[37] and the proarrhythmic effect of the stimulating was also found particularly in the acute myocardial ischemia model.[39–41] LCSD was able to increase the VF threshold, which is a quantitative marker of cardiac electrical instability, and to reduce the occurrence for VF.[42,43]

The initial clinical trial with LCSD in LQTS patients was performed by Schwartz and colleagues[44] in 1991. A 6-year worldwide investigation enrolled 85 patients with LQTS undergoing LCSD, and showed that LCSD reduced the number cardiac events from 99% to 45%, indicating that LCSD was an effective therapy in LQTS patients where β-blockers alone failed to effectively suppress VT/VF. Subsequently, in 2004, they published a larger clinical study enrolling 147 LQTS patients with high sudden death risks. The results showed that LCSD led to a 91% decrease in cardiac events and a mean QT interval shortening of 39 ms.[45]

LCSD has been used for patients with other channelopathies, such as catecholaminergic polymorphic VT.[46–48] Indeed, LCSD is considered an important adjunct therapy in patients with catecholaminergic polymorphic VT to prevent sympathetic surge that often triggers VT/VF. Although LCSD is an invasive surgical intervention and may result in complications, such as hemorrhage, pain and dry and warm left hand and forehead, and Horner syndrome, it has the potential of permanently suppressing the sympathetic outflow to the heart. Currently, most of LCSD is performed with video-assisted techniques, further reducing its complication rate.

Another important indication of LCSD is to treat electrical storm. A study by Bourke and colleagues[49] had shown that LCSD markedly reduced VT burden, indicating LCSD may be a potential adjunct for VT patients who were resistant to drug therapies. To evaluate the intermediate and long-term effects of cardiac sympathetic denervation (CSD), Vaseghi and colleagues[50] analyzed the burden of implantable cardioverter-defibrillation (ICD) shock in patients after LCSD or bilateral CSD. Results showed that in 90% patients, the number of ICD shocks was significantly decreased (19.6 ± 19 preprocedure vs 2.3 ± 2.9 post-procedure) in the following year, and 48% patients were 1-year freedom from shocks, indicating bilateral CSD in the successful management of electrical storm. Furthermore, they accessed the value of bilateral CSD and the characteristics of clinical outcomes in those patients (**Fig. 3**).[51] Data revealed that patients with advanced heart failure or longer VT cycle lengths before surgery, or receiving only LCSD, trended to the worse outcomes.

The different outcome of left and right stellate ganglionectomy were shown by Yanowitz and colleagues,[35] and such differences may be associated with the distribution of right and left stellate innervation to the ventricles. It was reported that the left and right ventricle were innervated predominantly by left and right cardiac sympathetic nerves, respectively,[35] but the norepinephrine release of left-sided are more than the right-side, which could be the major reason for the prone of LCSD. Vaseghi and colleagues[52] evaluated the activation recovery interval (ARI) and norepinephrine of the anterior left ventricle during left or right stellate ganglion stimulation, and results showed that left and right stellate ganglion stimulation shortens ARI and increases norepinephrine concentrations, but left stimulation induced a more significant increase in ARI dispersion, indicating the beneficial effects of left sympathectomy and the additional role of right sympathectomy. To date, the contribution of the right and left stellate ganglion to the genesis and maintenance of VT/VF remains controversial. Therefore, to perform LCSD or LCSD + right CSD to treat patients in electrical storm remains controversial.

Compared with surgical LCSD, SGB is a less invasive treatment to reduce cardiac sympathetic activity. This therapy was firstly used in patients with depression, dementia, and psychosis as early as the 1940s.[53,54] In 1976, Grossman[55] found that 15 mL of 1% lidocaine injection into the LSG was capable of abolishing VT in a patient with a ruptured congenital aneurysm of the basilar artery. In 2000, Nademanee and colleagues[56] demonstrated the antiarrhythmic effects of SGB in patients with

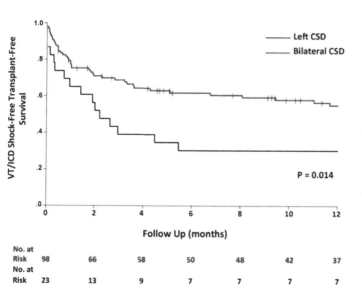

Fig. 3. The effects of LCSD versus bilateral CSD on electrical storm. Differences between LCSD and bilateral CSD in the combined end point. (*Reprinted from* Journal of the American College of Cardiology, Volume 69, Vaseghi M, Barwad P, Malavassi Corrales FJ, Tandri H, Mathuria N, Shah R, Sorg JM, Gima J, Mandal K, Saenz Morales LC, Lokhandwala Y and Shivkumar K, Cardiac Sympathetic Denervation for Refractory Ventricular Arrhythmias., Pages No 3070-3080, Copyright (2019), with permission from Elsevier.)

electrical storm. Subsequently, similar results were reported by others.[57–63] In a rabbit model, 0.5 mL of 0.25% bupivacaine significantly prolonged the 90% of monophasic action potential duration (APD), reduced the transmural dispersion of repolarization, and increased the effective refractory period (ERP) and the VF threshold. These findings indicate that SGB is an effective therapy to treat patients in electrical storm.

Moreover, there is an emerging, less invasive technique of SGB. The SGB is achieved by light irradiation, not local anesthetic injection. The types of light used in studies include low-level laser therapy, xenon light therapy, and linear-polarized near-infrared ray therapy.[64–66] Although it is mainly used in pain conditions, the noninvasive idea should be introduced into the SGB therapy for VT.

THE EFFECTS OF RENAL SYMPATHETIC DENERVATION TO TREAT VENTRICULAR TACHYARRHYTHMIA

Targeting the renal sympathetic nervous system is a potential therapeutic approach to treat VT. In

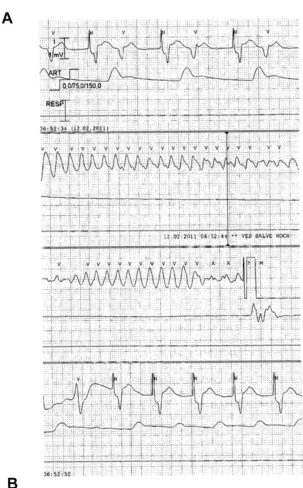

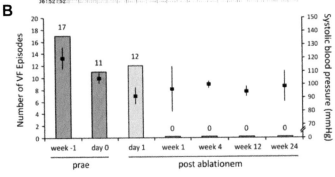

Fig. 4. The effects of RDN on VT storm. Tracing of a polymorphic VT via electrocardiogram and blood pressure (*A*). Number of VF episodes before and after RDN (*B*). (*Reprinted from* Clinical Research in Cardiology, Volume 101, Huang B, Scherlag BJ, Yu L, Lu Z, He B, Jiang H,Renal sympathetic denervation for treatment of ventricular arrhythmias: a review on current experimental and clinical findings, Pages No 535-543, Copyright (2019), with permission from Springer.)

1934, RDN was first used in humans with uncontrolled hypertension[67,68]; later RDN was used as an extracardiac therapeutic option for VT.[69-72] A proof-of-principle trial enrolling 50 patients showed that RDN reduced renal noradrenaline spillover, which verified the effectiveness of RDN.[3] Preclinical studies also demonstrate that RDN could significantly reduce the episodes of ventricular arrhythmias during 1 hour of acute myocardial ischemia, increase the ventricular ERP and APD, decrease the maximal slope of the restitution curve, inhibit APD alternans, and decrease the incidence of spontaneous ventricular arrhythmia. These results suggest that RDN can stabilize ventricular electrophysiologic properties.[27] Compared with CSD, RDN had similar effects on ventricular electrophysiologic properties, such as a significant decrease in heart rate and an increase in the ventricular ERP and APD in a canine model.[73] A study by Linz and colleagues[74] showed that RDN decreased the occurrence of ventricular arrhythmias in pigs subjected to 20 minutes of acute ventricular ischemia induced by left anterior descending artery occlusion followed by reperfusion. Dai and colleagues[75] demonstrated that RDN was able to inhibit ventricular substrate remodeling in a long-term rapid pacing model.

In 2012, Ukena and colleagues[72] published the results of RSD on two heart failure patients with VT storm. RDN was able to reduce the incidence of ventricular tachyarrhythmias acutely and chronically (**Fig. 4**).

In cardiomyopathy patients with electrical storm, the effectiveness and safety of RDN were also demonstrated.[70,71,76] Evranos and colleagues[77] enrolled 32 patients suffering from refractory VT with dilated cardiomyopathy to undergo RDN as an adjuvant therapy to ICD and they reported encouraging results that RDN may suppress electrical storm. Moreover, Armaganijan and colleagues[69] did a 6-month follow-up in patients with ICDs who underwent RDN for refractory VT, and found that RDN reduced the median number VT/VF and appropriate ICD therapies, suggesting that RDN was capable of reducing arrhythmic burden. To date, all the clinical studies of using RSD to treat ventricular tachyarrhythmia were small case series. Large randomized clinical trials are needed to verify the efficacy of RSD in treating VT/VF.

SUMMARY

There is a strong association between the autonomic nervous system and VT. Sympathetic denervation is an emerging therapy to prevent or treat ventricular tachyarrhythmias by rebalancing the sympathetic and parasympathetic activity. Large randomized clinical trials are needed to verify the efficacy of sympathetic denervation in treating VT/VF.

ACKNOWLEDGMENTS

This study was supported by the National Natural Science Foundation of China (No.81871486, 81570463).

REFERENCES

1. Estes EH Jr, Izlar HL Jr. Recurrent ventricular tachycardia. A case successfully treated by bilateral cardiac sympathectomy. Am J Med 1961;31:493–7.
2. Zipes DP, Festoff B, Schaal SF, et al. Treatment of ventricular arrhythmia by permanent atrial pacemaker and cardiac sympathectomy. Ann Intern Med 1968;68:591–7.
3. Krum H, Schlaich M, Whitbourn R, et al. Catheter-based renal sympathetic denervation for resistant hypertension: a multicentre safety and proof-of-principle cohort study. Lancet 2009;373:1275–81.
4. Maling HM, Moran NC. Ventricular arrhythmias induced by sympathomimetic amines in unanesthetized dogs following coronary artery occlusion. Circ Res 1957;5:409–13.
5. Han J, Garciadejalon P, Moe GK. Adrenergic effects on ventricular vulnerability. Circ Res 1964;14: 516–24.
6. Hockman CH, Mauck HP Jr, Hoff EC. ECG changes resulting from cerebral stimulation. II. A spectrum of ventricular arrhythmias of sympathetic origin. Am Heart J 1966;71:695–700.
7. Armour JA, Hageman GR, Randall WC. Arrhythmias induced by local cardiac nerve stimulation. Am J Physiol 1972;223:1068–75.
8. Kliks BR, Burgess MJ, Abildskov JA. Influence of sympathetic tone on ventricular fibrillation threshold during experimental coronary occlusion. Am J Cardiol 1975;36:45–9.
9. Janse MJ, Schwartz PJ, Wilms-Schopman F, et al. Effects of unilateral stellate ganglion stimulation and ablation on electrophysiologic changes induced by acute myocardial ischemia in dogs. Circulation 1985;72:585–95.
10. Liu YB, Wu CC, Lu LS, et al. Sympathetic nerve sprouting, electrical remodeling, and increased vulnerability to ventricular fibrillation in hypercholesterolemic rabbits. Circ Res 2003;92:1145–52.
11. Swissa M, Zhou S, Gonzalez-Gomez I, et al. Long-term subthreshold electrical stimulation of the left stellate ganglion and a canine model of sudden cardiac death. J Am Coll Cardiol 2004;43:858–64.
12. Zhou S, Jung BC, Tan AY, et al. Spontaneous stellate ganglion nerve activity and ventricular arrhythmia in

a canine model of sudden death. Heart Rhythm 2008;5:131–9.

13. Wang M, Li S, Zhou X, et al. Increased inflammation promotes ventricular arrhythmia through aggravating left stellate ganglion remodeling in a canine ischemia model. Int J Cardiol 2017;248:286–93.

14. Yu L, Wang Y, Zhou X, et al. Leptin injection into the left stellate ganglion augments ischemia-related ventricular arrhythmias via sympathetic nerve activation. Heart Rhythm 2018;15:597–606.

15. Shusterman V, Aysin B, Gottipaty V, et al. Autonomic nervous system activity and the spontaneous initiation of ventricular tachycardia. ESVEM Investigators. Electrophysiologic Study versus Electrocardiographic Monitoring Trial. J Am Coll Cardiol 1998;32:1891–9.

16. Cao JM, Fishbein MC, Han JB, et al. Relationship between regional cardiac hyperinnervation and ventricular arrhythmia. Circulation 2000;101:1960–9.

17. Cao JM, Chen LS, KenKnight BH, et al. Nerve sprouting and sudden cardiac death. Circ Res 2000;86:816–21.

18. Ng GA, Brack KE, Patel VH, et al. Autonomic modulation of electrical restitution, alternans and ventricular fibrillation initiation in the isolated heart. Cardiovasc Res 2007;73:750–60.

19. Ng GA, Mantravadi R, Walker WH, et al. Sympathetic nerve stimulation produces spatial heterogeneities of action potential restitution. Heart Rhythm 2009;6:696–706.

20. Hayashi H, Fujiki A, Tani M, et al. Role of sympathovagal balance in the initiation of idiopathic ventricular tachycardia originating from right ventricular outflow tract. Pacing Clin Electrophysiol 1997;20: 2371–7.

21. Yu L, Zhou L, Cao G, et al. Optogenetic modulation of cardiac sympathetic nerve activity to prevent ventricular arrhythmias. J Am Coll Cardiol 2017;70: 2778–90.

22. Schlaich MP, Sobotka PA, Krum H, et al. Renal denervation as a therapeutic approach for hypertension: novel implications for an old concept. Hypertension 2009;54:1195–201.

23. Tsioufis C, Dimitriadis K, Tsioufis P, et al. ConfidenHT system for diagnostic mapping of renal nerves. Curr Hypertens Rep 2018;20:49.

24. Tellez A, Rousselle S, Palmieri T, et al. Renal artery nerve distribution and density in the porcine model: biologic implications for the development of radiofrequency ablation therapies. Transl Res 2013;162: 381–9.

25. Sakakura K, Ladich E, Cheng Q, et al. Anatomic assessment of sympathetic peri-arterial renal nerves in man. J Am Coll Cardiol 2014;64:635–43.

26. Yu L, Huang B, Wang Z, et al. Impacts of renal sympathetic activation on atrial fibrillation: the potential role of the autonomic cross talk between kidney and heart. J Am Heart Assoc 2017;6.

27. Huang B, Yu L, He B, et al. Renal sympathetic denervation modulates ventricular electrophysiology and has a protective effect on ischaemia-induced ventricular arrhythmia. Exp Physiol 2014;99:1467–77.

28. Yu L, Huang B, Zhou X, et al. Renal sympathetic stimulation and ablation affect ventricular arrhythmia by modulating autonomic activity in a cesium-induced long QT canine model. Heart Rhythm 2017;14:912–9.

29. Yu L, Li X, Huang B, et al. Atrial fibrillation in acute obstructive sleep apnea: autonomic nervous mechanism and modulation. J Am Heart Assoc 2017;6 [pii:e006264].

30. Huang B, Yu L, Scherlag BJ, et al. Left renal nerves stimulation facilitates ischemia-induced ventricular arrhythmia by increasing nerve activity of left stellate ganglion. J Cardiovasc Electrophysiol 2014;25: 1249–56.

31. Pokushalov E, Romanov A, Corbucci G, et al. A randomized comparison of pulmonary vein isolation with versus without concomitant renal artery denervation in patients with refractory symptomatic atrial fibrillation and resistant hypertension. J Am Coll Cardiol 2012;60:1163–70.

32. Pokushalov E, Romanov A, Katritsis DG, et al. Renal denervation for improving outcomes of catheter ablation in patients with atrial fibrillation and hypertension: early experience. Heart Rhythm 2014;11:1131–8.

33. Schwartz PJ. The rationale and the role of left stellectomy for the prevention of malignant arrhythmias. Ann N Y Acad Sci 1984;427:199–221.

34. Burnett CF Jr, Evans JA. Follow-up report on resection of the anginal pathway in thirty-three patients. J Am Med Assoc 1956;162:709–12.

35. Yanowitz F, Preston JB, Abildskov JA. Functional distribution of right and left stellate innervation to the ventricles. Production of neurogenic electrocardiographic changes by unilateral alteration of sympathetic tone. Circ Res 1966;18:416–28.

36. Moss AJ, McDonald J. Unilateral cervicothoracic sympathetic ganglionectomy for the treatment of long QT interval syndrome. N Engl J Med 1971; 285:903–4.

37. Schwartz PJ, Malliani A. Electrical alternation of the T-wave: clinical and experimental evidence of its relationship with the sympathetic nervous system and with the long Q-T syndrome. Am Heart J 1975; 89:45–50.

38. Schwartz PJ. Idiopathic long QT syndrome: progress and questions. Am Heart J 1985;109: 399–411.

39. Harris AS, Otero H, Bocage AJ. The induction of arrhythmias by sympathetic activity before and after occlusion of a coronary artery in the canine heart. J Electrocardiol 1971;4:34–43.

40. Schwartz PJ, Vanoli E. Cardiac arrhythmias elicited by interaction between acute myocardial ischemia

and sympathetic hyperactivity: a new experimental model for the study of antiarrhythmic drugs. J Cardiovasc Pharmacol 1981;3:1251–9.

41. Schwartz PJ, Vanoli E, Zaza A, et al. The effect of antiarrhythmic drugs on life-threatening arrhythmias induced by the interaction between acute myocardial ischemia and sympathetic hyperactivity. Am Heart J 1985;109:937–48.

42. Schwartz PJ, Snebold NG, Brown AM. Effects of unilateral cardiac sympathetic denervation on the ventricular fibrillation threshold. Am J Cardiol 1976;37:1034–40.

43. Odero A, Bozzani A, De Ferrari GM, et al. Left cardiac sympathetic denervation for the prevention of life-threatening arrhythmias: the surgical supraclavicular approach to cervicothoracic sympathectomy. Heart Rhythm 2010;7:1161–5.

44. Schwartz PJ, Locati EH, Moss AJ, et al. Left cardiac sympathetic denervation in the therapy of congenital long QT syndrome. A worldwide report. Circulation 1991;84:503–11.

45. Schwartz PJ, Priori SG, Cerrone M, et al. Left cardiac sympathetic denervation in the management of high-risk patients affected by the long-QT syndrome. Circulation 2004;109:1826–33.

46. Wilde AA, Bhuiyan ZA, Crotti L, et al. Left cardiac sympathetic denervation for catecholaminergic polymorphic ventricular tachycardia. N Engl J Med 2008;358:2024–9.

47. Roses-Noguer F, Jarman JW, Clague JR, et al. Outcomes of defibrillator therapy in catecholaminergic polymorphic ventricular tachycardia. Heart Rhythm 2014;11:58–66.

48. De Ferrari GM, Dusi V, Spazzolini C, et al. Clinical management of catecholaminergic polymorphic ventricular tachycardia: the role of left cardiac sympathetic denervation. Circulation 2015;131:2185–93.

49. Bourke T, Vaseghi M, Michowitz Y, et al. Neuraxial modulation for refractory ventricular arrhythmias: value of thoracic epidural anesthesia and surgical left cardiac sympathetic denervation. Circulation 2010;121:2255–62.

50. Vaseghi M, Gima J, Kanaan C, et al. Cardiac sympathetic denervation in patients with refractory ventricular arrhythmias or electrical storm: intermediate and long-term follow-up. Heart Rhythm 2014;11:360–6.

51. Vaseghi M, Barwad P, Malavassi Corrales FJ, et al. Cardiac sympathetic denervation for refractory ventricular arrhythmias. J Am Coll Cardiol 2017;69:3070–80.

52. Vaseghi M, Zhou W, Shi J, et al. Sympathetic innervation of the anterior left ventricular wall by the right and left stellate ganglia. Heart Rhythm 2012;9:1303–9.

53. Karnosh LJ, Gardner WJ. The effects of bilateral stellate ganglion block on mental depression; report of 3 cases. Cleve Clin Q 1947;14:133–8.

54. Karnosh LJ, Gardner WJ. Observations on mood after stellate ganglionectomy. South Med J 1948;41:631–6.

55. Grossman MA. Cardiac arrhythmias in acute central nervous system disease. Successful management with stellate ganglion block. Arch Intern Med 1976;136:203–7.

56. Nademanee K, Taylor R, Bailey WE, et al. Treating electrical storm : sympathetic blockade versus advanced cardiac life support-guided therapy. Circulation 2000;102:742–7.

57. Cardona-Guarache R, Padala SK, Velazco-Davila L, et al. Stellate ganglion blockade and bilateral cardiac sympathetic denervation in patients with life-threatening ventricular arrhythmias. J Cardiovasc Electrophysiol 2017;28:903–8.

58. Fudim M, Boortz-Marx R, Patel CB, et al. Autonomic modulation for the treatment of ventricular arrhythmias: therapeutic use of percutaneous stellate ganglion blocks. J Cardiovasc Electrophysiol 2017;28:446–9.

59. Hayase J, Patel J, Narayan SM, et al. Percutaneous stellate ganglion block suppressing VT and VF in a patient refractory to VT ablation. J Cardiovasc Electrophysiol 2013;24:926–8.

60. Hulata DF, Le-Wendling L, Boezaart AP, et al. Stellate ganglion local anesthetic blockade and neurolysis for the treatment of refractory ventricular fibrillation. A Case Rep 2015;4:49–51.

61. Rajesh MC, Deepa KV, Ramdas EK. Stellate ganglion block as rescue therapy in refractory ventricular tachycardia. Anesth Essays Res 2017;11:266–7.

62. Scanlon MM, Gillespie SM, Schaff HV, et al. Urgent ultrasound-guided bilateral stellate ganglion blocks in a patient with medically refractory ventricular arrhythmias. Crit Care Med 2015;43:e316–8.

63. Smith DI, Jones C, Morris GK, et al. Trial ultrasound-guided continuous left stellate ganglion blockade before surgical gangliolysis in a patient with a left ventricular assist device and intractable ventricular tachycardia: a pain control application to a complex hemodynamic condition. ASAIO J 2015;61:104–6.

64. Mii S, Kim C, Matsui H, et al. Increases in central retinal artery blood flow in humans following carotid artery and stellate ganglion irradiation with 0.6 to 1.6 microm irradiation. J Nippon Med Sch 2007;74:23–9.

65. Momota Y, Kani K, Takano H, et al. High-wattage pulsed irradiation of linearly polarized near-infrared light to stellate ganglion area for burning mouth syndrome. Case Rep Dent 2014;2014:171657.

66. Nakajima F, Komoda A, Aratani S, et al. Effects of xenon irradiation of the stellate ganglion region on fibromyalgia. J Phys Ther Sci 2015;27:209–12.

67. Page IH. The effect on renal efficiency of lowering arterial blood pressure in cases of essential hypertension and nephritis. J Clin Invest 1934;13:909–15.

68. Page IH, Heuer GJ. The effect of renal denervation on the level of arterial blood pressure and renal function in essential hypertension. J Clin Invest 1935;14:27–30.

69. Armaganijan LV, Staico R, Moreira DA, et al. 6-month outcomes in patients with implantable cardioverter-defibrillators undergoing renal sympathetic denervation for the treatment of refractory ventricular arrhythmias. JACC Cardiovasc Interv 2015;8:984–90.

70. Remo BF, Preminger M, Bradfield J, et al. Safety and efficacy of renal denervation as a novel treatment of ventricular tachycardia storm in patients with cardiomyopathy. Heart Rhythm 2014;11:541–6.

71. Scholz EP, Raake P, Thomas D, et al. Rescue renal sympathetic denervation in a patient with ventricular electrical storm refractory to endo- and epicardial catheter ablation. Clin Res Cardiol 2015;104:79–84.

72. Ukena C, Bauer A, Mahfoud F, et al. Renal sympathetic denervation for treatment of electrical storm: first-in-man experience. Clin Res Cardiol 2012;101:63–7.

73. Huang B, Yu L, He B, et al. Sympathetic denervation of heart and kidney induces similar effects on ventricular electrophysiological properties. EuroIntervention 2015;11:598–604.

74. Linz D, Wirth K, Ukena C, et al. Renal denervation suppresses ventricular arrhythmias during acute ventricular ischemia in pigs. Heart Rhythm 2013;10:1525–30.

75. Dai Z, Yu S, Zhao Q, et al. Renal sympathetic denervation suppresses ventricular substrate remodelling in a canine high-rate pacing model. EuroIntervention 2014;10:392–9.

76. Staico R, Armaganijan L, Moreira D, et al. Renal sympathetic denervation and ventricular arrhythmias: a case of electrical storm with multiple renal arteries. EuroIntervention 2014;10:166.

77. Evranos B, Canpolat U, Kocyigit D, et al. Role of adjuvant renal sympathetic denervation in the treatment of ventricular arrhythmias. Am J Cardiol 2016;118:1207–10.

Mapping and Ablation of Ventricular Arrhythmias in Cardiomyopathies

Henry H. Hsia, MD, FHRS[a],*, Nanqing Xiong, MD[b]

KEYWORDS

• Ventricular arrhythmia • Substrate • Cardiomyopathy • Mapping • Catheter ablation

KEY POINTS

• Nonischemic cardiomyopathies consist of heterogeneous patients with distinct and variable arrhythmia substrates, often located in midmyocardial or subepicardial myocardium.
• Preoperative imaging and real-time image integration to guide catheter ablation are feasible, with significant impacts on procedural management and improved outcomes, particularly in patients with dilated cardiomyopathy, arrhythmogenic right ventricular cardiomyopathy , or in those undergoing epicardial ablation.
• Inaccessibility of arrhythmogenic substrate and disease progression are important causes of ablation failure.
• Early referral for ventricular tachycardia ablation is associated with decreased arrhythmia recurrence and acute complication rate compared with late referrals.
• Adjunctive epicardial mapping/ablation along with novel ablation techniques may provide alternative options for refractory arrhythmias.

INTRODUCTION

Catheter ablation is an important therapy in the management of ventricular tachycardia (VT).[1] Multiple studies have shown the efficacy of catheter ablation in reducing VT recurrences[2,3] and that it is superior to antiarrhythmic drugs,[4] particularly in patients with postinfarct VTs. The annual VT ablation volumes have increased over the last decade (>4-fold from 2000 to 2012).[5–7] Freedom from recurrent arrhythmia in patients with structural heart disease is also strongly associated with an improved transplant-free survival, independent of cause of cardiomyopathies, ejection fraction (EF), or heart failure status (**Fig. 1**).[8]

However, despite advances in techniques and technologies, arrhythmia recurrence remains high,[7] particularly in patients with structural heart disease and large scars.[2,9] Compared with ischemic heart disease, the long-term success rates after catheter ablation in patients with nonischemic cardiomyopathies were significantly worse despite additional epicardial interventions

Disclosure: H.H. Hsia is on the Medtronic Advisory Board and Data Safety Monitoring Board (DSMB), the St Jude Medical Speakers Bureau, and the Biosense-Webster Speakers Bureau; is a consultant and member of DSMB for VytronUS; and is a consultant and member of DSMB for FaraPulse. There is no conflict or relationship with industry to disclose for Dr N. Xiong.
^a Cardiac Electrophysiology Service, University of California, San Francisco, MUE436, 400 Parnassus Avenue, San Francisco, CA 94143, USA; ^b Department of Cardiology, Husham Hospital Furan University, No.12 Wulumuqizhong Road, Shanghai 200040, China
* Corresponding author.
E-mail address: henry.hsia@ucsf.edu

Card Electrophysiol Clin 11 (2019) 635–655
https://doi.org/10.1016/j.ccep.2019.08.005
1877-9182/19/© 2019 Elsevier Inc. All rights reserved.

(Fig. 2).[10] Catheter ablation currently has a class IIa indication for reducing recurrent arrhythmias and implantable cardioverter-defibrillator shocks in patients with nonischemic structural heart diseases.[1]

PATHOLOGY/SUBSTRATE

Nonischemic cardiomyopathies represent a spectrum of heterogeneous myocardial diseases with distinct and variable pathologic processes and electroanatomic substrates. Common causes include dilated cardiomyopathy (DCM), hypertrophic cardiomyopathy (HCM), arrhythmogenic right ventricular cardiomyopathy (ARVC), cardiac sarcoidosis (CS), left ventricular noncompaction

(LVNC), and cardiomyopathy related to Lamin A/C mutation (LMNA).

Dilated Cardiomyopathy

In patients with left ventricle (LV) nonischemic DCM, the predominant arrhythmia mechanism is scar-based reentry, followed by abnormal automaticity, and Purkinje system–related arrhythmias.[11,12] Unlike ischemic cardiomyopathy with arrhythmogenic substrates located predominately near the subendocardial scar related to prior infarction, the locations of arrhythmogenic substrate in DCM do not follow any vascular distribution. Autopsy series of explanted hearts with DCM have shown a high incidence of interstitial and replacement

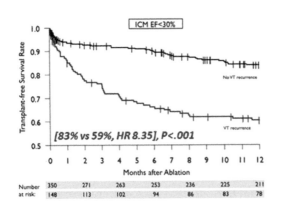

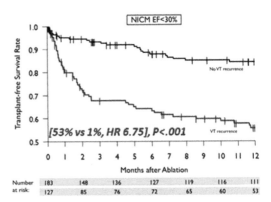

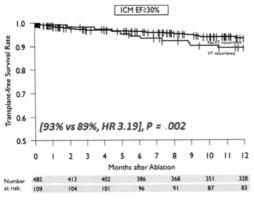

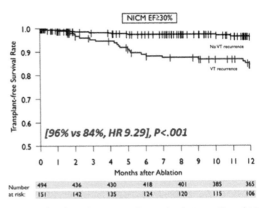

Fig. 1. Analysis of mortality by cardiomyopathy cause and ventricular function. Data from the International VT Ablation Center Collaborative (IVTCC) Group showed that successful VT ablation does not just reduce arrhythmia recurrence rate but is associated with a mortality benefit. Kaplan-Meier display of transplant-free survival by VT recurrence in patients with EF greater than or equal to 30% and less than 30%. Freedom from VT recurrence after catheter ablation is strongly associated with improved transplant-free survival, independent of left ventricular EF (LVEF). Successful VT ablation may have benefit beyond arrhythmia control, supporting a shift from its current role as a therapy of last resort. HR, hazard ratio; ICM, ischemic cardiomyopathy; NICM, nonischemic cardiomyopathy. (Adapted from Tung R, Vaseghi M, Frankel D, et al., Freedom from recurrent ventricular tachycardia after catheter ablation is associated with improved survival in patients with structural heart disease: An International VT Ablation Center Collaborative Group study. Heart Rhythm, 2015. 12: 1997-2007; with permission)

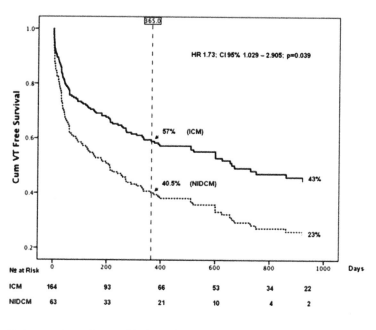

Fig. 2. Kaplan–Meier curves for ventricular tachycardia (VT)–free survival after a single procedure for nonischemic dilated cardiomyopathy (NIDCM) and ischemic cardiomyopathy (ICM) after correction for the relevant confounders. The bold curve represents the cumulative VT-free survival for ICM; the dotted curve, cumulative VT-free survival for NIDCM. At the end of the first year (represented with a perpendicular dotted line), the VT-free survival for ICM was 57% vs 40.5% for NIDCM. At the end of the follow-up period (days), the cumulative VT-free survival for ICM was 43% vs only 23% in NIDCM. The hazard ratio (HR) for VT-free survival was 1.73 (95% confidence interval [CI], 1.029–2.905; P=0.039). (*From* Dinov B, Fiedler L, Schönbauer R, et al., Outcomes in catheter ablation of ventricular tachycardia in dilated nonischemic cardiomyopathy compared with ischemic cardiomyopathy: Results from the Prospective Heart Centre of Leipzig VT (HELP-VT) Study. Circulation, 2014. 129: 728–736; with permission.)

myocardial fibrosis, despite a relative paucity of visible scar.[13,14]

Cardiac MRI (CMR) is a valuable diagnostic tool in patients with nonischemic cardiomyopathies presenting with ventricular arrhythmias. CMR resulted in a change in diagnosis in greater than 40% of the patients who underwent the standard diagnostic tests (echocardiography, stress test, and coronary angiography)[15] (**Fig. 3**). Late gadolinium-enhanced imaging further enhanced the performance of CMR in detecting arrhythmogenic substrates, particularly in patients with no prior history of structural heart disease with negative evaluations.

Electroanatomic mapping and MRI studies in patients with DCM showed a predilection of midwall or subepicardial scar, with relative endocardial sparing; however, significant variability exists among patients[12,16–21] (**Fig. 4**). Epicardial confluent abnormal low-voltage areas (<1.0 mV) commonly are located over the basal LV perivalvular regions, often characterized by wide (>80 milliseconds), split, and/or late potentials that might serve as a substrate for VT.[21]

Two preferential patterns of scar locations (anteroseptal [AS] and inferolateral [IL]) emerge in most patients with LV nonischemic DCM with nearly equal distribution.[22–24] Epicardial scar with late potentials are commonly observed in the basal IL LV subtype, with a higher prevalence of previous history of suspected myocarditis. Whereas intramural substrate predominates in the AS subtype, manifested as large unipolar endocardial low-voltage abnormalities at periaortic/AS regions (**Fig. 5**). The presence of AS substrate is also often associated with frequent arrhythmia recurrences, poorer outcomes, and a paucity of epicardial ablation targets[23,25] (**Fig. 6**).

Arrhythmogenic Right Ventricular Cardiomyopathy

ARVC is an inherited genetically determined myocardial dystrophy predominantly affecting the right ventricle (RV). It is characterized by progressive replacement of myocardium with fibrofatty infiltrate, starting from the epicardium or midmyocardium and then extending to become transmural, often leading to wall thinning and aneurysm formation. The pathologic findings typically are located at the inferior/peritricuspid annular, infundibular, and apical regions, the so-called triangle of dysplasia, the hallmark of ARVC.[26–28]

ARVC is a complex genetic disease with a heterogeneous clinical presentations and variable disease progression.[29,30] Causative mutations in genes encoding desmosomal proteins for cell-to-cell adhesions have been identified, with other

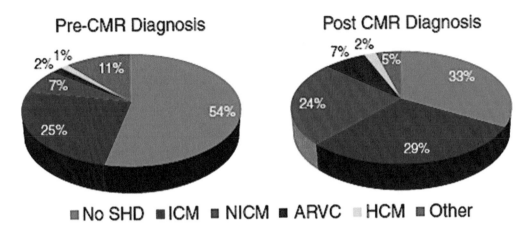

High Resolution Cardiac MRI
Identification of Substrate of Ventricular Arrhythmias

Pre-CMR Diagnosis

Post CMR Diagnosis

■ No SHD ■ ICM ■ NICM ■ ARVC ▪ HCM ■ Other

CMR modified the Dx in 48 patients (31% of all and 43% of those with no SHD):
No SHD (54→33%), Ischemic cardiomyopathy (25→29%), Non-ischemic cardiomyopathy
(7→24%), ARVC (2→7%), Hypertrophic cardiomyopathy (1→2%), and Other (11→5%)

LGE-CMR significantly increased the detection of SHD (17%→38%, P<.001).

Fig. 3. Utility of Cardiac Magnetic Resonance Imaging in Identification of Ventricular Arrhythmia Substrate. A total of 157 consecutive patients with ventricular arrhythmias were prospectively enrolled. Pre-CMR diagnosis was based on the standard diagnostic tests (echocardiography, stress test and coronary angiography). Cardiac MRI modified the diagnosis in 48 patients (31% of all cohorts and 43% of those with no SHD), particularly in those with non-ischemic cardiomyopathy (from 7% to 24%). Late gadolinium-enhanced (LGE) CMR imaging significantly increased the detection of SHD (17à38%, P <0.001), and further modified therapy in 12% patients. CMR, Cardiac MRI; NSVT, Nonsustained VT; VF, Ventricular fibrillation; SHD, Structural Heart Disease. (*Adapted from* Hennig A, Salel M, Sacher F, et al. Europace 2018, 20; (F12): f179–f191.)

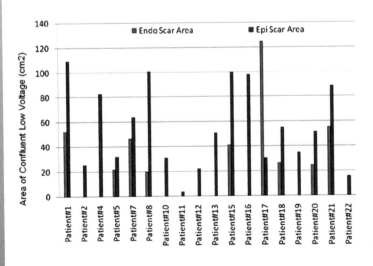

Fig. 4. Epicardial and Endocardial Area of Confluent Low Voltage in the 18 Patients With Epicardial VT. Epicardial (Epi) (red) and endocardial (Endo) (blue) area of confluent low voltage in the 18 patients with epicardial ventricular tachycardia (VT) identified on the basis of entrainment mapping, pacemapping, and successful elimination of VT with epicardial ablation. (*From* Cano O, Hutchinson M, Lin D, et al. Electroanatomic Substrate and Ablation Outcome for Suspected Epicardial Ventricular Tachycardia in Left Ventricular Nonischemic Cardiomyopathy. J Am Coll Cardiol 2009, 54(9): 799–808; with permission.)

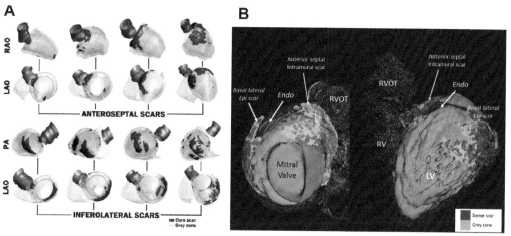

Fig. 5. (*A*) Typical examples of basal anteroseptal scars are shown in right anterior oblique (RAO) and left anterior oblique (LAO) views, typical inferolateral scars in posterioranterior (PA) and LAO views. Red indicates core scar; and yellow, gray zone. (*B*) Epicardial and intramural septal scar in nonischemic DCM. Delayed enhancement with high-resolution CT scan of a patient with nonischemic DCM with recurrent ventricular arrhythmias. The images showed the typical patterns of scar locations (AS and IL). The intramural AS scar is distributed along the interventricular septum and around the periaortic region. The IL scar is subepicardial and distant from the endocardial shell. RVOT, right ventricular outflow tract. (*From* [A] Piers S, Tao Q, van Huls van Taxis C, et al., Contrast-enhanced MRI-derived scar patterns and associated ventricular tachycardias in nonischemic cardiomyopathy: Implications for the ablation strategy. Circ Arrhythm Electrophysiol, 2013. 6: 875–883; with permission.)

mutations associated with more aggressive phenotypes of left-dominant arrhythmogenic cardiomyopathy and LV noncompaction.[31] ARVC is a major cause of sudden death in young people and athletes, and exercise restriction is critical in affected individuals and at-risk family members.

Electrical abnormalities with arrhythmia appear early in the ARVC phenotype, even in the absence of RV structural disease as defined

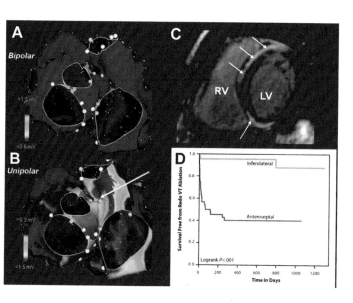

Fig. 6. Intramural septal substrate for VT in nonischemic DCM. Intramural septal scar in patients with nonischemic DCM. (*A*) Normal LV and RV endocardial bipolar voltage (0.5–1.5 mV) in the posteroanterior (PA) view. (*B*) Unipolar endocardial voltage maps showing septal low-voltage (<8.3 mV) area (*arrows*), suggestive of deeper intramural scar. (*C*) CMR showed extensive midmyocardial and intramural septal delayed gadolinium enhancement (*arrows*). (*D*) Kaplan-Meier curve comparing freedom from redo procedure according to scar location. RV, right ventricle. (*Adapted from* [A, B] Haqqani H, Tschabrunn C, Tzou W, et al., Isolated septal substrate for ventricular tachycardia in nonischemic dilated cardiomyopathy: Incidence, characterization, and implications. Heart Rhythm, 2011. 8: 1169–1176; [C] Hutchinson MD, et al. Card Electrophysiol Clin 2010; 2:93–103; and [D] Oloriz T, Silberbauer J, Maccabelli G, et al., Catheter ablation of ventricular arrhythmia in non-ischaemic cardiomyopathy: Anteroseptal versus inferolateral scar sub-types. Circ Arrhythm Electrophysiol, 2014. 7: 414-423; with permission.)

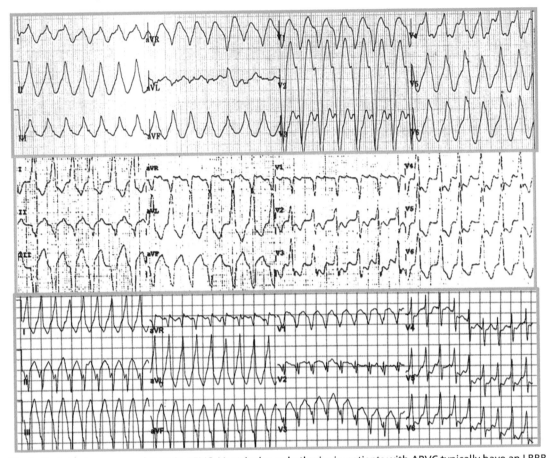

Fig. 7. Sustained monomorphic VT in ARVC. Ventricular arrhythmias in patients with ARVC typically have an LBBB QRS morphology. It may have an inferior frontal axis and positive precordial transition, mimicking idiopathic RVOT arrhythmias (*top*).

Table 1
Electrocardiogram arrhythmogenic right ventricular cardiomyopathy/dysplasia risk score

ECG Characteristic	Points
Anterior T-wave inversion (V_1-V_3) in sinus rhythm	3
VT/PVC Morphology	
Lead I QRS duration ≥120 ms	2
QRS notching (multiple leads)	2
V_5 transition or later	1
Maximum total score	8

An ECG score of 5 or greater correctly distinguishes arrhythmogenic right ventricular dysplasia/cardiomyopathy from idiopathic VT 93% of the time, with a sensitivity of 84%, specificity of 100%, positive predictive value of 100%, and negative predictive value of 91%.

(*Adapted from* Hoffmayer K, Bhave P, Marcus G, et al., An electrocardiographic scoring system for distinguishing right ventricular outflow tract arrhythmias in patients with arrhythmogenic right ventricular cardiomyopathy from idiopathic ventricular tachycardia. Heart Rhythm, 2013. 10: 477-482; with permission.)

by the modified 2010 task force criteria.[29] Ventricular arrhythmias in ARVC typically have a left bundle branch block (LBBB) morphology, which can mimic idiopathic right ventricular outflow tract (RVOT) VT. However, several electrocardiogram (ECG) characteristics help to distinguish ARVC from structurally normal hearts, including (1) VT/premature ventricular complexes (PVC) QRS duration in lead I of greater than or equal to 120 milliseconds, (2) QRS notching in multiple leads, (3) late precordial (≥V_5) transition, and (4) anterior T-wave inversions in leads V_1 to V_3 during sinus rhythm[32] (**Fig. 7**). An ECG risk score has been developed that correctly distinguishes ARVC from idiopathic RVOT ventricular arrhythmias 93% of the time, with 84% sensitivity and 100% specificity (**Table 1**).

In patients with the suspected or electrical form of ARVC, epicardial scar with late potentials predominate, and endocardium may only show unipolar low-voltage abnormality[33] (**Fig. 8**). In contrast, in the definitive or structural form of ARVC, greater endocardial scar burden was noted that extended to the basal midinferior and peritricuspid segments. These findings suggested progression of ARVC from an electrical arrhythmogenic form to an RV structural disease accompanied by the extension of substrate.[34]

Hypertrophic Cardiomyopathy

Malignant ventricular arrhythmias in patients with HCM stem from abnormal cellular hypertrophy, pathologic myocardial disarray, and disruption of cellular architecture,[35] which constitute the substrate for reentrant VT or ventricular fibrillation (VF). Myocardial scar detected by late gadolinium

enhancement (LGE) on CMR significantly correlated with both depolarizing and repolarizing abnormalities, with observed arrhythmias originated from the LGE-positive segments.[36] HCM myocardial scars were often patchy, focal or multifocal, and located at midmyocardial and epicardial regions, and were predictive of all-cause mortality.[37]

Patients with HCM with LV apical aneurysms are at a higher risk for arrhythmic sudden death and thromboembolic events, with an increased incidence of recurrent monomorphic VTs.[38,39] Transmural LGE along the aneurysmal rim often extend contiguously into adjacent LV walls and serve as the scar substrate for reentrant

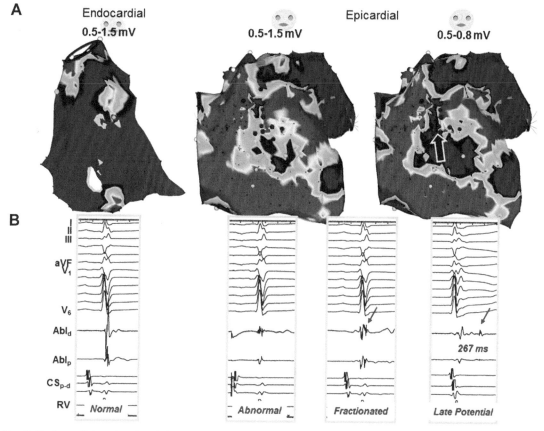

Fig. 8. Endocardial and epicardial voltage maps in a patient with ARVC and VT. Endocardial and epicardial maps with VT-related conducting channels in a patient with an ARVC and recurrent VTs. (A) Endocardial electroanatomic map showed a normal endocardial bipolar voltage profile displayed in standard color gradient: purple colored areas represent normal (amplitude ≥ 1.5 mV) endocardium with dense scar depicted as red (amplitude<0.5 mV). The border zone (amplitude 0.5–1.5 mV) is defined as areas with the color gradient between red and purple. There is minimal RV endocardial abnormality with a small low-voltage region at anterior RVOT, representing the area of prior failed endocardial ablations. Epicardial voltage maps over the RV in the left anterior oblique view showed extensive dense epicardial scar. A VT-related conducting channel within the epicardial scar substrate is visible after color threshold adjustment from 0.5 to 1.5 mV to 0.5 to 0.8 mV (arrow). (B) Electrogram recordings showed normal RV endocardial bipolar signal and abnormal, fractionated epicardial bipolar electrograms with late potential (arrows) recorded 267 milliseconds after onset of the surface QRS complex.

arrhythmias. Multiple VTs can be encountered, and circuits may be endocardial, epicardial, or intramural in location, requiring different approaches to eliminate VTs.[40]

Sarcoidosis

Sarcoidosis is a systemic inflammatory process of unknown cause, characterized by granulomatous infiltration, inflammation, and fibrosis. Clinically manifest cardiac involvement occurs in perhaps 5% of patients with sarcoidosis, resulting in focal or multifocal granulomas or inflammation. The 3 principal manifestations of CS are conduction abnormalities, ventricular arrhythmias, and heart failure.[41,42] An estimated 20% to 25% of patients with pulmonary/systemic sarcoidosis have asymptomatic cardiac involvement and there is a growing realization that CS may be the first manifestation of sarcoidosis. In patients with clinically manifest CS, the extent of LV dysfunction is the most important predictor of prognosis. Because of progressive, coexisting inflammation and replacement fibrosis, ventricular arrhythmias may arise from complex mechanisms that include abnormal automaticity, triggered activity, or scar-related reentry.

LGE on CMR and 18F-fluorodeoxyglucose (FDG) uptake on PET are useful to define the extent of myocardial scar and inflammation.[41,42] In patients with a diagnosis of CS based on established criteria and VT, MRI LGE was noted in nearly all (91%) patients and abnormal FDG-PET was found in 65% of the cases. Abnormal electrogram recordings correlated to myocardial segments with more scar transmurality (LGE) with less inflammation on PET.[43] The abnormal substrate had a predominant distribution in the basal perivalvular segments and interventricular septum, although patchy LV, anterior wall and confluent right ventricular involvement are also observed.[44]

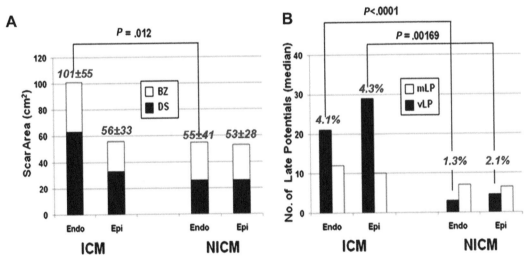

Fig. 9. Differences in substrates between nonischemic DCM and ICM. Differences in scar area and LPs between ICM and NICM substrate. (A) Endocardial scar area (101 ± 55 cm²) was twice the epicardial scar area (56 ± 33 cm²) in patients with ICM, whereas patients with NICM had equal extent of scar on the endocardium and epicardium (55 ± 41 cm² vs 53 ± 28 cm²). Less dense scar (DS) (*solid bars*) was observed in patients with NICM. Open bars indicate border zone (BZ). (B) Patients with NICM had significantly less slow conduction, with fewer LP recordings, than patients with ICM, particularly the vLPs. LP-targeted ablation was more effective in patients with ICM (82% nonrecurrence at 12 ± 10 months' follow-up) versus NICM with less favorable outcomes (50% at 15 ± 13 months' follow-up). (*Adapted from* Nakahara S, Tung R, Ramirez R, et al., Characterization of the arrhythmogenic substrate in ischemic and nonischemic cardiomyopathy: Implications for catheter ablation of hemodynamically unstable ventricular tachycardia. J Am Coll Cardiol, 2010. 55: 2355-2365; with permission.)

Despite limited data, if there is evidence of active inflammation, immunosuppression is the first suggested step, along with antiarrhythmic drug therapy. Catheter ablation is reasonable if VT cannot be controlled (expert consensus recommendations class IIa).[41,42]

Other Cardiomyopathies

LVNC is a heterogeneous myocardial disorder characterized by prominent LV wall trabeculae, a thin compacted layer, and deep intertrabecular recesses.[45,46] The morphologic abnormalities were usually defined by echocardiography, CMR, or computed tomography (CT). Its clinical features range from asymptomatic healthy subjects with normal LV function to thromboembolism, heart failure, arrhythmias, and sudden cardiac death. It is unclear whether LVNC is a distinct cardiomyopathy or a trait shared by different cardiac diseases.[47] However, genetics seem play an important role in LVNC, with nearly half of the patients with either known mutations or probable familial cardiomyopathy.[48]

Treatments focus on improvement of cardiac function and reduction of mechanical stress in patients with systolic dysfunction. The presence of ventricular arrhythmias is an independent risk factor for mortality.[46] Ventricular arrhythmias was reported in 38% to 47% of adult patients with LVNC and in 13% to 18% of those who die suddenly. Implantable cardioverter-defibrillators are effective in preventing sudden arrhythmic death in patients with LVNC, particularly in those with severe ventricular dysfunction, recurrent syncope, or a family history of sudden cardiac death.

Lamins are major architectural proteins that provide a platform for nuclear structure support, DNA repair, cellular signaling, and chromatin organization. Mutations in lamin A/C (LMNA) gene are associated with a wide spectrum of diseases (laminopathies) that include familial DCM, muscular dystrophies, and other multisystem diseases.[49] LMNA cardiomyopathy phenotype has a high penetrance and is characterized by DCM and conduction system disease. Cardiac symptoms usually occur in middle age, with progressive conduction disease, associated with a high incidence of sudden death (~30%) and heart failure (~30%).[49–51] Overall, the clinical course is more aggressive than other forms of dilated cardiomyopathy. Risk of malignant ventricular arrhythmia and sudden death is high and these may occur in the absence of significant ventricular dilatation/dysfunction.

Table 2
Ventricular tachycardia ablation in idiopathic dilated cardiomyopathy versus ischemic cardiomyopathy

	IDCM (n = 63)	ICM (n = 164)	P Value
Epicardial ablation, n (%)	19 (30.2)	2 (1.2)	.0001
Noninducible PES, n (%)	9 (15.8)	14 (9.9)	.360
Substrate mapping, n (%)	42 (66.7)	147 (89.6)	<.0001
VT induced (n/pt)	2.1 ± 1.2	2.2 ± 1.3	.744
VT mappable (n/pt)	1.61 ± 0.80	1.96 ± 0.80	.06
VT ablated (n/pt)	1.40 ± 1.11	1.64 ± 1.15	.168
Clinical VT CL (ms)	364 ± 86	385 ± 93	.133
Procedure time (min)	181 ± 63.6	155 ± 49	.003
Fluoroscopy time (min)	39 ± 22.4	26 ± 19	.0001
Failure, n (%)	7 (11.1)	8 (4.9)	.132

Abbreviations: CL, cycle lengths; ICM, ischemic cardiomyopathy; IDCM, idiopathic DCM; PES, programmed electrical stimulation; pt, patient.

Adapted from Dinov B, Fiedler L, Schönbauer R, et al., Outcomes in catheter ablation of ventricular tachycardia in dilated nonischemic cardiomyopathy compared with ischemic cardiomyopathy: Results from the Prospective Heart Centre of Leipzig VT (HELP-VT) Study. Circulation, 2014. 129: 728-736; with permission.

Multiple risk factors for ventricular arrhythmias in LMNA cardiomyopathy have been identified, including a prolonged PR interval, nonsustained VT, ventricular dysfunction (EF<45%), male gender, and nonmissense mutations.[52–54] Imaging studies have implicated midmyocardial basal septal fibrosis, detected as LGE on CMR, or reduced echocardiographic strain as a common pathogenic mechanism linking progressive conduction disease and substrate for scar-based reentrant VTs in this population.

MAPPING AND ABLATION
Dilated Cardiomyopathy

The arrhythmogenic substrate abnormalities differ significantly between ischemic and

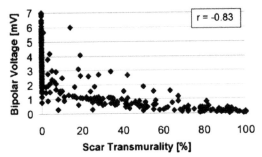

Fig. 10. Correlation of MRI scar transmurality and bipolar voltage. Increasing scar transmurality demonstrates a good correlation with decreasing bipolar voltage (Spearman rank correlation analysis). (*From* Dickfeld T, Tian J, Ahmad G, et al., MRI-guided ventricular tachycardia ablation: Integration of late gadolinium-enhanced 3D scar in patients with Implantable Cardioverter-Defibrillators. Circ Arrhythm Electrophysiol, 2011. 4: 172–184; with permission.)

nonischemic cardiomyopathies. In general, endocardial scar area is twice the epicardial scar area in patients with postinfarct cardiomyopathy, whereas patients with nonischemic DCM have near-equal extent of low-voltage scars on the endocardium and epicardium,[12,55] with a paucity of late-potential (LP) and very-late-potential (vLP) recordings (**Fig. 9**). Although ablation targeting such local abnormal ventricular activities (LAVAs) is an effective strategy,[56] mapping and ablation of VT in nonischemic DCM remains a challenge with limited success (see **Fig. 2**; **Table 2**).[10,55] In some patients with DCM who undergo endocardial/epicardial electroanatomic mapping, low-voltage scar areas with LAVAs may be present over the basal lateral perivalvular regions. An ablation strategy that targets these epicardial VTs and the VT substrate can result in intermediate-term arrhythmia control.[21]

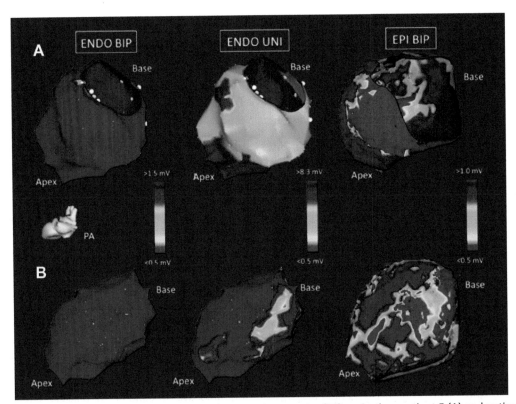

Fig. 11. Images taken from 2 EPI+ patients in the posterior-anterior (PA) projection: patient 5 (A) and patient 7 (B). The LV ENDO BIP voltage maps (left) are normal in both patients. Patient 5 has extensive LV ENDO UNI low voltage involving the entire lateral and inferior LV walls (A, middle). There is a large region of corresponding LV EPI BIP low voltage seen (A, right) corresponding spatially with the ENDO UNI abnormality. Patient 7 has 2 confluent low UNI voltage regions at the basal-mid lateral and apical LV segments (B, middle). The corresponding LV EPI BIP map shows 2 corresponding low-voltage areas (B, right). See text for further discussion. (*From* Hutchinson M, Gerstenfeld E, Desjardins B, et al., Endocardial unipolar voltage mapping to detect epicardial ventricular tachycardia substrate in patients with Nnonischemic left ventricular cardiomyopathy. Circ Arrhythm Electrophysiol, 2010. 4: 49–55; with permission.)

Increasing scar transmurality defined by MRI correlated with a decreasing endocardial bipolar voltage (**Fig. 10**); however, endocardial voltage mapping could identify scars only to a limited extent, especially in patient with nonischemic dilated cardiomyopathy. A viable endocardial layer (>2-mm thickness) may result in >1.5 mV recorded bipolar voltage during endocardial mapping despite up to 63% transmural, mid-myocardial or sub-epicardial scar.[22,57] Although imperfect, the use of endocardial unipolar electrogram recordings provides a wider field of view that may help to identify midwall or subepicardial scar (**Fig. 11**).[58–60] Abnormal low endocardial unipolar voltage (cutoff value of <8.3 mV) corresponded to the presence of epicardial scar with LAVAs in 82% of patients.[58]

Predominant AS and IL scar patterns are present in most patients with nonischemic DCM.

Distinct QRS patterns during VT as well as baseline ECG characteristics can be correlated to these different substrate locations with implications for ablation strategy.[22–24] VT with LBBB-inferior axis is predictive of AS scar (positive predictive value, 100%), whereas RBBB-superior axis is suggestive of an IL substrate with more epicardial involvement (positive predictive value, 89%). The extent of unipolar scar in the endocardial AS or epicardial IL area is significantly correlated with the following ECG parameters during sinus rhythm: PR interval, QRS duration, and the mean voltage in the limb leads (**Fig. 12**). A small r in V3, conduction disturbance/atrioventricular block (PR interval >230 milliseconds, QRS duration >170 milliseconds, or paced rhythm), has 92% and 81% sensitivity and specificity, respectively, in predicting AS scar pattern. A PR interval of less than 170 milliseconds and a low-

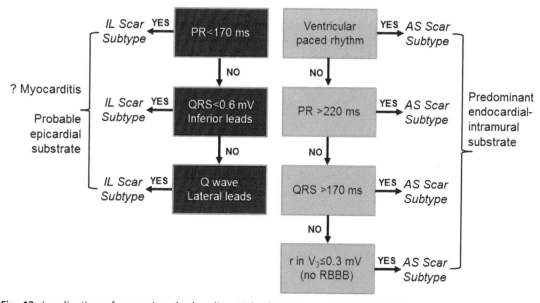

Fig. 12. Localization of scar using the baseline 12-lead ECG in nonischemic DCM in patients with ventricular arrhythmias. The extent and the scar subtype in patients with nonischemic DCM correlated with baseline ECG parameters during sinus rhythm: (1) PR interval, (2) QRS duration, and (3) mean voltage in the limb leads. A small r in V3, conduction disturbance/atrioventricular block (PR interval >230 milliseconds, QRS duration >170 milliseconds, or paced rhythm) have a 92% and 81% of sensitivity and specificity, respectively, in predicting AS intramural septal scar pattern. A PR interval of less than 170 milliseconds and a low-voltage q wave or fragmented QRS in the limb leads are more frequently observed in patients with the IL scar pattern with more epicardial involvement. (*Adapted from* Oloriz T, Wellens H, Santagostino G, et al., The value of the 12-lead electrocardiogram in localizing the scar in non-ischaemic cardiomyopathy. Europace, 2016. 18: 1850-1859; with permission.)

voltage q wave or fragmented QRS in the limb leads are more frequently observed in patients with an IL scar pattern.[24] Simple ECG analysis therefore can predict scar in most of these patients.

Coupled with unipolar endocardial voltage mapping, such ECG criteria are therefore helpful in identifying the potential arrhythmic substrate location, particularly in patients with AS intramural scar, in which epicardial mapping/ablation is of limited value. Overall, up to 60% of patients with nonischemic DCM with ventricular arrhythmias do not need an epicardial approach.[61,62] These findings have important practical implications for preprocedural planning and intraoperative ablation strategy.

Arrhythmogenic Right Ventricular Cardiomyopathy

In ARVC, replacement fibrofatty scars constitute the substrate for macroreentry VT circuits,

similar to those observed after myocardial infarction.[63] However, early arrhythmogenic substrate is predominantly epicardial.[34] Similar to nonischemic DCM, endocardial unipolar voltage mapping (cutoff value of <5.5 mV) may serve to detect epicardial scar substrate in ARVC (**Fig. 13**).[33,64]

Overall, CMR is less sensitive than three-dimensional (3D) electroanatomic mapping in detecting RV scar.[28] However, areas of hypoattenuation on contrast-enhanced multidetector CT (MDCT) identify myocardial fat distribution, with a good concordance to epicardial scar and abnormal electrogram recordings (LAVAs), which serves as substrate for VT in ARVC.[65,66]

Catheter ablation is an effective treatment of ventricular arrhythmias in patients with ARVC, with complete LP abolition being a strong predictor of good long-term outcome.[34] Meta-analysis showed that a combined endocardial-epicardial ablation strategy is associated with a

Endocardial Unipolar Voltage to Identify Epicardial Substrate in ARVC

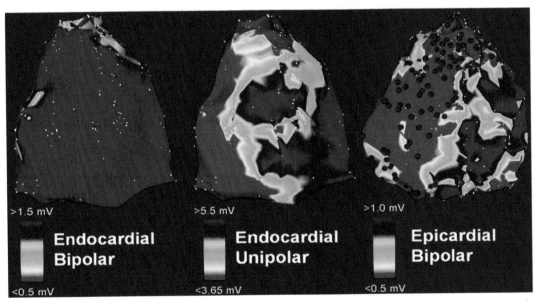

Fig. 13. Endocardial unipolar voltage mapping to detect epicardial scar substrate in ARVC. Unipolar endocardial electrograms defining the location and greater extent of epicardial bipolar electrogram abnormalities in a patient with ARVC. (*Left*) Endocardial bipolar voltage map shows a paucity of low-voltage regions. (*Center*) Endocardial unipolar voltage mapping reveals a much greater burden of abnormal myocardium (<5.5 mV) extending from the lateral tricuspid valve up to the pulmonic valve region and inferiorly across the RV free wall. (*Right*) Epicardial bipolar voltage map confirms the extensive area of abnormal epicardium. Black dots represent wide, split, and/or late epicardial electrograms and help to identify low-voltage areas consistent with scar versus fat. (*Adapted from* Polin G, Haqqani H, Tzou W, *et al.*, Endocardial unipolar voltage mapping to identify epicardial substrate in arrhythmogenic right ventricular cardiomyopathy/dysplasia. Heart Rhythm, 2011. 8: 76–83; with permission.)

lower risk of VT recurrence and subsequent mortality than endocardial-only ablation approach regardless of timing of the epicardial procedure (**Fig. 14**).[33,67–71]

Hypertrophic Cardiomyopathy

Management of ventricular arrhythmias in patients with HCM is challenging. Efficacy of catheter ablation may be limited by the thickness of the tissue and nonendocardial, septal substrate locations. Epicardial low-voltage area was identified in 80% of the patients and was more prevalent than endocardial scar, but some had intramural reentry.[40,72] Epicardial ablation was required in 59% of cases.[73] In patients with LV apical aneurysms, successful VT ablation can be achieved endocardially in the neck/rim of the aneurysm.

Small observational studies or case reports have shown the feasibility and safety of VT ablation in patients with HCM. With a combination of endo-and epicardial ablation, freedom from recurrent ventricular arrhythmia was achieved in a majority of the patients.[72,73] However, long-term risk of VT recurrence, heart

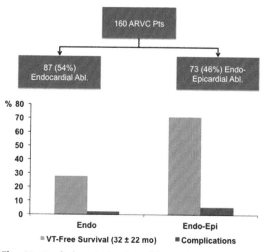

Pooled Analysis of VT Ablation in ARVC

Fig. 14. Pooled analysis of VT ablation (Abl.) results in ARVC. Pooled analysis of the available evidence on VT ablation in ARVC. Endocardial-epicardial mapping and ablation significantly improves long-term arrhythmia-free survival. Pts, patients. (St. Jude Medical is a trademark of Abbott or its related companies. Reproduced with permission of Abbott, © 2019. All rights reserved; and from Santangeli, et al. Current and future indications for ventricular tachycardia ablation: The evidence from clinical trials, in Ventricular Tachycardia Ablation: A Practical Guide S. Mahapatra, et al., Editors. 2014, CardioText Publishing.)

transplantation, and death is high after adjusting for potential covariates.[74]

Sarcoidosis

Catheter ablation of ventricular arrhythmias in patients with CS can be challenging because of the dynamic disease process, coexisting inflammation and fibrotic scars, and extensive multifocal substrate. Abnormal electrograms were recorded over multiple endocardial and epicardial segments. The most common endocardial LV involvements include basal, midseptum, and midanterior wall, whereas the most common RV regions include RVOT, free/septal wall, and midbasal septum. Epicardial electrogram abnormalities had a prevalent distribution over the RV free wall, anterior, and anterior-lateral basal LV[43] (**Fig. 15**). Abnormal endocardial low-voltage areas predominantly involved basal septum and perivalvular regions of either the RV or LV endocardium, whereas epicardial scars were more commonly located on the anterolateral basal wall. These findings were all consistent with CMR and PET images.

It is important to note that up to 40% of the abnormal electrogram recordings were located outside the bipolar low-voltage scar (<1.5 mV endocardium and <1.0 mV epicardium). Unipolar voltage mapping may be used to better identify regions that harbor abnormal electrical substrate as potential targets for substrate-based ablation.[43] However, despite the use of preprocedural imaging, use of adjunctive epicardial mapping, and experienced operators, the outcomes of catheter VT ablation were only modest because of extensive scarring and multiple inducible morphologies.[44,75] Although the overall VT-free survival was at best ~50% at 2-year follow-up, VT control was achievable in most patients.[42,75]

Other Cardiomyopathies

In a small series of patients with LVNC undergoing catheter ablation of drug-refractory sustained VTs, the abnormal electrophysiologic substrate typically involved the LV apical and midapical segments, corresponding to the noncompacted myocardium identified by imaging. In contrast with patients who present with focal PVCs, the ventricular ectopy often arises from LV basal-septal regions and/or papillary muscles. Catheter ablation is safe and effective in achieving good arrhythmia control over long-term follow-up in most patients.[76]

In patients with LMNA cardiomyopathy, midmyocardial basal septal fibrosis predominates but also involves basal inferior and subaortic, mitral annular regions. Multiple VTs were commonly observed. Catheter ablation is

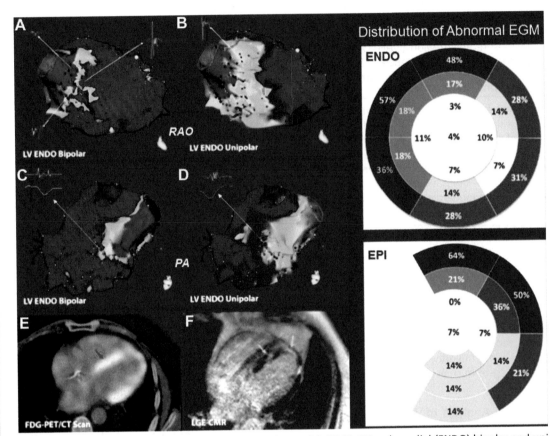

Fig. 15. Electroanatomic mapping and imaging in patients with LV CS. LV endocardial (ENDO) bipolar and unipolar voltage maps are shown. Maps showed a basal septal involvement (*A*) with extension to the inferior midseptum and inferior wall involvement (*C*). The ENDO unipolar maps (*B, D*) showed a more extensive involvement of the septum from the base toward the apex (*B*) as well as a basal IL wall (*D*). Abnormal fractionated, late, and split electrogram (EGM) (*black dots and arrows*) are often located outside the low bipolar voltage area. PET/CT scan (*E*) shows active inflammation of the inferior midbasal septum and IL basal wall (*red arrows*) and contrast-enhanced CMR (*F*) shows patchy areas of LGE on the midinferior and apical septum (*green arrows*). Bull's-eye maps of the distribution of fractionated, late, and split potentials among the LV endocardium and epicardium (EPI). Percentage of patients with involvement of each ventricular segment was shown. Darker colors represent greater degree of involvement. . RAO, right anterior oblique. (*Adapted from* Muser D, Santangeli P, Liang J, et al., Characterization of the electroanatomic substrate in cardiac sarcoidosis: Correlation with imaging findings of scar and inflammation. JACC Clin Electrophysiol, 2018. 4: 291-303; with permission.)

associated with a poor acute procedural success rate (25%), a high rate of complications (25%), and near-universal arrhythmia recurrence (91%).[54] A combination of intramural substrate, basal perivalvular scar, and disease progression may have contributed to poor ablation outcomes in this population.

IMAGING

Preprocedural imaging[20] or real-time image integration[77] to guide catheter ablation is feasible in large series of patients with scar-related VTs, with significant impacts on procedural management and improved outcomes (**Fig. 16**). The structural abnormalities may be segmented as areas of LGE on CMR, and areas of wall thinning or myocardial hypoattenuation on MDCT scans. Imaging integration provides detailed topographic substrate characteristics and important complementary information to electroanatomic mapping, particularly in patients with nonischemic DCM or ARVC, and in those undergoing epicardial approach.

OUTCOMES OF VENTRICULAR TACHYCARDIA ABLATION

The outcomes of catheter ablation in nonischemic cardiomyopathies depend on the causes of

Impact of Image Integration on VT Ablation Outcomes

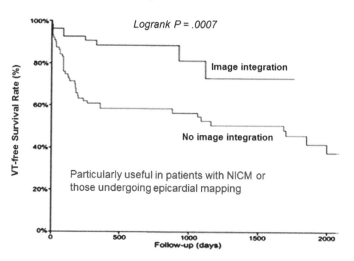

Logrank P = .0007

Image integration

No image integration

Particularly useful in patients with NICM or those undergoing epicardial mapping

Fig. 16. VT-free survival in ablation procedures with and without real-time image integration. Myocardial scar may be detected as wall thinning on MDCT or fibrosis characterized by late gadolinium enhancement on CMR in ICM and NICM. The extent of myocardial fatty infiltrate can be measured as hypoattenuation on MDCT for ARVC. The impact of image integration on procedural management was higher in ARVC/NICM than in ICM (*P*<.01), and higher in cases with epicardial approach (*P*<.0001). (*Adapted from* Yamashita S, Sacher F, Mahida S, et al., Image integration to guide catheter ablation in scar-related ventricular tachycardia. J Cardiovasc Electrophysiol, 2016. 27: 699-708; with permission.)

underlying heart disease and disease progression (**Fig. 17**).[74,78] Hypertrophic cardiomyopathy, valvular heart disease, and sarcoidosis have the highest risk of VT recurrences, often associated with midmyocardial scar deep within the interventricular septum or periaortic/LV summit regions.

Catheter ablation is a safe and effective approach in patients with nonischemic DCM and VT.[79,80] Epicardial ablation and other adjuvant ablation techniques (discussed later) may be required to provide arrhythmia control. However, despite advances in ablation technologies and techniques, there is no significant difference in the long-term procedural outcomes over the years (Muser and colleagues,[79] supplemental material), which may in part reflect the underlying disease progression.[81,82]

Adjusted VT Recurrence by Etiology

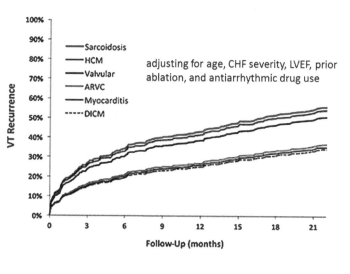

— Sarcoidosis
— HCM
— Valvular
— ARVC
— Myocarditis
····DICM

adjusting for age, CHF severity, LVEF, prior ablation, and antiarrhythmic drug use

Fig. 17. Outcomes of VT catheter ablation in nonischemic heart diseases. N = 780 patients (57 ± 14 years old, 18% women, LVEF 37% ± 13%). Patient characteristics and outcomes were noted for the 6 most common NICM causes (idiopathic DCM 66%, ARVC 13%, valvular cardiomyopathy 6%, myocarditis 6%, HCM 4%, sarcoidosis 3%). Multivariable Cox proportional hazards modeling was used to adjust for potential confounders. One-year freedom from VT was 69%, and freedom from VT, heart transplant, and death was 62%. After adjusting for comorbidities, including age, heart failure severity, EF, prior ablation, and antiarrhythmic medication use, myocarditis, ARVC, and dilated ischemic cardiomyopathy (DICM) showed similar outcomes, whereas HCM, valvular cardiomyopathy, and sarcoidosis had the highest risk of VT recurrence. CHF, congestive heart failure. (*Adapted from* Vaseghi M, Hu T, Tung R, et al., Outcomes of catheter ablation of ventricular tachycardia based on etiology in nonischemic heart disease: An International Ventricular Tachycardia Ablation Center Collaborative Study. JACC: Clin Electrophysiol, 2018. 4: 1141-1150; with permission.)

Disease progression, defined by (1) scar area enlargement and (2) ventricular remodeling with chamber dilatation or decreased systolic function, occurred in 75% of patients with ARVC and nonischemic DCM over a period of 28 ± 18 months.[82] Although individual variation existed, scar progressions were observed in ~50% of ARVC (57%) and nonischemic DCM (46%).[34,81,82] Worsening ventricular function and remodeling have been associated with higher rates of VT recurrence, mortality, and transplant. In a meta-analysis, early referral for VT ablation was associated with decreased VT recurrence and acute complications compared with late referral (**Fig. 18**).[83]

OTHER ABLATION TECHNIQUES/ TECHNOLOGIES

Although inaccessibility of arrhythmogenic substrate and disease progression are important causes of ablation failure, recurrent arrhythmias after failed ablation often originate from sites adjacent to prior lesions and successful reablation was performed predominately (70%) within the prior scar, strongly suggesting incomplete index ablation and the need for more durable lesion formation.[82]

Various adjunctive ablation technologies have recently been examined to fulfill this important and expanding niche. These technologies include (1) bipolar ablation,[84,85] (2) ablation using high-impedance irrigation (half-normal saline) to minimize energy loss,[86,87] (3) transcoronary alcohol interventions,[88,89] (4) noninvasive cardiac radiation using stereotactic body radiation therapy,[90] and (5) needle catheter ablation (**Fig. 19**).[91] These novel therapeutic paradigms have shown promise in elimination/control of arrhythmias with complex, deep intramural substrates.

Early vs Late Referral for Catheter VT Ablation in Patients with Structural Heart Disease

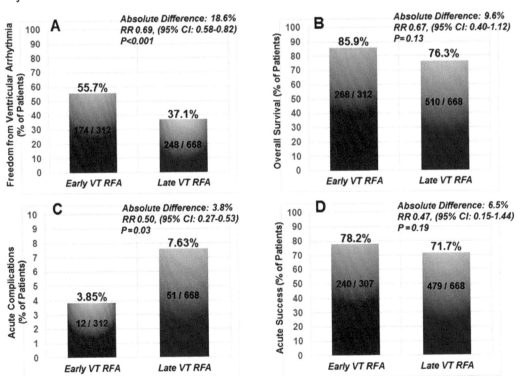

Fig. 18. Early versus late referral for catheter ablation of VT in patients with structural heart disease. Absolute and relative differences in outcomes in the early versus late referral groups. (*A*) VT recurrence. (*B*) Total mortality. (*C*) Acute complications. (*D*) Acute recurrence. Early referral for VT ablation was associated with decreased VT recurrence (relative risk (RR), 0.69 [95% CI, 0.58–0.82], *P*<.0001) and acute complications (RR, 0.50 [95% CI, 0.27–0.93], *P* = .03) compared with late referral. There was no significant difference between early and late referral for total mortality and acute procedural success. RFA, radiofrequency ablation. (*Adapted from* Romero J, Di Biase L, Diaz J, et al., Early versus late referral for catheter ablation of ventricular tachycardia in patients with structural heart disease: A systematic review and meta-analysis of clinical outcomes. JACC Clin Electrophysiol, 2018. 4: 374-382; with permission.)

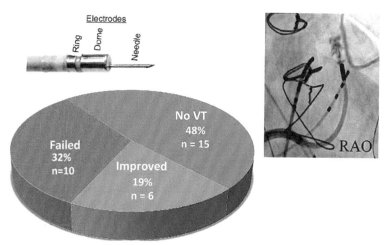

Fig. 19. Infusion needle radiofrequency ablation. A multicenter study of the efficacy of a novel infusion needle radiofrequency (RF) ablation in 31 patients (71% nonischemic) with refractory ventricular arrhythmias. Prior failed therapies included a median of 2 antiarrhythmic drugs and a median of 2 prior catheter ablation procedures (2 or more procedures in 71%), including epicardial procedures in 39% of patients. At potential target sites, the needle is inserted into the myocardium and electrogram recordings with pacing from the needle are used to determine the feasibility of RF energy delivery. If ablation is considered, 50:50 mix of radiographic contrast and saline is injected and the fluoroscopy assessed for evidence of tissue staining and needle position. The pie chart reflects the single-procedure outcomes. After a single procedure, the infusion needle catheter ablation resulted in an overall 68% improved outcome, with arrhythmia abolition in 48% and substantial improvement in an additional 19% of patients at a 6 months of follow-up. (*Adapted from* Stevenson W, Tedrow U, Reddy V, et al., Infusion needle radiofrequency ablation for treatment of refractory ventricular arrhythmias. J Am Coll Cardiol, 2019, 73(12): 1413-1425; with permission.)

SUMMARY

Mapping and ablation of ventricular arrhythmias in patients with nonischemic cardiomyopathies remain a major challenge because of the heterogeneous populations with distinct and variable arrhythmia substrates. The electroanatomic abnormalities are frequently distributed in midmyocardial and subepicardial layers, inaccessible to conventional endocardial ablations. Diagnostic diligence with a thorough understanding of the potential mechanisms/substrate, coupled with detailed electroanatomic mapping, is essential. Careful procedural planning, advanced imaging, and unipolar recordings help to formulate ablation strategy, facilitate work flow, and improve outcomes.

Inaccessibility of arrhythmogenic substrate and disease progression are important causes of ablation failure. Early intervention may help to improve outcomes and minimize complications. In addition to epicardial approach, several novel adjunctive ablation techniques are capable of serving as alternative options in refractory cases.

REFERENCES

1. Al-Khatib S, Stevenson WG, Ackerman M, et al. 2017 AHA/ACC/HRS Guideline for management of patients with ventricular arrhythmias and the prevention of sudden cardiac death: executive summary: a report of the American College of Cardiology/American Heart Association Task Force on Clinical Practice Guidelines and the Heart Rhythm Society. Heart Rhythm 2018;15: e190–252.

2. Stevenson W, Wilber D, Natale A, et al. Irrigated radiofrequency catheter ablation guided by electroanatomic mapping for recurrent ventricular tachycardia after myocardial infarction: the multicenter thermocool ventricular tachycardia ablation trial. Circulation 2008;118:2773–82.

3. Marchlinski F, Haffajee C, Beshai J, et al. Long-term success of irrigated radiofrequency catheter ablation of sustained ventricular tachycardia. J Am Coll Cardiol 2016;67:674–83.

4. Sapp J, Wells G, Parkash R, et al. Ventricular tachycardia ablation versus escalation of antiarrhythmic drugs. N Engl J Med 2016;375:111–21.

5. Palaniswamy C, Kolte D, Harikrishnan P, et al. Catheter ablation of post infarction ventricular tachycardia: Ten-year trends in utilization, in-hospital complications, and in-hospital mortality in the United States. Heart Rhythm 2014;11: 2056–63.

6. Briceño D, Gupta T, Romero J, et al. Catheter ablation of ventricular tachycardia in nonischemic cardiomyopathy: a propensity score-matched

analysis of in-hospital outcomes in the United States. J Cardiovasc Electrophysiol 2018;29: 771–9.

7. Yousuf O, Zusterzeel R, Sanders W, et al. Trends and outcomes of catheter ablation for ventricular tachycardia in a community cohort. JACC Clin Electrophysiol 2018;4:1189–99.

8. Tung R, Vaseghi M, Frankel D, et al. Freedom from recurrent ventricular tachycardia after catheter ablation is associated with improved survival in patients with structural heart disease: an International VT Ablation Center Collaborative Group study. Heart Rhythm 2015;12:1997–2007.

9. Yokokawa M, Desjardins B, Crawford T, et al. Reasons for recurrent ventricular tachycardia after catheter ablation of post-infarction ventricular tachycardia. J Am Coll Cardiol 2013;61:66–73.

10. Dinov B, Fiedler L, Schönbauer R, et al. Outcomes in catheter ablation of ventricular tachycardia in dilated nonischemic cardiomyopathy compared with ischemic cardiomyopathy: Results from the Prospective Heart Centre of Leipzig VT (HELP-VT) Study. Circulation 2014;129:728–36.

11. Delacretaz E, Stevenson W, Ellison K, et al. Mapping and radiofrequency catheter ablation of the three types of sustained monomorphic ventricular tachycardia in nonischemic heart disease. J Cardiovasc Electrophysiol 2000;11:11–7.

12. Soejima K, Stevenson W, Sapp J, et al. Endocardial and epicardial radiofrequency ablation of ventricular tachycardia associated with dilated cardiomyopathy: the importance of low-voltage scars. J Am Coll Cardiol 2004;43:1834–42.

13. Unverferth D, Baker P, Swift S, et al. Extent of myocardial fibrosis and cellular hypertrophy in dilated cardiomyopathy. Am J Cardiol 1986;57: 816–20.

14. Roberts W, Siegel R, McManus B. Idiopathic dilated cardiomyopathy: analysis of 152 necropsy patients. Am J Cardiol 1987;60:1340–55.

15. Hennig A, Salel M, Sacher F, et al. High-resolution three-dimensional late gadolinium-enhanced cardiac magnetic resonance imaging to identify the underlying substrate of ventricular arrhythmia. Europace 2018;20:f179–91.

16. McCrohon JA, Moon JC, Prasad SK, et al. Differentiation of heart failure related to dilated cardiomyopathy and coronary artery disease using gadolinium-enhanced cardiovascular magnetic resonance. Circulation 2003;108:54–9.

17. Nazarian S, Bluemke D, Lardo A, et al. Magnetic resonance assessment of the substrate for inducible ventricular tachycardia in nonischemic cardiomyopathy. Circulation 2005;112(18):2821–5.

18. Bogun F, Desjardins B, Good E, et al. Delayed-enhanced magnetic resonance imaging in nonischemic cardiomyopathy: utility for identifying the ventricular arrhythmia substrate. J Am Coll Cardiol 2009;53:1138–45.

19. Hsia H, Callans D, Marchlinski F. Characterization of endocardial electrophysiological substrate in patients with nonischemic cardiomyopathy and monomorphic ventricular tachycardia. Circulation 2003; 108:704–10.

20. Siontis K, Kim H, Sharaf Dabbagh G, et al. Association of preprocedural cardiac magnetic resonance imaging with outcomes of ventricular tachycardia ablation in patients with idiopathic dilated cardiomyopathy. Heart Rhythm 2017;14:1487–93.

21. Cano O, Hutchinson M, Lin D, et al. Electroanatomic substrate and ablation outcome for suspected epicardial ventricular tachycardia in left ventricular nonischemic cardiomyopathy. J Am Coll Cardiol 2009;54:799–808.

22. Piers S, Tao Q, van Huls van Taxis C, et al. Contrast-enhanced MRI-derived scar patterns and associated ventricular tachycardias in nonischemic cardiomyopathy: implications for the ablation strategy. Circ Arrhythm Electrophysiol 2013;6: 875–83.

23. Oloriz T, Silberbauer J, Maccabelli G, et al. Catheter ablation of ventricular arrhythmia in non-ischaemic cardiomyopathy: anteroseptal versus inferolateral scar sub-types. Circ Arrhythm Electrophysiol 2014; 7:414–23.

24. Oloriz T, Wellens H, Santagostino G, et al. The value of the 12-lead electrocardiogram in localizing the scar in non-ischaemic cardiomyopathy. Europace 2016;18:1850–9.

25. Haqqani H, Tschabrunn C, Tzou W, et al. Isolated septal substrate for ventricular tachycardia in nonischemic dilated cardiomyopathy: incidence, characterization, and implications. Heart Rhythm 2011; 8:1169–76.

26. Basso C, Corrado D, Marcus F, et al. Arrhythmogenic right ventricular cardiomyopathy. Lancet 2009;373:1289–300.

27. Basso C, Corrado D, Bauce B, et al. Arrhythmogenic right ventricular cardiomyopathy. Circ Arrhythm Electrophysiol 2012;5:1233–46.

28. Marra M, Leoni L, Bauce B, et al. Imaging study of ventricular scar in arrhythmogenic right ventricular cardiomyopathy: comparison of 3D standard electroanatomical voltage mapping and contrast-enhanced cardiac magnetic resonance. Circ Arrhythm Electrophysiol 2012;5:91–100.

29. Marcus F, McKenna W, Sherrill D, et al. Diagnosis of arrhythmogenic right ventricular cardiomyopathy/ dysplasia: proposed modification of the task force criteria. Circulation 2010;121:1533–41.

30. Wang W, James C, Calkins H. Diagnostic and therapeutic strategies for arrhythmogenic right ventricular dysplasia/cardiomyopathy patient. Europace 2019; 21:9–21.

31. López-Ayala J, Gómez-Milanés I, Sánchez Muñoz J, et al. Desmoplakin truncations and arrhythmogenic left ventricular cardiomyopathy: characterizing a phenotype. Europace 2014;16:1838–46.

32. Hoffmayer K, Bhave P, Marcus G, et al. An electrocardiographic scoring system for distinguishing right ventricular outflow tract arrhythmias in patients with arrhythmogenic right ventricular cardiomyopathy from idiopathic ventricular tachycardia. Heart Rhythm 2013;10:477–82.

33. Garcia F, Bazan V, Zado E, et al. Epicardial substrate and outcome with epicardial ablation of ventricular tachycardia in arrhythmogenic right ventricular cardiomyopathy/dysplasia. Circulation 2009;120: 366–75.

34. Kirubakaran S, Bisceglia C, Silberbauer J, et al. Characterization of the arrhythmogenic substrate in patients with arrhythmogenic right ventricular cardiomyopathy undergoing ventricular tachycardia ablation. Europace 2017;19:1049–62.

35. Tomaselli G, Marbán E. Electrophysiological remodeling in hypertrophy and heart failure. Cardiovasc Res 1999;42:270–83.

36. Sakamoto N, Kawamura Y, Sato N, et al. Late gadolinium enhancement on cardiac magnetic resonance represents the depolarizing and repolarizing electrically damaged foci causing malignant ventricular arrhythmia in hypertrophic cardiomyopathy. Heart Rhythm 2015;12:1276–84.

37. Adabag A, Maron B, Appelbaum E, et al. Occurrence and frequency of arrhythmias in hypertrophic cardiomyopathy in relation to delayed enhancement on cardiovascular magnetic resonance. J Am Coll Cardiol 2008;51:1369–74.

38. Furushima H, Chinushi M, Iijima K, et al. Ventricular tachyarrhythmia associated with hypertrophic cardiomyopathy: incidence, prognosis, and relation to type of hypertrophy. J Cardiovasc Electrophysiol 2010;21:991–9.

39. Rowin E, Maron B, Haas T, et al. Hypertrophic cardiomyopathy with left ventricular apical aneurysm: implications for risk stratification and management. J Am Coll Cardiol 2017;69:761–73.

40. Inada K, Seiler J, Roberts-Thomson K, et al. Substrate characterization and catheter ablation for monomorphic ventricular tachycardia in patients with apical hypertrophic cardiomyopathy. J Cardiovasc Electrophysiol 2011;22:41–8.

41. Birnie D, Sauer W, Bogun F, et al. HRS expert consensus statement on the diagnosis and management of arrhythmias associated with cardiac sarcoidosis. Heart Rhythm 2014;11:1305–23.

42. Birnie D, Nery P, Ha A, et al. Cardiac sarcoidosis. J Am Coll Cardiol 2016;68:411–21.

43. Muser D, Santangeli P, Liang J, et al. Characterization of the electroanatomic substrate in cardiac sarcoidosis: correlation with imaging findings of scar and inflammation. JACC Clin Electrophysiol 2018;4:291–303.

44. Kumar S, Barbhaiya C, Nagashima K, et al. Ventricular tachycardia in cardiac sarcoidosis: characterization of ventricular substrate and outcomes of catheter ablation. Circ Arrhythm Electrophysiol 2015;8:87–93.

45. Arbustini E, Favalli V, Narula N, et al. Left ventricular noncompaction: a distinct genetic cardiomyopathy? J Am Coll Cardiol 2016;68:949–66.

46. Towbin J, Lorts A, Jefferies J. Left ventricular noncompaction cardiomyopathy. Lancet 2015;386: 813–25.

47. Arbustini E, Weidemann F, Hall J. Left ventricular noncompaction: a distinct cardiomyopathy or a trait shared by different cardiac diseases? J Am Coll Cardiol 2014;64:1840–50.

48. van Waning J, Caliskan K, Hoedemaekers Y, et al. Genetics, clinical features, and long-term outcome of noncompaction cardiomyopathy. J Am Coll Cardiol 2018;71:711–22.

49. Wang X, Zabell A, Koh W, et al. Lamin A/C cardiomyopathies: current understanding and novel treatment strategies. Curr Treat Options Cardiovasc Med 2017;19:21. https://doi.org/10.1007/s11936-017-0520-z.

50. Taylor M, Fain P, Sinagra G, et al. Natural history of dilated cardiomyopathy due to lamin A/C gene mutations. J Am Coll Cardiol 2003;41(5):771–80.

51. Hasselberg N, Haland T, Saberniak J, et al. Lamin A/C cardiomyopathy: young onset, high penetrance, and frequent need for heart transplantation. Eur Heart J 2018;39:853–60.

52. van Rijsingen I, Arbustini E, Elliott P, et al. Risk factors for malignant ventricular arrhythmias in lamin a/c mutation carriers: a European cohort study. J Am Coll Cardiol 2012;59:493–500.

53. Hasselberg N, Edvardsen T, Petri H, et al. Risk prediction of ventricular arrhythmias and myocardial function in Lamin A/C mutation positive subjects. Europace 2014;16:563–71.

54. Kumar S, Androulakis A, Sellal J, et al. Multicenter experience with catheter ablation for ventricular tachycardia in Lamin A/C cardiomyopathy. Circ Arrhythm Electrophysiol 2016;9 [pii:e004357].

55. Nakahara S, Tung R, Ramirez R, et al. Characterization of the arrhythmogenic substrate in ischemic and nonischemic cardiomyopathy: implications for catheter ablation of hemodynamically unstable ventricular tachycardia. J Am Coll Cardiol 2010;55:2355–65.

56. Jaïs P, Maury P, Khairy P, et al. Elimination of local abnormal ventricular activities: a new end point for substrate modification in patients with scar-related ventricular tachycardia. Circulation 2012;125: 2184–96.

57. Dickfeld T, Tian J, Ahmad G, et al. MRI-guided ventricular tachycardia ablation: integration of late

gadolinium-enhanced 3D scar in patients with implantable cardioverter-defibrillators. Circ Arrhythm Electrophysiol 2011;4:172–84.

58. Hutchinson M, Gerstenfeld E, Desjardins B, et al. Endocardial unipolar voltage mapping to detect epicardial ventricular tachycardia substrate in patients with Nnonischemic left ventricular cardiomyopathy. Circ Arrhythm Electrophysiol 2010;4:49–55.

59. Tokuda M, Tedrow U, Inada K, et al. Direct comparison of adjacent endocardial and epicardial electrograms: implications for substrate mapping. J Am Heart Assoc 2013;2:e000215. https://doi.org/10.1161/JAHA.113.000215.

60. Glashan C, Androulakis A, Tao Q, et al. Whole human heart histology to validate electroanatomical voltage mapping in patients with non-ischaemic cardiomyopathy and ventricular tachycardia. Eur Heart J 2018;39:2867–75.

61. Sacher F, Roberts-Thomson K, Maury P, et al. Epicardial VT ablation: a multicenter safety study. J Am Coll Cardiol 2010;55:2366–72.

62. Andreu D, Ortiz-Pérez J, Boussy T, et al. Usefulness of contrast-enhanced cardiac magnetic resonance in identifying the ventricular arrhythmia substrate and the approach needed for ablation. Eur Heart J 2014;35:1316–26.

63. Corrado D, Wichter T, Link M, et al. Treatment of arrhythmogenic right ventricular cardiomyopathy/dysplasia: an international task force consensus statement. Circulation 2015;132:441–53.

64. Polin G, Haqqani H, Tzou W, et al. Endocardial unipolar voltage mapping to identify epicardial substrate in arrhythmogenic right ventricular cardiomyopathy/dysplasia. Heart Rhythm 2011;8:76–83.

65. Komatsu Y, Jadidi A, Sacher F, et al. Relationship between MDCT-imaged myocardial fat and ventricular tachycardia substrate in arrhythmogenic right ventricular cardiomyopathy. J Am Heart Assoc 2014;3. https://doi.org/10.1161/JAHA.114.000935 [pii:e000935].

66. Cochet H, Denis A, Komatsu Y, et al. Automated quantification of right ventricular fat at contrast-enhanced cardiac multidetector CT in arrhythmogenic right ventricular cardiomyopathy. Radiology 2015;275:683–91.

67. Santangeli P, DiBiase L, Hsia H, et al. Current and future indications for ventricular tachycardia ablation: the evidence from clinical trials. In: Mahapatra S, et al, editors. Ventricular tachycardia ablation: a practical guide. Minneapolis (MN): CardioText Publishing; 2014. p. 41–61.

68. Romero J, Cerrud-Rodriguez R, Di Biase L, et al. Combined endocardial-epicardial versus endocardial catheter ablation alone for ventricular tachycardia in structural heart disease: a systematic review and meta-analysis. JACC Clin Electrophysiol 2019;5:13–24.

69. Bai R, Di Biase L, Shivkumar K, et al. Ablation of ventricular arrhythmias in arrhythmogenic right ventricular dysplasia/cardiomyopathy: arrhythmia-free survival after endo-epicardial substrate based mapping and ablation. Circ Arrhythm Electrophysiol 2011;4:478–85.

70. Berruezo A, Fernández-Armenta J, Mont L, et al. Combined endocardial and epicardial catheter ablation in arrhythmogenic right ventricular dysplasia incorporating scar dechanneling technique. Circ Arrhythm Electrophysiol 2012;5:111–21.

71. Philips B, Madhavan S, James C, et al. Outcomes of catheter ablation of ventricular tachycardia in arrhythmogenic right ventricular dysplasia/cardiomyopathy. Circ Arrhythm Electrophysiol 2012;5:499–505.

72. Dukkipati S, d'Avila A, Soejima K, et al. Long-term outcomes of combined epicardial and endocardial ablation of monomorphic ventricular tachycardia related to hypertrophic cardiomyopathy. Circ Arrhythm Electrophysiol 2011;4:185–94.

73. Santangeli P, Di Biase L, Lakkireddy D, et al. Radiofrequency catheter ablation of ventricular arrhythmias in patients with hypertrophic cardiomyopathy: safety and feasibility. Heart Rhythm 2010;7:1036–42.

74. Vaseghi M, Hu T, Tung R, et al. Outcomes of catheter ablation of ventricular tachycardia based on etiology in nonischemic heart disease: an international ventricular tachycardia ablation center collaborative study. JACC Clin Electrophysiol 2018;4:1141–50.

75. Muser D, Santangeli P, Pathak R, et al. Long-term outcomes of catheter ablation of ventricular tachycardia in patients with cardiac sarcoidosis. Circ Arrhythm Electrophysiol 2016;9(8). https://doi.org/10.1161/CIRCEP.116.004333 [pii:e004333].

76. Muser D, Liang J, Witschey W, et al. Ventricular arrhythmias associated with left ventricular noncompaction: electrophysiologic characteristics, mapping, and ablation. Heart Rhythm 2017;14:166–75.

77. Yamashita S, Sacher F, Mahida S, et al. Image integration to guide catheter ablation in scar-related ventricular tachycardia. J Cardiovasc Electrophysiol 2016;27:699–708.

78. Tokuda M, Tedrow U, Kojodjojo P, et al. Catheter ablation of ventricular tachycardia in nonischemic heart disease. Circ Arrhythm Electrophysiol 2012;5:992–1000.

79. Muser D, Santangeli P, Castro S, et al. Long-term outcome after catheter ablation of ventricular tachycardia in patients with nonischemic dilated cardiomyopathy. Circ Arrhythm Electrophysiol 2016;9 [pii:e004328].

80. Tzou W, Rothstein P, Cowherd M, et al. Repeat ablation of refractory ventricular arrhythmias in patients

with nonischemic cardiomyopathy: impact of mid-myocardial substrate and role of adjunctive ablation techniques. J Cardiovasc Electrophysiol 2018;29: 1403–12.

81. Liuba I, Frankel D, Riley M, et al. Scar progression in patients with nonischemic cardiomyopathy and ventricular arrhythmias. Heart Rhythm 2014;11:755–62.

82. Berte B, Sacher F, Venlet J, et al. VT recurrence after ablation: incomplete ablation or disease progression? A multicentric European study. J Cardiovasc Electrophysiol 2016;27:80–7.

83. Romero J, Di Biase L, Diaz J, et al. Early versus late referral for catheter ablation of ventricular tachycardia in patients with structural heart disease: a systematic review and meta-analysis of clinical outcomes. JACC Clin Electrophysiol 2018;4:374–82.

84. Koruth J, Dukkipati S, Miller M, et al. Bipolar irrigated radiofrequency ablation: a therapeutic option for refractory intramural atrial and ventricular tachycardia circuits. Heart Rhythm 2012;9:1932–41.

85. Sauer P, Kunkel M, Nguyen D, et al. Successful ablation of ventricular tachycardia arising from a mid-myocardial septal outflow tract site utilizing a simplified bipolar ablation setup. HeartRhythm Case Rep 2019;5:105–8.

86. Nguyen D, Gerstenfeld E, Tzou W, et al. Radiofrequency ablation using an open irrigated electrode cooled with half-normal saline. JACC Clin Electrophysiol 2017;3:1103–10.

87. Nguyen D, Tzou W, Sandhu A, et al. Prospective multicenter experience with cooled radiofrequency ablation using high impedance irrigant to target deep myocardial substrate refractory to standard ablation. JACC Clin Electrophysiol 2018;4:1176–85.

88. Tokuda M, Sobieszczyk P, Eisenhauer AK, et al. Transcoronary ethanol ablation for recurrent ventricular tachycardia after failed catheter ablation: an update. Circ Arrhythm Electrophysiol 2011;4:889–96.

89. Kreidieh B, Rodríguez-Mañero M, Schurmann P, et al. Retrograde coronary venous ethanol infusion for ablation of refractory ventricular tachycardia. Circ Arrhythm Electrophysiol 2016;9 [pii:e004352].

90. Cuculich P, Schill M, Kashani R, et al. Noninvasive cardiac radiation for ablation of ventricular tachycardia. N Engl J Med 2017;377:2325–36.

91. Stevenson W, Tedrow U, Reddy V, et al. Infusion needle radiofrequency ablation for treatment of refractory ventricular arrhythmias. J Am Coll Cardiol 2019;73:1413–25.

Substrate Mapping in Ventricular Arrhythmias

Roderick Tung, MD

KEYWORDS

- Ventricular tachycardia • Electroanatomic mapping • Voltage mapping • Bipolar • Isochronal
- Electrograms

KEY POINTS

- Ventricular tachycardia is typically hemodynamically unstable and strategies to target the arrhythmogenic substrate during sinus rhythm are essential for therapeutic ablation.
- Electroanatomic mapping is the cornerstone of substrate-based strategies; ablation can be directed within a delineated scar region defined by low voltage.
- Bipolar voltage mapping has inherent limitations; electrogram amplitudes are intimately related to the electrode area of the recording catheter and orientation of the activation wavefront.
- Specific electrogram characteristics, such as local uncoupling, fractionation, and evidence of slow conduction, may improve the specificity of localizing the most arrhythmogenic regions within the substrate.
- Deceleration zones during sinus rhythm are niduses for reentry and can be identified by isochronal late activation mapping, which is a functional analysis of substrate propagation with local annotation to electrogram offset.

RATIONALE FOR DEFINING THE SUBSTRATE

During catheter ablation of arrhythmias, it is not a common requirement to map during ongoing tachycardia because slow pathway modification and accessory pathway elimination are typically guided by electroanatomy and electrogram timing, respectively. There is much debate as to how atrial fibrillation (AF) should be mapped and no consensus exists to date, because the cornerstone of AF ablation revolves around ablation of triggers during sinus rhythm, which predominantly resided within in the region of the pulmonary veins. In this regard, perhaps atrial flutter is the only arrhythmia that is best suited for mapping during tachycardia, because it may be explored by activation and entrainment mapping.

Scar-related ventricular tachycardia (VT) is similar to atrial flutter; reentry is the most common mechanism, except that hemodynamic instability is the rule, because the majority of patients have structural heart disease with left ventricular systolic dysfunction. Therefore, methods to target VT without requiring long sustained periods of tachycardia are necessary in clinical practice. Before the advent of electroanatomic mapping systems, ablation of scar-related VT was guided by limited entrainment mapping and pace mapping within low-voltage regions under fluoroscopic navigation.[1,2] Because surgical therapies for VT such as encircling ventriculotomy[3] or subendocardial resection[4] were shown to result in improved freedom from recurrent VT, early strategies with catheter ablation required delineation of the scar boundaries by electroanatomic voltage mapping to define the margin in which therapy was directed to mimic surgery[5] (**Fig. 1**). For this reason, the use of electroanatomic mapping to define scar became essential to treat VT with an anatomic approach during sinus rhythm.

Disclosures/Conflicts of Interest: Speaking honorarium for Boston Scientific, Abbott, Biosense Webster.
Department of Medicine, Section of Cardiology, The University of Chicago Medicine, Center for Arrhythmia Care, Pritzker School of Medicine, 5841 South Maryland Avenue, MC 6080, Chicago, IL 60637, USA
E-mail address: rodericktung@uchicago.edu

Card Electrophysiol Clin 11 (2019) 657–663
https://doi.org/10.1016/j.ccep.2019.08.009
1877-9182/19/© 2019 Elsevier Inc. All rights reserved.

cardiacEP.theclinics.com

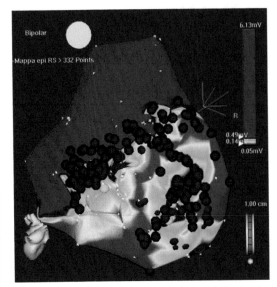

Fig. 1. Electroanatomic map with low voltage in the inferior apex (posterior view). The voltage setting is less than 0.5 mV, which displays dense scar. The ablation lesions (*red circles*) are directed at the superior border zone and a T-shaped lesion is created to connect the scar border toward the center of the scar.

WHAT IS MEANT BY A SUBSTRATE-BASED APPROACH?

The definition of substrate-based ablation approaches varies widely across centers, but typically signifies that voltage mapping is performed within the chamber of interest and techniques such as pace mapping, entrainment, or activation mapping are used within the low-voltage region identified. Once areas of functional significance are determined by these techniques, an ablation lesion set is delivered to target these regions within low-voltage regions that represent scar during sinus rhythm, rather than VT. In this regard, any ablation directed toward low-voltage regions constitutes substrate modification, because this procedure may decrease the arrhythmogenicity of the scar.

A pure substrate-based approach typically describes a strategy in which VT mapping is not performed and, in some practices, VT is never induced.[6] Instead, ablation is performed within low-voltage regions with the assumption that the VT of interest originates with scar regions. However, in patients with structural heart disease, up to 20% of patients may have idiopathic VTs that do not emanate from the scar substrate.[7,8] Therefore, it is our opinion that VT induction should be performed at some point during the procedure to confirm that the morphology and site or origin is likely to be eliminated by modification of the substrate defined by electroanatomic mapping.

DEFINING SCAR: MAPPING SYSTEMS AND CATHETERS

Delineation of scar by low-voltage regions identified by contact mapping was first validated by Callans and associates[9] and Marchlinski and associates[5] in a porcine postinfarction model and in human controls, respectively. In the late 1990s, these authors reported a strong correlation between bipolar amplitudes of less than 1.5 mV with gross anatomic scar. These seminal studies were performed with large-tip (Navistar, 4 mm) ablation catheters and a magnetically based electroanatomic mapping system (CARTO, Biosense Webster, Diamond Bar, CA) and the thresholds proposed from these studies continue to be universally implemented to represent scar regions, where dense scar was defined as less than 0.5 mV and border zone was defined as 0.5 to 1.5 mV. It is important to emphasize that scar is electrically inert and does not have a voltage, but the scar identified by contact voltage mapping represents relative degrees of the admixture between collagen and surviving tissue, where dense scar has the greatest concentration and confluence of fibrosis.

Although voltage mapping with by single-point acquisition continues to be the most traditional method, multielectrode catheters have gained popularity because they increase the speed of mapping with simultaneous acquisition of multiple points for a given catheter position.[10,11] As a result, substrate mapping is achieved with higher density and higher resolution in the present era (**Fig. 2**). Ultra-high-density mapping (>1000 mapping points) of the ventricle with smaller electrodes and tighter interelectrode spacing has been validated in preclinical and human cases using linear multielectrode catheters with electrofield navigation (NavX, Abbott, Abbott Park, IL)[12,13] and basket configurations with printed minielectrodes (Rhythmia, Boston Scientific, Inc, Marlborough, MA).[14,15]

For all mapping strategies, the density of mapping is critically important to optimize the accuracy of scar delineation. Scar is often patchy and inhomogenous and the identification of tissue heterogeneity is predicated on the resolution of the mapping technique.[16,17] Interpolation is a setting during voltage mapping that interprets missing data points as the most adjacent value acquired and large degrees of interpolation may compromise the accuracy of maps and sensitivity to detect pathologic areas. Although multielectrode catheters allow for higher density acquisition, it is important to ensure that contact is optimally uniform on the recording electrodes. With the majority

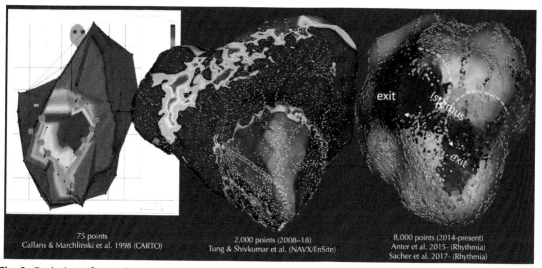

Fig. 2. Evolution of mapping systems with improvement in system resolution owing to multielectrode catheter acquisition. Initial validation of CARTO was performed with 75 points, whereas use of duodecapolar linear catheter increase mapping density of more than 1000 points with the NAVX system. The Rhythmia system has the highest resolution, with a basket-shaped catheter and minielectrodes.

of mapping systems, electrodes that are outside of a prespecified range from the eternal shell of geometry are excluded from representation.

ROLE OF EPICARDIAL APPROACH

Although endocardial mapping frequently identifies the postinfarct substrate, epicardial substrate may be present in a significant proportion of patients with ischemic cardiomyopathy. Estimates for the prevalence of arrhythmogenic epicardial substrate range across various reports from 10% to 75%.[18–20] A recent meta-analysis suggested that a combined epicardial–endocardial approach for ischemic cardiomyopathy might improve survival.[21] Nonischemic etiologies have a propensity toward epicardial locations and the percutaneous technique described by Sosa and colleagues[22] has become invaluable to for patients that have incomplete substrate identification and/or modification with endocardial approach alone. Prior endocardial failure, cardiac MRI, and unipolar mapping may be useful predictors of significant epicardial substrates.[23]

Myocardial scar is architecturally complex and exists in a 3-dimensional realm with variable transmurality. Representation of the low-voltage substrate based on the surface mapped with an electroanatomic mapping system oversimplifies the scar as a 2-dimensional or planar depiction. Simultaneous epicardial–endocardial mapping may provide greater insight into the substrate with a 3-dimensional perspective during sinus rhythm, as well as VT, where activation gaps

can be interpreted as indirect evidence of intramural activation remote from the surface recorded.

LIMITATIONS OF BIPOLAR VOLTAGE MAPPING

Contact voltage mapping can be conceptualized as taking an electrical biopsy of the myocardial surface, where the size of the recording instrument (antenna) determines the mass sampled. A greater amount of myocardium sampled results in a larger bipolar voltage recording, which highlights the critical relationship between electrogram amplitude and electrode area. An electrogram cannot be dissociated from the instrument used to record it. Electrode areas are determined by 2 factors: (1) electrode size (2) interelectrode spacing.[24] An increase in interelectrode spacing has clearly been shown to have a linear relationship with bipolar amplitude recorded and unipolar recordings, which do not have a finite interelectrode distance, are the largest in voltage[25] (**Fig. 3**). For this reason, unipolar mapping has been shown to provide voltage information at a greater depth (midmyocardial or epicardial) in patients with a paucity of endocardial scar.[26]

Because there is currently a multitude of catheter configurations that are used in clinical practice, it is important to emphasize that voltage thresholds ought to be tailored to specific catheters based on size, electrode distances, and configuration[27] (**Box 1**). Therefore, a universal threshold of less than 1.5 mV to define myocardial

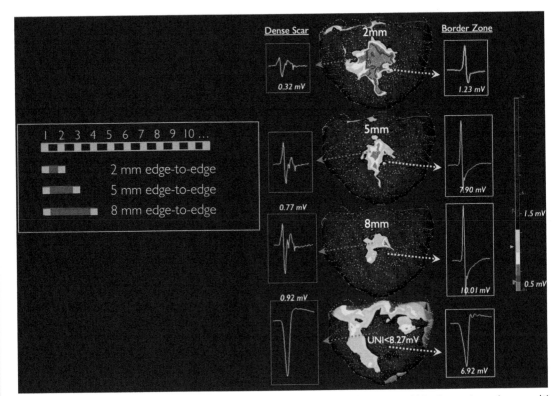

Fig. 3. Impact of electrode spacing on low-voltage detection. Progressively increased bipole spacing using a multi-electrode catheter shows a decrease in scar area with wide spacing at a fixed threshold of less than 1.5 mV. The scar area is critically dependent upon the size of the bipole recording and adjustments in the thresholds should be made based on the electrode area. (*Adapted from* Tung R, Kim S, Yagishita D, Vaseghi M, Ennis DB, Ouadah S, Ajijola OA, Bradfield JS, Mahapatra S, Finn P, Shivkumar K. Scar Voltage Threshold Determination Using Ex Vivo MRI Integration in a Porcine Infarct Model Heart Rhythm. 2016. pii: S1547-5271(16):3504-5; with permission.)

scar may not be optimal if applied across all mapping catheters and systems. For this reason, complementary information such as electrogram characteristics and functional propagation may be useful to define the pathologic substrate for VT.

Bipolar electrogram amplitude is also intimately related to the orientation of the electrode pair to the angle of the incident wavefront.[24] In theory, a wavefront that propagates perpendicularly toward both electrodes of a bipolar pair would be canceled, because the same unipolar amplitude is seen each electrode. The most optimal wavefront recorded by a bipole is one that runs parallel to the orientation to sense a directionality as it passes 1 electrode toward the other, resulting in a difference in unipolar activation. Significant variation in both unipolar and bipolar scar areas may result with differing activation wavefronts[28] **(Fig. 4)**. Discordance in low-voltage substrate identification is more common in mixed scar and septal locations and alternative wavefront mapping may be useful in selected cases in which substrate is not overt.

LOCAL ABNORMAL ELECTROGRAMS CHARACTERISTICS

Because voltage mapping has inherent limitations, an emphasis of local electrogram characteristics may improve the specificity of localizing the most arrhythmogenic zones. The presence of uncoupled or late potentials has been shown to be more predictive of critical sites for reentry than voltage-based channels.[29,30] Although late potentials have been shown to useful surrogates for isthmus sites during sinus rhythm, the activation wavefront may alter the degree of conduction delay observed for a given electrogram. Electrogram characteristics such as width or fractionation are useful because they signify local uncoupling of electrical activation, which are conducive for reentry. Local abnormal ventricular activities may be activated coincident with the timing of the far-field activation and extrastimuli and attention to high-frequency components is important to identify arrhythmogenic signals.[31–33]

More recently extensive ablation, or homogenization, aimed to target all local abnormal ventricular activities or abnormal electrograms within low-voltage regions has been shown to improve freedom from VT recurrence compared with incomplete elimination and/or more limited strategies.[31,34] These strategies require thorough delineation of the substrate because the ablation lesions set is completely determined by the extent and location of the abnormalities mapped.

FUNCTIONAL SUBSTRATE MAPPING: ANALYSIS OF PROPAGATION FOR WAVEFRONT DISCONTINUITIES

Whether sites of reentry can be predicted during sinus rhythm has been historically debated. If ventricular reentry responsible for VT is purely functional, reentrant patterns would not be predicted by or possess any resemblance to discontinuities during sinus rhythm. At our institution, we continue to perform a systemic analysis of sinus rhythm propagation to assess whether wavefront discontinuities are predictive of critical site for reentry.[35] An isochronal late activation map with local annotation to the last electrogram deflection allows for a visually friendly mapping display to rapidly identify late activated regions distinct from slow conduction regions, which are represented by isochronal crowding (**Fig. 5**).

Traditional annotation of local electrogram timing selects either the peak amplitude or maximal dV/dT, which does not incorporate late information or delayed local activation (final component of split or late electrogram).[36] Slow conduction regions, or deceleration zones, seem to harbor higher arrhythmogenicity than regions

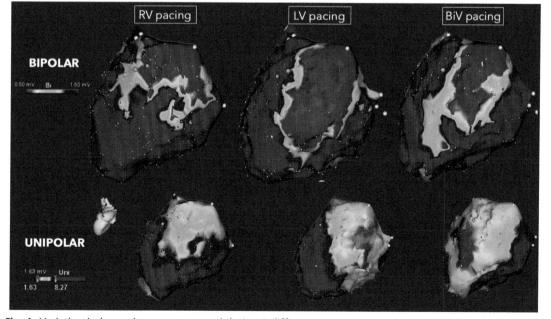

Fig. 4. Variation in low voltage scar mapped during 3 different activation wavefronts: right ventricle (RV), left ventricle (LV), biventricular (BiV) pacing. Both bipolar and unipolar scar areas differ as electrogram amplitudes are influenced by directionality.

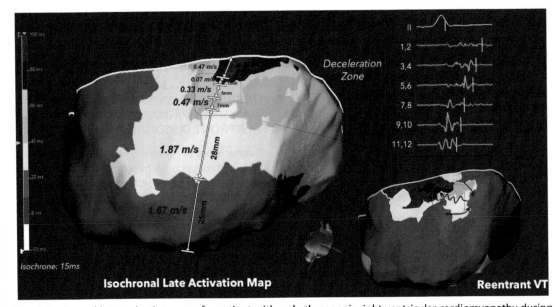

Fig. 5. Isochronal late activation map of a patient with arrhythmogenic right ventricular cardiomyopathy during epicardial mapping. The deceleration zone is defined as a region with isochronal crowding, where conduction velocity slows. Representative electrograms are shown. The reentrant VT circuit correlates with the deceleration zone rather than the latest isochrone of activation (*purple*) during sinus rhythm. (*Adapted from*: Raiman M, Tung R. Automated isochronal late activation mapping to identify deceleration zones: Rationale and methodology of a practical electroanatomic mapping approach for ventricular tachycardia ablation. *Comput Biol Med.* 2018; with permission.)

with latest activation, which provides evidence that the latest late potentials may be not be functionally relevant to reentry.

An isochronal late activation map may be complementary to voltage mapping and allows for a functional prioritization of local abnormal ventricular activities based on identifying the basis for late activation, which typically results from a wavefront discontinuity around a line of conduction block or conduction delay. The correlation between deceleration zones and the critical sites suggest that fixed anatomic boundaries evident during sinus are present may define the reentrant path. Prospective multicenter studies are necessary and planning is underway.

REFERENCES

1. Morady F, Harvey M, Kalbfleisch SJ, et al. Radiofrequency catheter ablation of ventricular tachycardia in patients with coronary artery disease. Circulation 1993;87:363–72.
2. Morady F, Kadish A, Rosenheck S, et al. Concealed entrainment as a guide for catheter ablation of ventricular tachycardia in patients with prior myocardial infarction. J Am Coll Cardiol 1991;17:678–89.
3. Guiraudon G, Fontaine G, Frank R, et al. Encircling endocardial ventriculotomy: a new surgical treatment for life-threatening ventricular tachycardias resistant to medical treatment following myocardial infarction. Ann Thorac Surg 1978;26:438–44.
4. Harken AH, Josephson ME, Horowitz LN. Surgical endocardial resection for the treatment of malignant ventricular tachycardia. Ann Surg 1979;190:456–60.
5. Marchlinski FE, Callans DJ, Gottlieb CD, et al. Linear ablation lesions for control of unmappable ventricular tachycardia in patients with ischemic and nonischemic cardiomyopathy. Circulation 2000;101:1288–96.
6. Di Biase L, Burkhardt JD, Lakkireddy D, et al. Ablation of stable VTs versus substrate ablation in ischemic cardiomyopathy: the VISTA randomized multicenter trial. J Am Coll Cardiol 2015;66:2872–82.
7. Ellis ER, Shvilkin A, Josephson ME. Nonreentrant ventricular arrhythmias in patients with structural heart disease unrelated to abnormal myocardial substrate. Heart Rhythm 2014;11:946–52.
8. Das MK, Scott LR, Miller JM. Focal mechanism of ventricular tachycardia in coronary artery disease. Heart Rhythm 2010;7:305–11.
9. Callans DJ, Ren JF, Michele J, et al. Electroanatomic left ventricular mapping in the porcine model of healed anterior myocardial infarction. Correlation with intracardiac echocardiography and pathological analysis. Circulation 1999;100:1744–50.
10. Tung R, Ellenbogen KA. Emergence of multielectrode mapping: on the road to higher resolution. Circ Arrhythm Electrophysiol 2016;9 [pii:e004281].
11. Acosta J, Penela D, Andreu D, et al. Multielectrode vs. point-by-point mapping for ventricular tachycardia substrate ablation: a randomized study. Europace 2018;20:512–9.

12. Tung R, Nakahara S, Maccabelli G, et al. Ultra high-density multipolar mapping with double ventricular access: a novel technique for ablation of ventricular tachycardia. J Cardiovasc Electrophysiol 2011;22: 49–56.

13. Nakahara S, Tung R, Ramirez RJ, et al. Characterization of the arrhythmogenic substrate in ischemic and nonischemic cardiomyopathy implications for catheter ablation of hemodynamically unstable ventricular tachycardia. J Am Coll Cardiol 2010;55:2355–65.

14. Anter E, Tschabrunn CM, Buxton AE, et al. High-resolution mapping of postinfarction reentrant ventricular tachycardia: electrophysiological characterization of the circuit. Circulation 2016;134:314–27.

15. Martin R, Maury P, Bisceglia C, et al. Characteristics of scar-related ventricular tachycardia circuits using ultra-high-density mapping. Circ Arrhythm Electrophysiol 2018;11:e006569.

16. Nakahara S, Tung R, Ramirez RJ, et al. Distribution of late potentials within infarct scars assessed by ultra high-density mapping. Heart Rhythm 2010;7(12): 1817–24.

17. Ashikaga H, Sasano T, Dong J, et al. Magnetic resonance-based anatomical analysis of scar-related ventricular tachycardia: implications for catheter ablation. Circ Res 2007;101:939–47.

18. Tung R, Michowitz Y, Yu R, et al. Epicardial ablation of ventricular tachycardia: an institutional experience of safety and efficacy. Heart Rhythm 2013;10:490–8.

19. Schmidt B, Chun KR, Baensch D, et al. Catheter ablation for ventricular tachycardia after failed endocardial ablation: epicardial substrate or inappropriate endocardial ablation? Heart Rhythm 2010;7: 1746–52.

20. Sacher F, Roberts-Thomson K, Maury P, et al. Epicardial ventricular tachycardia ablation a multicenter safety study. J Am Coll Cardiol 2010;55:2366–72.

21. Romero J, Cerrud-Rodriguez RC, Di Biase L, et al. Combined endocardial-epicardial versus endocardial catheter ablation alone for ventricular tachycardia in structural heart disease: a systematic review and meta-analysis. JACC Clin Electrophysiol 2019;5:13–24.

22. Sosa E, Scanavacca M, d'Avila A, et al. A new technique to perform epicardial mapping in the electrophysiology laboratory. J Cardiovasc Electrophysiol 1996;7:531–6.

23. Boyle NG, Shivkumar K. Epicardial interventions in electrophysiology. Circulation 2012;126:1752–69.

24. Anter E, Josephson ME. Substrate Mapping for Ventricular Tachycardia: Assumptions and Misconceptions. JACCCEP 2015;1:341–52.

25. Tung R, Kim S, Yagishita D, et al. Scar voltage threshold determination using ex vivo magnetic resonance imaging integration in a porcine infarct model: influence of interelectrode distances and three-dimensional spatial effects of scar. Heart Rhythm 2016;13:1993–2002.

26. Hutchinson MD, Gerstenfeld EP, Desjardins B, et al. Endocardial unipolar voltage mapping to detect epicardial ventricular tachycardia substrate in patients with nonischemic left ventricular cardiomyopathy. Circ Arrhythm Electrophysiol 2011;4:49–55.

27. Berte B, Relan J, Sacher F, et al. Impact of electrode type on mapping of scar-related VT. J Cardiovasc Electrophysiol 2015;26(11):1213–23.

28. Tung R, Josephson ME, Bradfield JS, et al. Directional Influences of ventricular activation on myocardial scar characterization: voltage mapping with multiple wavefronts during ventricular tachycardia ablation. Circ Arrhythm Electrophysiol 2016;9 [pii:e004155].

29. Bogun F, Good E, Reich S, et al. Isolated potentials during sinus rhythm and pace-mapping within scars as guides for ablation of post-infarction ventricular tachycardia. J Am Coll Cardiol 2006;47:2013–9.

30. Arenal A, Glez-Torrecilla E, Ortiz M, et al. Ablation of electrograms with an isolated, delayed component as treatment of unmappable monomorphic ventricular tachycardias in patients with structural heart disease. J Am Coll Cardiol 2003;41:81–92.

31. Jais P, Maury P, Khairy P, et al. Elimination of local abnormal ventricular activities: a new end point for substrate modification in patients with scar-related ventricular tachycardia. Circulation 2012; 125:2184–96.

32. Porta-Sanchez A, Jackson N, Lukac P, et al. Multicenter study of ischemic ventricular tachycardia ablation with decrement-evoked potential (DEEP) mapping with extra stimulus. JACC Clin Electrophysiol 2018;4:307–15.

33. Acosta J, Andreu D, Penela D, et al. Elucidation of hidden slow conduction by double ventricular extrastimuli: a method for further arrhythmic substrate identification in ventricular tachycardia ablation procedures. Europace 2018;20:337–46.

34. Vergara P, Trevisi N, Ricco A, et al. Late potentials abolition as an additional technique for reduction of arrhythmia recurrence in scar related ventricular tachycardia ablation. J Cardiovasc Electrophysiol 2012;23:621–7.

35. Irie T, Yu R, Bradfield JS, et al. Relationship between sinus rhythm late activation zones and critical sites for scar-related ventricular tachycardia: systematic analysis of isochronal late activation mapping. Circ Arrhythm Electrophysiol 2015;8: 390–9.

36. Raiman M, Tung R. Automated isochronal late activation mapping to identify deceleration zones: rationale and methodology of a practical electroanatomic mapping approach for ventricular tachycardia ablation. Comput Biol Med 2018;102: 336–40.

Mapping and Ablation of Arrhythmias from Uncommon Sites (Aortic Cusp, Pulmonary Artery, and Left Ventricular Summit)

Santhisri Kodali, MD, Pasquale Santangeli, MD, PhD, Fermin C. Garcia, MD*

KEYWORDS

• Outflow tract • Pulmonary artery • Left ventricular summit • Catheter ablation

KEY POINTS

• Challenging sites for catheter ablation of idiopathic ventricular arrhythmias encompass the aortic cusps, pulmonary artery, and notably the left ventricular summit.
• A systematic approach should be used to direct mapping efforts between endocardial, coronary venous, and epicardial sites.
• Foci at the left ventricular summit, particularly intraseptal and at the inaccessible region, remain difficult to reach.
• When percutaneous techniques fail, surgical ablation remains an option, but with the risk of late coronary artery stenosis.

INTRODUCTION

Catheter ablation is routinely used to treat patients with symptomatic premature ventricular contractions (PVCs) or ventricular tachycardia (VT) of an idiopathic nature that fail or are intolerant to antiarrhythmic drugs for control, and those with PVC-induced cardiomyopathy. Very frequently, the ventricular arrhythmias (VAs) arise from the right ventricular outflow tract (RVOT) and left ventricular outflow tract (LVOT)[1–3] and their supporting structures. However, at present, certain locations remain challenging areas of ectopic foci to target and a cohesive understanding of the underlying complex anatomy is pivotal to optimizing ablation success. We herein present the relevant anatomy, electrocardiogram (ECG) features, and challenges related to mapping and ablation of idiopathic VAs (after exclusion of structural heart disease by imaging techniques including echocardiography and cardiac magnetic resonance imaging) from the aortic cusps, pulmonary artery (PA), and left ventricular summit (LVS).

GENERAL APPROACH TO MAPPING OF IDIOPATHIC PREMATURE VENTRICULAR CONTRACTIONS

Before bringing the patient to the electrophysiology laboratory, antiarrhythmic drugs should be discontinued 5 half-lives before the procedure. Mapping should be performed under as minimal sedation as possible to avoid VA suppression. Rarely, even systemic absorption from subcutaneous lidocaine can suppress VAs. The 12-lead ECG of the spontaneous VA should be acquired while the patient is on the table before administration of any sedation. Beta-adrenergic agonists such

Disclosures: The authors have no relevant financial disclosures or conflicts of interest.
Cardiac Electrophysiology, Hospital of the University of Pennsylvania, 3400 Spruce Street, 9 Founders Pavilion, Philadelphia, PA 19104, USA
* Corresponding author.
E-mail address: fermin.garcia@uphs.upenn.edu

Card Electrophysiol Clin 11 (2019) 665–674
https://doi.org/10.1016/j.ccep.2019.08.012
1877-9182/19/© 2019 Elsevier Inc. All rights reserved.

as isoproterenol (1–3 μg/min) and burst ventricular or atrial pacing is sometimes helpful to manifest the clinical VA. By accessing the femoral vessels, mapping may be accomplished via a retrograde aortic approach or less commonly, an antegrade trans-septal approach (directed at the anterior and inferior aspect of the interatrial septum). We perform all PVC/VT ablation procedures at our institution with the use of intracardiac echocardiography (ICE) to facilitate direct visualization of structures, catheter positioning, and monitor for potential complications. A 3-dimensional electroanatomic map is constructed of the outflow tracts, ventricles, and course of the coronary arteries (if visualized) and displayed via the CartoSound module (Biosense Webster, Diamond Bar, CA), accounting for interindividual variability in cardiac rotation and axis within the thorax for the most accurate online attitudinal orientation. Before ablation, the proximity of the coronary ostia must be verified by either ICE or via coronary arteriography; the former does not require radiation and avoids the risks of contrast, an additional arterial access, and the possibility of coronary artery air embolism. but does necessitate greater operator experience and adds substantive cost.

AORTIC CUSPS
Anatomic Considerations and Prevalence

To fully appreciate the challenges related to mapping and ablation of aortic cusp VAs, one must understand the surrounding complex anatomy. The aortic root is centrally located in the heart and intimately connected to the left ventricular (LV) ostium at the fibrous aortoventricular membrane (penetrated by the aorta anteriorly and mitral valve posteriorly).[4] The aortic sinuses of Valsalva support the right coronary cusp (RCC), left coronary cusp (LCC), and noncoronary cusp (NCC), which are attached to the LV ostium via independent membranous attachments.[4,5] The RCC is situated anteriorly, the LCC laterally and superior to the RCC, and the NCC posteriorly. The interleaflet triangles are extensions of thin, fibrous tissue, a consequence of the semilunar contour of the aortic valve leaflets, arising from the ventricular aspect of the aortic root and bounded superiorly by the sinotubular junction and elsewhere between the aortic sinuses. The interleaflet triangle confined between the right and left coronary sinuses is the smallest and lies posterior to the subpulmonary infundibulum.[4,5] The base of the NCC contains mainly fibrous tissue owing to its proximity to the aortomitral continuity. The RCC contains LV myocardial fibers that are oriented in a parallel fashion to the base of the RCC. The LCC interfaces with the LV myocardium for a significantly shorter segment relative to the RCC,[5] with its posterior aspect in apposition to the left fibrous trigone. **Fig. 1** illustrates the structures comprising the aortic root.

Aortic root VAs constitute 15% to 17% of idiopathic outflow tract VAs. The LCC is the most common site of origin (SOO), followed by the RCC, and then by the RCC–LCC junction.[1,6–9] Myocardial extensions have been observed traversing the ventriculoarterial junction above the aortic valve, contiguous with the subvalvular myocardium, and past the level of attachment of the RCC (most frequent), LCC, and the NCC. On rare occasions, myocardial sleeves were seen to extend directly into the RCC and even the NCC (total 2.2%).[10,11] Additionally, the interventricular septum has been very infrequently observed to harbor myocardial extensions.[11,12] These findings may account for rare reported cases of successful VA ablation performed from the NCC.[8,12]

Salient Electrocardiographic Features

The first step of 12-lead ECG analysis is to distinguish between VAs of RVOT versus aortic cusp

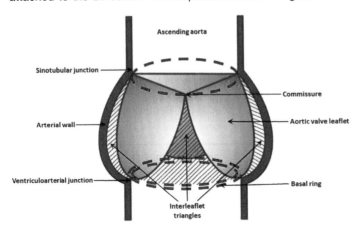

Fig. 1. Anatomy of the aortic root.

Ascending aorta

Sinotubular junction

Commissure

Aortic valve leaflet

Arterial wall

Ventriculoarterial junction

Basal ring

Interleaflet triangles

origin. Both exhibit a left bundle branch block (LBBB) pattern with an inferior axis and a dominantly negative QRS morphology in leads AVR and AVL. However, aortic cusp VAs have been shown to display an earlier R/S transition that occurs at or before lead V3. Ouyang and colleagues[1] demonstrated that an aortic cusp origin was favored over an RVOT origin when a greater R/S amplitude ratio and R wave duration was seen in leads V1 or V2, explained by the more posterior and rightward orientation of the aortic cusp region relative to the RVOT. Lin and colleagues[13] applied the results of pace mapping guided by ICE and electroanatomic mapping to define salient features of aortic cusp PVCs. The findings yielded a precordial R/S transition seen by lead V2 for LCC PVCs and by lead V3 for RCC PVCs.

Two other studies focused on VA SOO from the RCC–LCC junction and found that either a QS morphology in lead V1 or a QRS morphology in leads V1 to V3 was often seen.[14,15] Betensky and colleagues[16] determined that in situations where the R/S transition occurred at lead V3 and baseline LBBB was not present, a V2 transition ratio of 0.6 or greater or a transition that occurred earlier during the PVC relative to sinus rhythm were predictive of LVOT origin. LCC VAs are often characterized by negativity in lead I, whereas RCC VAs exhibit a positive component.[17] Additionally, VAs arising from below rather than within the aortic sinuses of Valsalva are more likely to exhibit an S wave of greater depth and duration in lead I and an AVL/AVR Q wave ratio of greater than 1.45.[18]

Mapping and Catheter Ablation

The general approach to mapping and catheter ablation of VAs was discussed elsewhere in this article. In localizing the PVC/VT, activation mapping should reveal a unipolar QS electrogram morphology with maximum negative dV/dt and corresponding maximum bipolar electrogram amplitude (typically 20–40 ms before the PVC) at the SOO. However, unipolar morphology should be used only as an adjunct given that many sites within the LVOT also yield a unipolar QS recording owing to the relative position within the heart. Pace mapping represents another strategy for localizing idiopathic VAs and a 12/12 match of all ECG leads should be sought, including both amplitude and notching. On occasion, a VA origin may be within the aortic cusp region, but exhibit an early breakout site in the RVOT owing to preferential conduction via an insulated fiber (earlier activation in the aortic cusp but a better pace map with a shorter stimulus-to-QRS interval in the RVOT); as

such, the successful ablation site may be from the adjacent RVOT.[19] Effectiveness of pace mapping from the aortic cusps in particular is reduced by a smaller and nonuniformly distributed myocardial mass available for electrical capture. This in turn, requires higher output pacing, which can produce imperfect pace maps even at the true SOO owing to an enlarged virtual electrode and far-field capture.[20] Accuracy of pace mapping may also be diminished by preferential conduction, particularly in the region of the RCC, capturing the conduction system. Activation mapping is preferable to pace mapping but may be impractical in cases where the frequency of PVCs/VT is low in the electrophysiology laboratory.

Radiofrequency (RF) energy is the standard used for ablation of aortic cusp VAs. Irrigated ablation catheters are often used for easier energy delivery and reduced risk of coagulum formation. At our institution, ablation within the aortic root is started at 20 Watts with titration up to 40 Watts, goal impedance drop of 10 to 15 Ohms, and duration of 60 to 120 seconds. To prevent collateral injury, ablation should be kept at minimum more than 5 mm away from the coronary ostia.[1,7,17] ICE is valuable in confirming a safe distance away from the coronary arteries and to avoid inadvertent immobilization of aortic valve structures before RF delivery. If ablation within the aortic cusps is ineffective or proximity to the coronary ostia too close, adjacent sites, including the subvalvular LV myocardium, should be mapped. **Fig. 2** illustrates an example of PVC ablation from the RCC–LCC junction.

PULMONARY ARTERY
Anatomic Considerations and Prevalence

Among patients with structurally normally hearts, the prevalence of VAs originating from the main PA has been reported at less than 5%, emphasizing the infrequent nature of supravalvular VAs.[2,3,10,21] The RVOT courses leftward and anterior to the LVOT, with the posterior RVOT subjacent to the LCC and the posterior RV infundibulum overlying the RCC.[11] The region between the RV infundibulum and the pulmonic valve comprises the distal aspect of the RVOT.[11] The pulmonic annulus is cephalad and leftward of the aortic annulus. Analogous to the aortic root, the pulmonary root is composed of the sinuses of Valsalva, semilunar pulmonic leaflets, interleaflet triangles, and the subpulmonic infundibulum. The pulmonic sinuses of Valsalva accommodate the right, left, and anterior cusps and, unlike the aortic cusps, the pulmonic cusps are circumferentially supported by RV infundibular myocardial fibers.

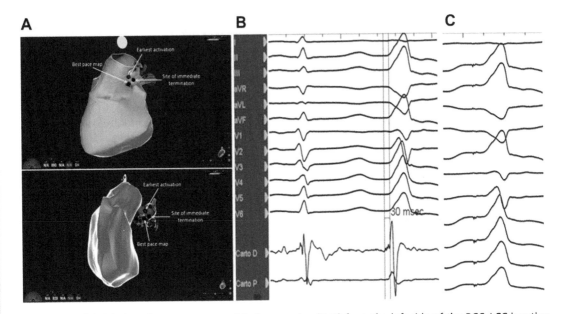

Fig. 2. Successful ablation of a premature ventricular complex (PVC) from the left side of the RCC–LCC junction. (*A*) Three-dimensional anatomic reconstruction of the left ventricle and aortic cusps shown in 2 views with the dark blue dot denoting the site of the best pace map, the pink dot denoting the site of earliest activation, and the maroon dot denoting the site of immediate termination of the PVC with RF delivery. (*B*) Intracardiac electrograms corresponding to the site of earliest bipolar activation (−30 ms). (*C*) Best pace map obtained with pacing from the ablator with 99% PASO match.

The left cusp lies inferiorly to the right and anterior cusps.[22] Beyond the sinotubular junction lies the pulmonary trunk and artery. The left main coronary artery and LCC are situated adjacent to and behind the posterior PA.

RV myocardial extensions past the ventriculoarterial junction and into the PA were noted by Hasdemir and colleagues[10] in 22% of cases. In another study, RV myocardial extensions to the PA were seen in 74% of autopsied hearts extending in either a supracuspal or intercuspal manner and relatively symmetric between the right, left, and anterior cusps. Similar to the aortic cusps, direct myocardial extension into the pulmonic cusps was rare at 1.7% (most frequent in the anterior cusp and never seen to involve the right cusp).[11]

Salient Electrocardiographic Features

Prior studies have elucidated the typical ECG characteristics of RVOT Vas, which comprise an LBBB pattern with an inferior axis, QS morphology in leads AVR and AVL, and precordial transition at lead V3 or later.[23–25] A precordial transition later during the VA relative to sinus rhythm has been shown to be more consistent with an RVOT origin.[16] An incomplete right bundle branch block morphology may also be seen particularly if the VA focus is from a posterior site or if the origin is supravalvular.[26] Relative to endocardial RVOT origin, supravalvular PA VAs are more likely to display a greater AVL/AVR Q wave amplitude ratio and a greater lead V2 R/S ratio. Supravalvular PA VAs will also exhibit a stronger inferior axis with tall R waves (lead III > II), an rS pattern in lead V1, and a QS (rS) pattern in lead I owing to a leftward and more cephalad orientation.[21,25] In the study by Liao and colleagues,[22] lead I frequently exhibited a large R wave amplitude and commonly, more notching, and a longer duration of the R wave was seen in right cusp arrhythmias relative to the other pulmonic cusps. Another more recent investigation also demonstrated VAs arising from the right cusp to demonstrate a significantly greater R wave amplitude in lead I as well as a higher degree of notching in the inferior leads; however, no observations were seen consistently to discriminate left versus anterior cusp origin.[27] It should be noted that these latter 2 studies were limited by unavailability of ICE. Application of these ECG criteria to distinguish endocardial RVOT locations from PA sites of VAs may be affected by individual variability in cardiac rotation and axis within the thorax.

Mapping and Catheter Ablation

Activation and pace mapping may both be used to localize VA origin and is usually accomplished via a transfemoral venous approach. The use of a long deflectable sheath is advisable to facilitate catheter positioning and stability. The catheter may then be deflected into a reverse U curve to map the PA.

PA VAs may be targeted at the SOO in the PA, via the preferential pathway of conduction or site of RV myocardial insertion.[22] It is also possible that RVOT VAs may be the true SOO and ablation from the pulmonic cusps, especially the right cusp, may simply represent another route of ablation. Relative to the RVOT, electrical capture within the PA is more difficult owing to a smaller myocardial mass rendering pace mapping less reliable. Pacing should be performed at threshold and higher levels of output and at a similar cycle length/coupling interval as the clinical VA, because the amount of the myocardial sleeve captured can affect the paced QRS morphology.[28] In supravalvular locations such as the PA, both near-field (representing the myocardial extension) and far-field (representing subvalvular myocardium) bipolar potentials are often recorded. A late near-field potential during sinus rhythm that during VA reverses to become early and precedes the far-field ventricular signal with an intervening isoelectric segment is indicative of the arrhythmia source (sometimes also seen in aortic cusp VAs). Meticulous attention must be paid to mapping as electrical noise can obscure near-field recordings. If, however, any component of the far-field signal is earlier than the near-field signal during both sinus rhythm and VA (even if near-field signal reversal is seen), the recording site is not the actual origin of the VA.

It is probably best to limit both power ($\leq$30 Watts) and the duration of each RF application in the PA to avoid impedance increases and steam pops. The left main coronary artery can course within 2 mm of the PA, as shown in 43% of cases in 1 study.[29] However, coronary arterial injury has not been reported thus far, likely owing to high coronary flow facilitating convective heat loss. PA stenosis has not been reported either, presumably owing to a larger vessel diameter and differences in connective tissue distribution relative to pulmonary veins. If early termination of the VA during ablation does not occur, the LVOT and great cardiac vein/anterior interventricular vein (GCV/AIV) should be explored. **Figs. 3** and **4** illustrate an example of catheter ablation of PVCs from the PA and a suggested mapping approach to outflow tract VAs when the 12-lead ECG is not consistent with a classic RVOT pattern, respectively.

LEFT VENTRICULAR SUMMIT
Anatomic Considerations and Prevalence

Owing to anatomic constraints, one of the most challenging regions to ablate VAs from is the

LVS. The LVS is the superior most aspect of the epicardial LV, lying above the aortic portion of the LVOT, and was first termed by McAlpine.[4] It is approximated as a triangular region bounded by the bifurcation of the left main coronary artery into the left anterior descending (LAD) and left circumflex arteries until the level of the first septal perforator. The junction of the GCV with the AIV further transects this region into a medial and superior region inaccessible to epicardial ablation (owing to overlying epicardial fat and proximity of coronary arteries), and a lateral and inferior accessible region. VAs arising from the LVS may be targeted from the accessible region, the underlying LV endocardium, and LCC and comprise 14.5% of all LV VAs.[30] The AIV generally arises between the middle and lower thirds of the anterior interventricular groove and courses with the LAD, most often to the left of it. LAD septal perforators and septal veins draining into the AIV may provide avenues for mapping and ablation of LVS VAs.

Salient Electrocardiographic Features

VT arising from the LVS is generally characterized by a right bundle branch block pattern and an inferior axis (R waves in lead III > II). However, an LBBB pattern with an inferior axis may also be seen, exhibiting an R/S transition at either lead V2 or V3.[30–32] ECG clues to epicardial origin comprise a maximal deflection index of 0.55 or greater, a pseudodelta wave of 34 ms or greater, an intrinsicoid deflection time of 85 ms or greater, a shortest RS complex of 121 ms or greater,[33] and a QS pattern in lead I,[34] although these intervals may be artificially prolonged by antiarrhythmic drugs such as amiodarone. A pattern break in lead V2 (loss of R wave from lead V1 to V2 followed by recovery of the R wave in V3) is suggestive of a septal LVS origin and is more likely to be successfully targeted from the endocardial LVS.[35] Successful epicardial ablation is predicted when at least 2 of the following morphologic criteria are met: (1) AVL/AVR Q wave ratio of greater than 1.85; (2) V1 R/S ratio of greater than 2; and (3) absence of Q waves in V1.[32] This underscores the importance of anticipating a possible epicardial strategy, associated with its own risks and potential complications.

Mapping and Catheter Ablation

When VA origin from the LVS is suspected, it is helpful to first sample the coronary venous signals to more efficiently direct mapping. We typically use a long deflectable sheath (Agilis or Lamp 90, St. Jude Medical, St Paul, MN) to gain entry into the coronary sinus. A venogram using a balloon-

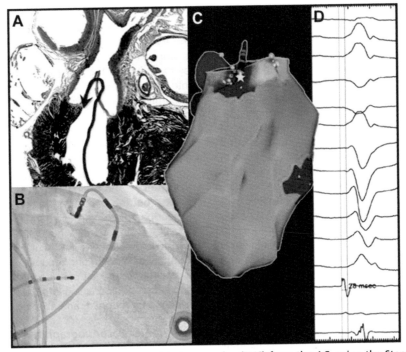

Fig. 3. Successful ablation of a premature ventricular complex (PVC) from the AC, using the Stereotaxis system, with immediate suppression. (*A*) Histology with arrow illustrating myocardium at the pulmonic sinus base. (*B*) Right anterior oblique fluoroscopic view demonstrating the ablation catheter at the site of earliest activation in the AC. (*C*) Three-dimensional anatomic reconstruction of the right ventricle, RVOT, and aortic cusps, with the yellow star denoting the site of earliest activation at the AC. (*D*) Intracardiac electrograms corresponding to the site of earliest bipolar activation (–28 ms). AC = anterior cusp. (*From* Anderson et al. The anatomic substrates for outflow tract arrhythmias. Heart Rhythm. 2019;16(2):290–97; with permission.)

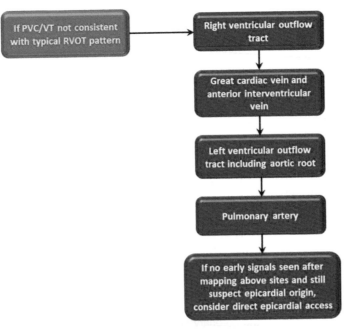

Fig. 4. Suggested order of mapping in the circumstance where the clinical VA is not consistent with a classical RVOT ECG pattern.

tipped catheter is performed to delineate the GCV, AIV, and septal perforators. If a branch of sufficient caliber is identified, a small catheter (eg, a 3F Map-It, Access Point Technologies, Rogers, MN) or a coated wire (Visionwire, Biotronik, Berlin, Germany) may be advanced and connected in a unipolar configuration to obtain activation and pace mapping data from the intramural septal LV. Pace mapping is preferably performed at threshold output to minimize the virtual electrode. A good pace map (>95% match) is frequently attainable from the GCV/AIV. We often use a long SL1 or SL0 sheath to optimize catheter stability and minimize flinging out of the subvalvular LVOT when mapping near the LVS. If the earliest activation (should be >20 ms presystolic) is seen in the distal GCV/proximal AIV, an epicardial origin is implied, and if the septal venous perforator demonstrates earliest activation, an intramural septal focus is suggested. **Fig. 5** illustrates a case of a successful endocardial LVS PVC ablation. Frequently, ablation from the AIV is precluded by proximity of the LAD. This consequently requires reinterrogation of the LVOT endocardium directly opposite to the earliest GCV/AIV site (marked by the mapping wire/catheter), LCC, and the septal and most leftward aspect of the RVOT as seen on left anterior oblique projection and ICE. We have reported 2 cases of successful ablation from the RVOT and distance from the AIV may be as near as within 10 mm.[36] Moreover, there is

even an anecdotal report of successful ablation from the left atrial appendage tip, which often lies near the leftmost RVOT.[37]

Because coronary veins are low-resistance conduits, the use of irrigated ablation catheters are necessary to achieve sufficient power delivery (20–40 Watts). Obstacles to ablation include high temperature or impedance increases, limiting power delivery, propinquity to coronary arteries, or venous branches of insufficient caliber to accommodate the ablation catheter. In such cases, ablation performed from structures in anatomic juxtaposition even if activation and pace mapping is slightly worse than the GCV/AIV may prove efficacious in over half of cases.[31] Sometimes, RF applications of 3 or more minutes and titration of power to 40 Watts are needed to penetrate transmurally. When only minimally early and/or far-field signals (gradual dV/dt) are seen, an intramural focus is implied (thus, higher pacing output is often needed to obtain an adequate pace map) and may need to be surrounded with lesions from multiple endocardial structures in apposition. Alternate percutaneous strategies include sequential (limited when endocardial and epicardial sites >8 mm apart) and simultaneous unipolar RF ablation, bipolar ablation (limited when impedance mismatch present between both electrodes), use of half-normal saline irrigant, and retrograde alcohol ablation.[38–41] A technique of using a system normally used to treat chronic total occlusions

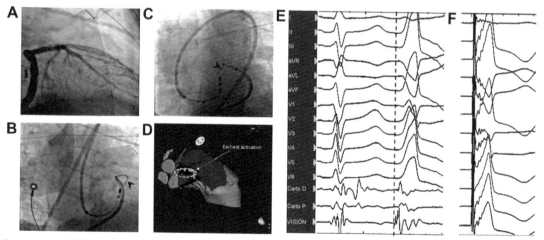

Fig. 5. Successful ablation of a LVS premature ventricular complex (PVC) from the basal LV endocardium. (*A*) Initial coronary sinus venogram. (*B, C*) Position of catheters in right anterior oblique and left anterior oblique fluoroscopic views, respectively. A unipolar wire (*arrowhead*) was advanced into a septal venous perforator and the ablation catheter was positioned at the LV endocardium, opposite to the site of earliest activation, where RF delivery eliminated the PVC. (*D*) Three-dimensional anatomic reconstruction of the left ventricle and aortic cusps showing the site of earliest activation along with the lesion set. (*E*) Electrograms recorded from the unipolar wire (−30 ms pre-PVC and earlier than GCV/AIV and endocardial sites, implying an intramural origin) and the ablation catheter. (*F*) Best pace map obtained by pacing from the unipolar wire.

of the coronary artery to achieve targeted ablation to the midmyocardium has also been described.[42] Intramyocardial needle catheter ablation has been performed to treat refractory VAs,[43] but efficacy in abolishing LVS VAs is not certain. Complications include significant myocardial injury, complete heart block, coronary venous dissection, cardiac tamponade, coronary artery thrombosis, aortic valve injury, and embolic events.

If elimination of the VA is unsuccessful or unfeasible from the coronary venous system or endocardial routes, a direct percutaneous epicardial approach may be tried, particularly if origin is suspected from the accessible region, despite poorer outcomes. The phrenic nerve must be carefully delineated via high output pacing (20 mA at maximal pulse width). Coronary angiography, notably in the left anterior oblique caudal view, best defines the coronary artery anatomy, which precludes ablation two-thirds of the time.[32] Last, if all percutaneous routes of LVS ablation fail, a surgical approach may be considered, although this may be associated with risk of late coronary artery stenosis.[44,45]

SUMMARY

The abolition of VAs from the aortic cusps, PA, and LVS still poses challenges despite advances in technology and our understanding of their complex anatomy. Notably, deep intramural foci within the LVS are among the most difficult areas to successfully ablate, owing to the myocardial thickness and proximity to multiple delicate structures. Especially when the ECG is not consistent with a classic RVOT origin, a systematic approach to mapping should be undertaken. As newer techniques make their way down the pipeline, the success and outcomes of percutaneous catheter ablation of VAs at challenging sites will continue to improve and in more patients, obviating the need for surgical ablation.

REFERENCES

1. Ouyang F, Fotuhi P, Ho SY, et al. Repetitive monomorphic ventricular tachycardia originating from the aortic sinus cusp: electrocardiographic characterization for guiding catheter ablation. J Am Coll Cardiol 2002;39(3):500–8.
2. Lerman BB, Stein KM, Markowitz SM. Idiopathic right ventricular outflow tract tachycardia: a clinical approach. Pacing Clin Electrophysiol 1996;19(12 Pt 1):2120–37.
3. Tada H, Tadokoro K, Miyaji K, et al. Idiopathic ventricular arrhythmias arising from the pulmonary artery: prevalence, characteristics, and topography of the arrhythmia origin. Heart Rhythm 2008;5(3):419–26.
4. McAlpine WA. Heart and coronary arteries. New York: Springer-Verlag; 1975.
5. Yamada T, Litovsky SH, Kay GN. The left ventricular ostium: an anatomic concept relevant to idiopathic ventricular arrhythmias. Circ Arrhythm Electrophysiol 2008;1(5):396–404.
6. Kanagaratnam L, Tomassoni G, Schweikert R, et al. Ventricular tachycardias arising from the aortic sinus of Valsalva: an under-recognized variant of left outflow tract ventricular tachycardia. J Am Coll Cardiol 2001;37(5):1408–14.
7. Hachiya H, Aonuma K, Yamauchi Y, et al. How to diagnose, locate, and ablate coronary cusp ventricular tachycardia. J Cardiovasc Electrophysiol 2002;13(6):551–6.
8. Yamada T, McElderry HT, Doppalapudi H, et al. Idiopathic ventricular arrhythmias originating from the aortic root prevalence, electrocardiographic and electrophysiologic characteristics, and results of radiofrequency catheter ablation. J Am Coll Cardiol 2008;52(2):139–47.
9. Tanaka Y, Tada H, Ito S, et al. Gender and age differences in candidates for radiofrequency catheter ablation of idiopathic ventricular arrhythmias. Circ J 2011;75(7):1585–91.
10. Hasdemir C, Aktas S, Govsa F, et al. Demonstration of ventricular myocardial extensions into the pulmonary artery and aorta beyond the ventriculo-arterial junction. Pacing Clin Electrophysiol 2007;30(4):534–9.
11. Gami AS, Noheria A, Lachman N, et al. Anatomical correlates relevant to ablation above the semilunar valves for the cardiac electrophysiologist: a study of 603 hearts. J Interv Card Electrophysiol 2011;30(1):5–15.
12. Yamada T, Lau YR, Litovsky SH, et al. Prevalence and clinical, electrocardiographic, and electrophysiologic characteristics of ventricular arrhythmias originating from the noncoronary sinus of Valsalva. Heart Rhythm 2013;10(11):1605–12.
13. Lin D, Ilkhanoff L, Gerstenfeld E, et al. Twelve-lead electrocardiographic characteristics of the aortic cusp region guided by intracardiac echocardiography and electroanatomic mapping. Heart Rhythm 2008;5(5):663–9.
14. Bala R, Garcia FC, Hutchinson MD, et al. Electrocardiographic and electrophysiologic features of ventricular arrhythmias originating from the right/left coronary cusp commissure. Heart Rhythm 2010;7(3):312–22.
15. Yamada T, Yoshida N, Murakami Y, et al. Electrocardiographic characteristics of ventricular arrhythmias originating from the junction of the left and right coronary sinuses of Valsalva in the aorta: the activation pattern as a rationale for the electrocardiographic characteristics. Heart Rhythm 2008;5(2):184–92.

16. Betensky BP, Park RE, Marchlinski FE, et al. The V(2) transition ratio: a new electrocardiographic criterion for distinguishing left from right ventricular outflow tract tachycardia origin. J Am Coll Cardiol 2011; 57(22):2255–62.

17. Callans DJ. Catheter ablation of idiopathic ventricular tachycardia arising from the aortic root. J Cardiovasc Electrophysiol 2009;20(8):969–72.

18. Kamioka M, Mathew S, Lin T, et al. Electrophysiological and electrocardiographic predictors of ventricular arrhythmias originating from the left ventricular outflow tract within and below the coronary sinus cusps. Clin Res Cardiol 2015;104(7):544–54.

19. Yamada T, Murakami Y, Yoshida N, et al. Preferential conduction across the ventricular outflow septum in ventricular arrhythmias originating from the aortic sinus cusp. J Am Coll Cardiol 2007;50(9):884–91.

20. Fedida J, Strisciuglio T, Sohal M, et al. Efficacy of advanced pace-mapping technology for idiopathic premature ventricular complexes ablation. J Interv Card Electrophysiol 2018;51(3):271–7.

21. Sekiguchi Y, Aonuma K, Takahashi A, et al. Electrocardiographic and electrophysiologic characteristics of ventricular tachycardia originating within the pulmonary artery. J Am Coll Cardiol 2005;45(6): 887–95.

22. Liao Z, Zhan X, Wu S, et al. Idiopathic ventricular arrhythmias originating from the pulmonary sinus cusp: prevalence, electrocardiographic/electrophysiological characteristics, and catheter ablation. J Am Coll Cardiol 2015;66(23):2633–44.

23. Dixit S, Gerstenfeld EP, Callans DJ, et al. Electrocardiographic patterns of superior right ventricular outflow tract tachycardias: distinguishing septal and free-wall sites of origin. J Cardiovasc Electrophysiol 2003;14(1):1–7.

24. Lee SH, Tai CT, Chiang CE, et al. Determinants of successful ablation of idiopathic ventricular tachycardias with left bundle branch block morphology from the right ventricular outflow tract. Pacing Clin Electrophysiol 2002;25(9):1346–51.

25. Asirvatham SJ. Correlative anatomy for the invasive electrophysiologist: outflow tract and supravalvar arrhythmia. J Cardiovasc Electrophysiol 2009; 20(8):955–68.

26. Suleiman M, Asirvatham SJ. Ablation above the semilunar valves: when, why, and how? Part I. Heart Rhythm 2008;5(10):1485–92.

27. Zhang J, Tang C, Zhang Y, et al. Pulmonary sinus cusp mapping and ablation: a new concept and approach for idiopathic right ventricular outflow tract arrhythmias. Heart Rhythm 2018;15(1):38–45.

28. Srivathsan KS, Bunch TJ, Asirvatham SJ, et al. Mechanisms and utility of discrete great arterial potentials in the ablation of outflow tract ventricular arrhythmias. Circ Arrhythm Electrophysiol 2008;1(1): 30–8.

29. Walsh KA, Fahy GJ. Anatomy of the left main coronary artery of particular relevance to ablation of left atrial and outflow tract arrhythmias. Heart Rhythm 2014;11(12):2231–8.

30. Yamada T, McElderry HT, Doppalapudi H, et al. Idiopathic ventricular arrhythmias originating from the left ventricular summit: anatomic concepts relevant to ablation. Circ Arrhythm Electrophysiol 2010;3(6): 616–23.

31. Jauregui Abularach ME, Campos B, Park KM, et al. Ablation of ventricular arrhythmias arising near the anterior epicardial veins from the left sinus of Valsalva region: ECG features, anatomic distance, and outcome. Heart Rhythm 2012;9(6):865–73.

32. Santangeli P, Marchlinski FE, Zado ES, et al. Percutaneous epicardial ablation of ventricular arrhythmias arising from the left ventricular summit: outcomes and electrocardiogram correlates of success. Circ Arrhythm Electrophysiol 2015;8(2): 337–43.

33. Berruezo A, Mont L, Nava S, et al. Electrocardiographic recognition of the epicardial origin of ventricular tachycardias. Circulation 2004;109(15): 1842–7.

34. Bazan V, Gerstenfeld EP, Garcia FC, et al. Site-specific twelve-lead ECG features to identify an epicardial origin for left ventricular tachycardia in the absence of myocardial infarction. Heart Rhythm 2007;4(11):1403–10.

35. Hayashi T, Santangeli P, Pathak RK, et al. Outcomes of catheter ablation of idiopathic outflow tract ventricular arrhythmias with an R wave pattern break in lead V2: a distinct clinical entity. J Cardiovasc Electrophysiol 2017;28(5):504–14.

36. Frankel DS, Mountantonakis SE, Dahu MI, et al. Elimination of ventricular arrhythmias originating from the GCV with ablation in the right ventricular outflow tract. Circ Arrhythm Electrophysiol 2014;7(5):984–5.

37. Benhayon D, Cogan J, Young M. Left atrial appendage as a vantage point for mapping and ablating premature ventricular contractions originating in the epicardial left ventricular summit. Clin Case Rep 2018;6(6):1124–7.

38. Teh AW, Reddy VY, Koruth JS, et al. Bipolar radiofrequency catheter ablation for refractory ventricular outflow tract arrhythmias. J Cardiovasc Electrophysiol 2014;25(10):1093–9.

39. Yamada T, Maddox WR, McElderry HT, et al. Radiofrequency catheter ablation of idiopathic ventricular arrhythmias originating from intramural foci in the left ventricular outflow tract: efficacy of sequential versus simultaneous unipolar catheter ablation. Circ Arrhythm Electrophysiol 2015;8(2):344–52.

40. Sandhu A, Schuller JL, Tzou WS, et al. Use of half-normal saline irrigant with cooled radiofrequency ablation within the great cardiac vein to ablate premature ventricular contractions arising from the left

ventricular summit. Pacing Clin Electrophysiol 2019; 42(3):301–5.

41. Kreidieh B, Rodriguez-Manero M, Schurmann P, et al. Retrograde coronary venous ethanol infusion for ablation of refractory ventricular tachycardia. Circ Arrhythm Electrophysiol 2016;9(7). https://doi.org/10.1161/CIRCEP.116.004352.

42. Romero J, Diaz JC, Hayase J, et al. Intramyocardial radiofrequency ablation of ventricular arrhythmias using intracoronary wire mapping and a coronary reentry system: description of a novel technique. HeartRhythm Case Rep 2018;4(7):285–92.

43. Sapp JL, Beeckler C, Pike R, et al. Initial human feasibility of infusion needle catheter ablation for refractory ventricular tachycardia. Circulation 2013; 128(21):2289–95.

44. Choi EK, Nagashima K, Lin KY, et al. Surgical cryoablation for ventricular tachyarrhythmia arising from the left ventricular outflow tract region. Heart Rhythm 2015;12(6):1128–36.

45. Aziz Z, Moss JD, Jabbarzadeh M, et al. Totally endoscopic robotic epicardial ablation of refractory left ventricular summit arrhythmia: first-in-man. Heart Rhythm 2017;14(1):135–8.

Mapping and Ablation of Unmappable Ventricular Tachycardia, Ventricular Tachycardia Storm, and Those in Acute Myocardial Infarction

Josef Kautzner, MD, PhD*, Petr Peichl, MD, PhD

KEYWORDS

- Ventricular tachycardia • Ventricular fibrillation • Arrhythmia substrate • Electroanatomic mapping
- Cardiac imaging • Mechanical circulatory support • Catheter ablation

KEY POINTS

- Mapping of arrhythmogenic substrate supported by cardiovascular imaging is the most used strategy for catheter ablation of unmappable ventricular tachycardias.
- The value of percutaneous mechanical circulatory support to enable mapping during unmappable ventricular tachycardias remains unanswered, because it does not seem to improve outcome.
- Catheter ablation in an electrical storm has been shown effective in abolishing the storm and improving the prognosis of certain subsets of patients.
- Focally triggered ventricular fibrillation in the subacute phase of myocardial infarction is amenable to catheter ablation, which can be considered as a life-saving procedure.

INTRODUCTION

Conventional mapping techniques in scar-related ventricular tachycardia (VT) include activation sequence mapping, pace mapping, and entrainment mapping, all now supported by a three-dimensional (3-D) electroanatomic mapping.[1,2] In stable VT, activation mapping and entrainment mapping are the most important strategies to determine the reentrant circuit and its critical components. In many patients, however, VT is either noninducible or hemodynamically unstable and, thus, unmappable.

In recent years, several technological advances have broadened significantly ablation options in unmappable VTs. In principle, new approaches focus on better identification of scar tissue or fibrosis on one side and conduction abnormalities on the other. Such detailed description of the arrhythmogenic substrate allows substantial modification in sinus rhythm or during device pacing without hemodynamic compromise to the patient. In some cases, however, the substrate is not well defined by mapping in sinus rhythm. In those cases, hemodynamic support may allow mapping during ongoing VT and entrainment

Relationship with Industry: Dr J. Kautzner has received speaker honoraria from Boehringer Ingelheim, Biosense Webster, Biotronik, Boston Scientific, Daiichi Sankyo, EPIX, Medtronic, Merck Sharp & Dohme, Pfizer, and St. Jude Medical;, and has served as a consultant for Bayer, Boehringer Ingelheim, Biosense Webster, Boston Scientific, EPIX, Medtronic, MicroPort, and St. Jude Medical (Abbott). Dr P. Peichl has received speaker honoraria from St Jude Medical (Abbott) and has served as a consultant for Biotronik and Boston Scientific.
Department of Cardiology, Institute for Clinical and Experimental Medicine (IKEM), Videnska 1958/9, Prague 14021, Czech Republic
* Corresponding author.
E-mail address: josef.kautzner@ikem.cz

cardiacEP.theclinics.com

mapping. All these approaches could be particularly useful in subjects with an electrical storm (ES).

Acute myocardial infarction is a different category, because ischemia may trigger ventricular fibrillation (VF) in the acute phase regardless of any substrate. In a subacute phase, however, polymorphic VT or ventricular fibrillation (VF) may be triggered by ectopic activity, usually from surviving conduction system of the left ventricle. In such a scenario, the focal ablation of a trigger may be a life-saving procedure.

This article describes novel options for catheter ablation of unmappable VTs and VTs in an ES and acute myocardial infarction more in detail.

HOW TO APPROACH UNMAPPABLE VENTRICULAR TACHYCARDIAS

Two strategies have been developed in recent years. Substrate identification in sinus rhythm and/or during short mapping in VT and its modification can be considered standard of care today. The alternative approach comprises mapping during VT with hemodynamic support—a strategy that is still investigational.

Substrate Identification and Modification

The advent of the electroanatomic mapping system allowed for the first time identifying scar as an area of low voltage.[3] New developments in substrate identification include imaging and the use of novel mapping tools. Some of these approaches are discussed briefly.

Preprocedural imaging

Preprocedural imaging of the myocardial substrate becomes more and more important in planning the ablation procedure, especially in nonischemic cardiomyopathies. Several imaging techniques could be used and provide important anatomic information, often supplemented by an assessment of myocardial function. These include echocardiography, nuclear imaging, computed tomography (CT), and/or magnetic resonance imaging (MRI). MRI, in particular, allows the most detailed description of the location and architecture of the myocardial scar and/or fibrosis.[4–6] Some researchers even suggest that MRI could be used to display individual channels of slow conduction within the scar tissue.[7] Although this might be a too ambitious expectation, the arrangement of the scar tissue may provide important information about the most arrhythmogenic region of the substrate[8] (**Fig. 1**). Other groups proposed the use of CT angiography with segmentation of left ventricular wall thinning and subsequent image integration with 3-D electroanatomic mapping system for guiding the ablation procedure.[9–12] In addition, CT may recognize fatty tissue in arrhythmogenic right ventricular cardiomyopathy.[13] Therefore, CT may be used alternatively prior to ablation in subjects who have a contraindication to MRI or who are claustrophobic. Finally, some groups used image-based simulation to estimate potential ablation targets of scar-related VT.[14] This method focuses on identification of the heterogeneous zone within the scar, which is interspersed with normal myocardium and forms the substrate for slowly conducting tissue as a prerequisite for reentry.

Intraprocedural imaging

Despite the potential promise of intraprocedural MRI for the guidance of catheter ablation, the use of this strategy is far from being established for daily routine.[15] On the other hand, intracardiac echocardiography (ICE) has been available for many years for intraprocedural imaging and guidance. It provides real-time information about cardiac anatomy and allows assessment of catheter location and catheter-tissue contact and monitoring of energy delivery to minimize the risk of pop formation and/or potential complications. It enables near-zero or zero fluoroscopy, especially together with the use of 3-D electroanatomic mapping system. The most sophisticated modality links directly ICE with electroanatomic mapping system CARTO (CARTOSOUND, Biosense Webster, Irvine, CA, USA) and through the magnetic sensor in the ICE catheter allows registration of structures visible on ICE directly in CARTO system (**Fig. 2**).

For VT ablation, ICE has been demonstrated to be useful to guide ablation on the papillary muscles, within the aortic cusps, and/or around the old thrombus.[16] It allows imaging of the scar tissue, its extent, and location (endocardial, midmyocardial, or epicardial). Some studies attempted to demonstrate the correlation between akinetic and thinned areas on ICE and scar defined by electroanatomic mapping.[17,18] Similarly, regions of increased echogenicity corresponded to electroanatomically described substrate.[19] The authors' experience confirms these observations, and location of the substrate on ICE corresponds to its electrophysiologic characteristics (**Fig. 3**). It is difficult, however, to quantify the extent and location of scar tissue from ICE images and evaluate reproducibility. First, the quality of images depends not only on the operator but also on individual anatomy of the heart and its arrangement within the chest. Second, the two-dimensional nature of the image prevents easily assessing 3-D characteristics of the scar tissue.

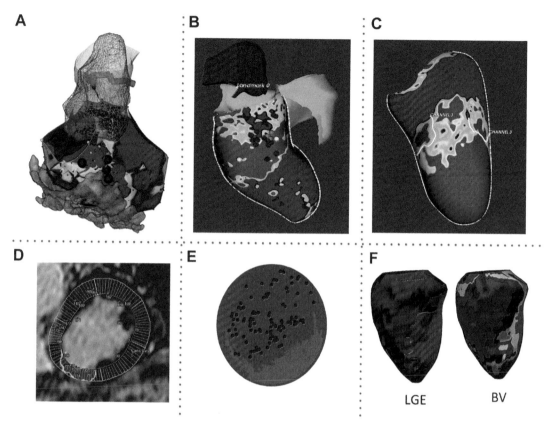

Fig. 1. Various examples of image integration of MRI with electroanatomic mapping. (*A*) Real-time integration of late gadolinium enhancement (LGE)-MRI with CARTO map. A 3-D mesh of MRI-derived scar (*yellow-brown color*) merged with the CARTO map. More extensive MRI-derived (midwall) scar compared with low-voltage area detected by endocardial mapping can be appreciated. (*B*) Layer-based processing of LGE-MRI integrated with projected CARTO points of interest. The figure shows VT-related sites located at the border of dense and heterogeneous scar. (*C*) Visualization of channels of heterogeneous scar within dense scar detected by layer-based processing of LGE-MRI. These areas may contain VT-related sites. (*D*) CARTO points projected onto a short-axis LGE-MRI slice. Radial chords are used to pair the CARTO points with underlying image characteristics (such as scar transmurality or wall thickness). (*E*) CARTO points projected on a bull's-eye plot representation of LGE-MRI of the left ventricle to appreciate spatial distribution of and density of the CARTO points. (*F*) LGE-MRI derived scar projected onto the same LV shell as a CARTO map can be used to directly compare extent of scar defined by various voltage cutoffs with MRI-derived scar. BV, bipolar voltage. (*Courtesy* of MUDr. Marek Sramko, Ph.D., FESC, Prague, Czech Republic).

Conventional Substrate Mapping

There are many well-established techniques for substrate mapping. The initial description was based on the identification of low-voltage areas using arbitrary voltage value derived from experimental work and from the mapping of a small series of patients and controls.[3,20] For endocardial mapping, areas with a bipolar voltage greater than 1.5 mV are considered to be normal, whereas regions with bipolar voltage less than 0.5 mV are areas of a dense scar. Ablation across the border zones allowed the abolition of VT in a majority of cases. Later, adjustments of voltage to identify channels of relatively preserved myocardium within low-voltage scar

were suggested.[21] Such channels have been shown to be poorly specific, however, when no characteristic local electrograms were observed.[22] In addition, correlation studies with MRI and voltage mapping in postinfarction substrates revealed that unless the scar involves at least 75% of the wall, the bipolar voltage could be higher than commonly used 1.5-mV limit.[23] Not surprisingly, many complementary strategies of voltage mapping were advocated in order to identify more precisely the myocardial substrate. One of them relies on recording late potentials and their subsequent elimination.[24,25] Another strategy focuses on the assessment of local abnormal ventricular activities. Ablation aimed at the elimination of all local abnormal

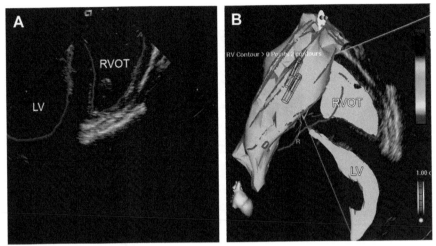

Fig. 2. An example of endocardial mapping with the CARTOSound Module that enables integration of ICE in the electroanatomic mapping system. (*A*) shows delineation of the endocardial contours (*green lines*). These are then used for 3-D reconstruction of cardiac chambers before entering them by the mapping catheter (*B*). LV, left ventricle; RVOT, right ventricular outflow tract.

ventricular activities has shown fewer VT recurrences and improved outcomes.[26,27] Pacing at 10 mV within the low-voltage regions to delineate islands of noncapture and channels of slow conduction in-between also can be used.[28] Different approach is to use pace mapping complemented with software that matches on-line QRS morphology during VT with paced morphology, demonstrating that critical isthmus of slow conduction can be identified as the site with the perfect match adjacent to the site with worst one.[29] Alternatively, a simplified approach has been advocated, modifying extensively all low-voltage areas by ablation lesions.[30,31] Even such a simplified strategy was associated with decreased VT recurrence and fewer hospitalizations.

Ultra–High-density Mapping

Advances in mapping systems in the past decade have allowed rapid creation of very high-density and high-resolution maps using multiple electrograms recorded by the multielectrode catheters and automatic annotation the voltage and timing from each electrode that is in the contact with the tissue. The obtained maps contain several thousands of points[25,32,33] and may display more late potentials. Small interelectrode distances also have potential to identify abnormal electrograms within presumably normal voltage areas.[34,35] Such a mapping strategy is considered more specific for the evaluation of substrate and yields usually a smaller area of the scar compared with conventional ablation catheter.[36]

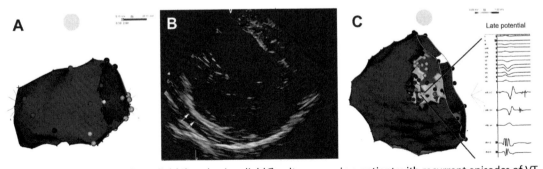

Fig. 3. The figure shows endocardial (*A*) and epicardial (*C*) voltage map in a patient with recurrent episodes of VT (posterior view). Although the endocardial voltage map showed normal electrograms, ICE revealed an area of high echogenicity on the epicardium of the left lateral wall and midmyocardially (*arrows* [*B*]). Subsequently, the patient underwent epicardial mapping and low voltage, fragmented and delayed electrograms were located in that region (late potentials). Ablation across the area resulted in noninducibility of VTs and prevented further arrhythmia episodes.

Multielectrode catheters also may offer a better characterization of reentrant circuits during VT when used with mapping systems to provide rapid automated interpretation.[37,38] Examples include Intellimap Orion (Rhythmia, Boston Scientific, Marlborough, MA, USA), PentaRay Nav (CARTO 3, Biosense Webster, Irvine, CA, USA) and Advisor HD GRID (EnSite Precision, Abbott, Santa Clara, CA, USA). Some published cases definitely expanded knowledge of VT circuits and their functional components. On the other hand, data are still lacking on how this strategy improves ablation outcomes. In addition, not all investigators share the enthusiasm for the use of high-density mapping for many other reasons. First, it increases the complexity of the procedure and prudent manipulation is necessary. There have been some cases of entanglement of the catheter in the chordae tendineae. Second, the mapping catheter may induce ectopy and this could make mapping during ongoing VT difficult because ectopy often terminates the arrhythmia. Third, using ICE to navigate during mapping, the authors could observe repeatedly difficulties with mapping the entire endocardial surface with these catheters (**Fig. 4**). Fourth, the interpretation of the circuit is often not trivial and often visual without standardization. The authors tend to use the multipolar mapping catheter positioned in the critical part of the substrate, mainly to help to see disappearance of the pathologic electrograms during ablation (**Fig. 5**).

Mapping of Omnipolar Electrograms

Because bipolar (and unipolar) electrogram amplitudes are significantly influenced by the direction of the activation wave front, the orientation of the catheter to the tissue, and interelectrode distance, new mapping strategies are being explored. In an attempt to improve the specificity and reproducibility of bipolar voltage mapping, the use of omnipolar electrograms has been introduced.[39] Using an array of small electrodes with known distances, an electrode orientation-independent mapping can determine the net direction of the wave fronts beat to beat. As a result, bipolar voltage amplitude can be obtained that is independent of orientation, collision, and fractionation influence. Omnipolar voltages may provide more physiologically relevant substrate characterization and, thus, result in more efficacious catheter ablation of VT.[40,41] Further clinical validation of this technology is ongoing, with continuing development and refinement of specialized multipolar grid catheters and integrated software.

Decrement-evoked Potentials Mapping

In an attempt to evaluate a more precisely functional component of the substrate in structural heart disease, a technique evaluating the so-called decrement-evoked potentials (DEEP) has been introduced.[42] These are progressively delayed abnormal potentials due to decremental conduction in a response to extra stimulus pacing. Their use is based on a hypothesis that areas of decremental conduction would precede unidirectional block and thus create the necessary slow conduction for reentry of ventricular tachycardia. Therefore, the strategy attempts to prioritize local electrograms during sinus, which are more likely to participate in ventricular tachycardia without VT induction. Pilot studies suggest that DEEP

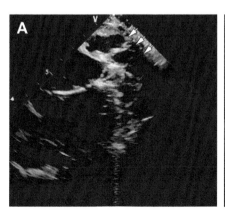
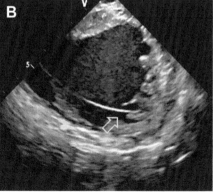

Fig. 4. (*A*) ICE imaging demonstrating limitations of endocardial mapping of the left ventricle with a mini-basket mapping catheter in a patient with ischemic cardiomyopathy and exaggerated trabeculation. Many areas of the endocardial surface cannot be mapped with the catheter (*arrows*). (*B*) ICE image of another patient with more pronounced trabecularization showing the advantage of mapping with conventional tip catheter under visual navigation ([*arrow*] catheter entering one of the fissures between trabeculae). ([A] *Courtesy of* Boston Scientific, Inc., Marlborough, MA.)

A

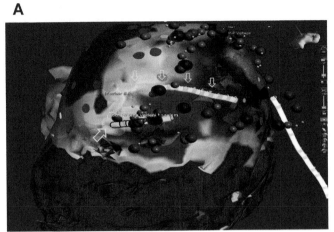

B

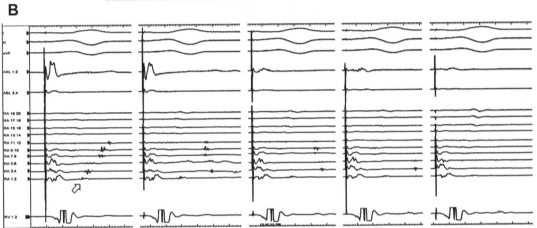

Fig. 5. (*A*) Electroanatomic voltage map of the left ventricle (tilted left oblique view) in a patient after anterior myocardial infarction, showing a large area of low voltage (*yellow and red colors*) and/or dense scar (*gray color*). Multipolar mapping catheter is placed across the center of the aneurysm (*small arrows*) to record abnormal potentials and their disappearance during catheter ablation around the scar (*brown points*). (*B*) Corresponding intracardiac electrograms from the ablation catheter (ABL 1.2 and ABL 3.4), multipolar mapping catheter (RA 1.2–19.20) and quadripolar catheter in the right ventricular apex (RV 1.2). Arrow depicts late potentials which are almost invisible in the ablation catheter and their gradual disappearance during ongoing ablation. ([A] *Courtesy of* Abbott, Inc., Abbott Park, IL.)

mapping could be more specific than late potential mapping in identifying areas critical for VT reentry. In addition, DEEP seem to correlate better with the location of diastolic channels or even critical isthmuses during VT than late potentials. It is encouraging that these data obtained in an operation theater seem replicated in the electrophysiology laboratory with electroanatomic mapping system.[43] In the multicenter study with 20 patients, DEEP substrate mapping identified the functional substrate critical for VTs with high specificity compared with late potentials. The most important question remains whether this rather time-consuming strategy requiring repeated programmed stimulation would increase procedural efficiency and efficacy.

Ripple Mapping

Software for ripple mapping enables to display both voltage and activation on the same electroanatomic map, where each local electrogram potential is shown in a dynamic bar on the map surface.[44] Each such bar projects outward in a proportion to the voltage amplitude at the time point at the current position, over the entirety of the electrogram's duration. The activation wave front appears as propagating waves of bars. This helps to identify areas of delayed local activation and display diastolic pathways and channels within the scar area. A recent feasibility study limited scar ablation within conduction channels resulted in 70% of patients being free of ventricular tachycardia recurrence at 6 months.[45] Promising data were obtained also in subjects with arrhythmogenic right ventricular cardiomyopathy and complete elimination of channels identified by ripple mapping was associated with freedom from VT.[46]

Epicardial Mapping

Because some substrates are localized predominantly epicardial or intramural, epicardial mapping has become an important strategy, especially in subjects with nonischemic cardiomyopathies and/or with Chagas disease.[47] Pericardial access for epicardial mapping of a substrate in Chagas disease was described by Sosa and colleagues[48] in 1996 and today it is an indispensable strategy in expert centers. In a recent multicenter study, the overall prevalence of epicardial circuits in patients referred for VT ablation was 13% (121 of 913 procedures).[49] Principles of analysis of the epicardial substrate are analogical to endocardial mapping.

More recently, epicardial mapping and ablation were described in patients with Brugada syndrome. In a seminal article, Nademanee and colleagues[50] reported on the epicardial mapping of the right ventricular outflow tract in 9 pts with type 1 Brugada electrocardiogram (ECG) pattern and previous history of cardiac arrest. Programmed electric stimulation induced VT/VF in all patients. Abnormal low-voltage areas with prolonged duration and delayed fragmented potentials around the anterior aspect of the right ventricular outflow tract epicardium were found in all subjects. Ablation targeted at the abnormal arrhythmogenic substrate in this location successfully abolished further arrhythmic episodes in all but 1 patient during a follow-up period of 20 months $\pm$ 6 months. The most interesting observation was that catheter ablation resulted in normalization of the Brugada ECG pattern (all had type 1 pattern preablation).

More recently, Pappone and colleagues[51] have introduced the concept of the dynamic substrate based on prospective evaluation in 191 consecutive patients with Brugada syndrome (103 had no documented VTs). At baseline, 53.4% of patients were inducible. Mapping of abnormal signals with manual determination of total signal duration was performed and color-coded maps were constructed showing regions of abnormal potentials: (1) a wide duration (>110 ms) with fragmented component (>3 distinct peaks); (2) late component of low-voltage amplitude ranging from 0.05 mV to 1.5 mV; (3) distinct and delayed component exceeding the end of the QRS complex; or (4) discrete double activity. A substrate size of 4 cm^2 best identified patients with inducible arrhythmias. Ajmaline increased inducibility rate in asymptomatic patients and ajmaline-induced type 1 ECG pattern was accompanied by a new appearance of abnormal potentials in the area of the right ventricular outflow tract (**Fig. 6**). Again, catheter ablation resulted in the abolition of these abnormal potentials and to normalization of the ECG pattern. Recently, Antzelevitch and colleagues[52] suggested how epicardial ablation exerts its ameliorative effect in the setting of Brugada syndrome by destroying the cells with the most prominent action potential notch, thus eliminating sites of abnormal repolarization and the substrate for VT or VF.

A

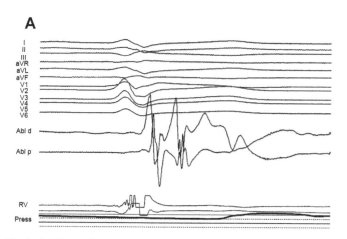

B

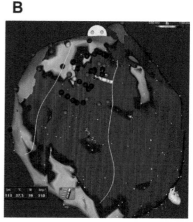

Fig. 6. (*A*) Shows fragmented late intracardiac electrograms (Abl d and Abl p) recorded on the epicardial surface of the right ventricular outflow tract in a patient with Brugada syndrome after administration of ajmaline. (*B*) Depicts the electroanatomic epicardial voltage map (anterior view) projected on endocardial contours of the right ventricle (*white lines*). Pink tags depict the area of fragmented potentials, dark red tags show ablation lesions. It is apparent that most of the epicardial surface shows practically normal voltage (*purple color*).

Mapping of Unmappable Ventricular Tachycardias With a Percutaneous Mechanical Circulatory Support

Technological advances in the field of mechanical circulatory support (MCS) enabled mapping during hemodynamically unstable VTs to identify the critical isthmus of the VT. The most common devices in this category include[53] (1) the percutaneous ventricular assist device (LVAD) (TandemHeart, Cardiac Assist, Pittsburgh, Pennsylvania), (2) the Impella microcirculatory axial blood flow pump (Abiomed, Danvers, Massachusetts), (3) venoarterial extracorporeal membrane oxygenation (ECMO), and (4) the intra-aortic balloon pump. There are inherent differences among them in the magnitude of hemodynamic support these systems provide.[54]

The first clinical series of mapping and ablation of hemodynamically unstable VTs with the use of hemodynamic support was published by Miller and colleagues.[55] A total of 10 VT mapping and ablation procedures were performed with the support of the Impella 2.5 MCS, and 13 procedures were performed either with an intra-aortic balloon pump (6 procedures) or with no device support (7 procedures). Although they showed that VTs can be mapped more successfully on MCS and more frequently terminated by ablation, no difference in number of inducible VTs at the end of the procedure or recurrent VTs at 3 months of follow-up was observed. On the other hand, the procedure duration was substantially longer on MCS (528.3 ± 105.5 vs 407.3 ± 62.1 min; $P = .01$). The first attempt to compare the results of VT ablation on MCS with substrate mapping was reported by Bunch and colleagues.[56] In a retrospective review of 13 consecutive patients with hemodynamically unstable VT who underwent TandemHeart-assisted ablation compared with 18 matched patients undergoing substrate-based VT ablation, they found a greater number of monomorphic VTs induced in the MCS group but no difference in inducibility after ablation. The freedom from ICD shocks/therapies for sustained VT was similar between groups. Again, the procedure on MCS was longer. Although the investigators claimed no difference in complication, MCS use was associated with complication in 31% versus substrate modification in 17%. Complications in prospective multicenter US registry of 66 patients was relatively high (36% for Impella and 19% for TandemHeart).[57]

A recent analysis of 1655 patients from the International VT Ablation Center Collaborative group described the results of 105 patients who received hemodynamic support.[58] These patients were sicker with multiple comorbidities. Acute procedural success was significantly lower (71.8 vs 73.7; $P = .04$) and complications were more frequent (12.5 vs 6.5; $P = .03$). Also, 1-year mortality was higher (34.7 vs 9.3%; $P < .001$). In a subgroup analysis of similarly sick patients (left ventricular ejection fraction [LVEF] ≤20% and New York Heart Association [NYHA] functional class III to IV), no difference was found in procedural success, complications and 1-year mortality between the groups of patients ablated on MCS or with substrate modification. Meta-analysis of available studies, involving 2026 patients with 284 of them undergoing ablation on MCS, showed again that patients receiving MCS during VT ablation were sicker with no significant difference in acute procedural success, VT recurrence, and mortality compared with patients ablated without MCS. MCS also was associated with higher complications and longer fluoroscopy and procedure time.[59] Although some investigators believe that a prospective randomized controlled trial would identify if the use of MCS in unstable patients undergoing VT ablation will have an impact on clinical outcomes, the authors feel that the outcome of such patients is mostly determined by the severity of underlying disease. Based on the authors' experience, such patients may more benefit from implantation of LVAD and/or heart transplantation. This was to some extent confirmed in a recent study in a series of patients with an ES and acute hemodynamic decompensation who underwent catheter ablation with ECMO support.[60] The outcome of these patients was poor and a majority died of refractory heart failure. On the other hand, the authors believe that MCS could have an impact in those patients who are not in advanced heart failure but have inadequately defined substrate by voltage and pace mapping strategies (Fig. 7). In these subjects, mapping during VT and the use of entrainment may help significantly in determination of a critical part of the circuit.

CATHETER ABLATION IN ELECTRICAL STORM

ES is defined as an occurrence of 3 or more distinct episodes of VT and/or VF within a 24-hour period, resulting in device intervention (either antitachycardia pacing and/or shock delivery). ES is a significant event that appears to be (based on existing evidence) associated with increased all-cause mortality and worse clinical outcomes.[61] Catheter ablation has become the therapy of choice in expert centers, although there are no data from randomized trials. Given the efficacy of ablation in terminating ES, however, this treatment option is used as an early treatment in

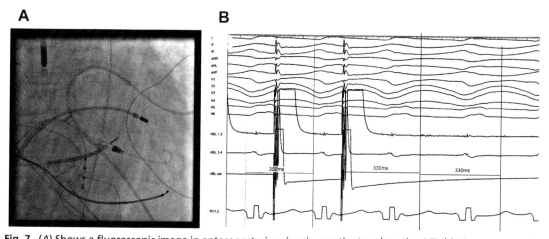

Fig. 7. (*A*) Shows a fluoroscopic image in anteroposterior view in a patient undergoing VT ablation supported by MCS Impella CP. Impella heart pump is introduced across the aortic valve using a retrograde approach, the ablation catheter is introduced into the left ventricle using a transseptal approach. Hemodynamic support by heart pump enabled mapping during ongoing VT. (*B*) Mid-diastolic potentials and concealed entrainment in the protected isthmus of slow conduction with matching postpacing interval. Radiofrequency ablation at this site resulted in the termination of arrhythmia. ([A] *Courtesy of* Abiomed, Danvers, CO.)

such condition. The principles of mapping are generally the same as discussed previously.

Data from the multicenter register showed that successful VT ablation in an ES reduces recurrences of arrhythmia and improves survival.[62] The authors' retrospective analysis of catheter ablation of VT in 328 patients (age: 63 years ± 12 years; 88% men; 72% ischemic cardiomyopathy; LVEF: 32% ± 12%) showed that ablation in ES was performed in 93 patients (28%). During the follow-up of 1088 days ± 779 days, 66.7% versus 60% patients (log rank $P = .053$) experienced VT/VF recurrence in ES versus non-ES group; and 40.9% versus 31.9% patients died (log rank $P = .02$), respectively.[63] In a multivariate analysis, ES was not an independent predictor of all-cause mortality but 5 other factors were identified: age greater than 70 years, NYHA class greater than or equal to 3, serum creatinine level greater than 115 μmol/L, LVEF less than or equal to 25%, and amiodarone therapy. When the population was dichotomized by the score of these risk factors, ES at index ablation remained a significant risk factor of total mortality only in the low-risk subgroup with only 1 risk factor.

Based on their experience, the authors have developed a stratified approach to ES (**Fig. 8**). Each patient is admitted to the acute cardiology unit and such admission is guaranteed similarly as for patients with ST-elevation myocardial infarction. A multidisciplinary team is involved. First, reversible causes are excluded. Second, the decision about the best treatment is made

depending on patient condition. If an arrhythmia is believed to be the primary cause of ES, ablation could be organized any time (24/7). The best examples are focally triggered VF or incessant VTs. In some subjects, arrhythmias are considered as secondary in severe heart failure. Then, therapy for heart failure is primary, often requiring implantation of LVAD. In less urgent cases, ablation is performed electively during a hospital stay.

Surgical ablation or implantation of a LVAD is indicated after failure of catheter ablation. When VT/VF recurs on LVAD, catheter ablation is successful and most of the arrhythmias are not related to inflow cannula but to the myocardial substrate.[64] A recent review of 18 available studies has confirmed initial observations.[65] Ablation allowed VT storm termination in 90% of cases.

VENTRICULAR TACHYCARDIAS IN ACUTE MYOCARDIAL INFARCTION

A majority of ventricular arrhythmias in acute myocardial infarction are of ischemic origin and, thus, polymorphic. Monomorphic VT in acute or subacute myocardial infarction is relatively rare and usually reflects the presence of the arrhythmogenic substrate from previous ischemic events (whether known or silent). There is 1 entity, however, which requires attention and which manifests usually during the subacute stage of myocardial infarction. It is VF triggered by monotopic ventricular ectopic beats.

Initially, focal triggering of VF from Purkinje fibers and successful elimination of the trigger by catheter ablation were described in patients with

Triage of patients with electrical storm

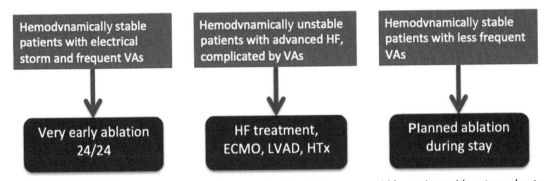

Fig. 8. Management algorithm for the ES. The example of the first group could be patient with a storm due to focally triggered VF—in this case, is ablation essential to abolish the arrhythmia. The middle group comprises patients in the terminal stage of heart failure with severe dysfunction where the authors prefer to treat primarily heart failure using mechanical support. The third group is the most frequent and catheter ablation is performed as an elective procedure. HF, heart failure; HTx, heart transplant; VAs, ventricular arrhythmias. (*Courtesy of* The Institute for Clinical and Experimental Medicine, Prague, Czech Republic; with permission.)

idiopathic VF.[66] Bansch and colleagues[67] reported for the first time their experience of catheter ablation in 4 patients with focally triggered VF after acute myocardial infarction. Again, the triggering foci were located within the Purkinje system, specifically in the left posterior fascicle. Catheter ablation of the triggering premature ectopic beats successfully controlled ES and none of the 4 patients experienced further episodes of VF within the follow-up period ranging between 5 months and 33 months. The investigators estimated that the scenario occurs relatively rarely in patients after acute myocardial infarction. In their experience, catheter ablation was only required in 4 reported patients out of a total of 2340 postinfarction patients (ie, 0.17% of cases). A similar observation was published by Enjoji and colleagues,[68] who reported experience with catheter ablation of triggering premature ventricular contractions in 4 patients with the acute coronary syndrome and low ejection fraction who suffered from multiple VF or VT episodes, despite successful revascularization.

Recently, the authors published experience with catheter ablation of triggering foci of VF after myocardial infarction, reporting on 9 subjects (mean age 62 yeras ± 7 years; 2 women; between 3 days and 171 months; mean LVEF 25% ± 7%).[69] In 6 of them (67%), the ablation procedure was performed on mechanical ventilation. Catheter ablation was successful in 8 patients. During a follow-up of 13 months ± 7 months, 2 patients died of progressive heart failure without any recurrence of ventricular arrhythmias. Another patient had a recurrence of focally triggered VF from the

other fascicle. The other had a recurrence of ES due to monomorphic VT that was successfully reablated by substrate modification. The authors' data from ablation of ES due to focally triggered VF in 22 subjects with ischemic heart disease show high acute success (86%) with relatively high early recurrences (36%) from a different part of Purkinje system. In the long term, 77% is without recurrences of ES.[70]

Available clinical data suggest that the trigger originates predominantly in the Purkinje fibers within myocardial necrosis and/or scar. This view is supported by some experimental data showing the survival of the Purkinje fibers in the region of myocardial infarction.[71,72] These cells are more resistant and, therefore, can survive even severe ischemia. They also can be nourished by retrograde perfusion through various ventricular sinusoidal channels, through the left atrial venous system or simply by diffusion of oxygen from ventricular cavity blood through the endocardium. These surviving Purkinje fibers crossing the border zone of the myocardial infarction demonstrate heightened automaticity, triggered activity, and supernormal excitability.

From a practical point of view, the authors recommend using the electroanatomic mapping system for ablation of triggering foci in post–myocardial infarction patients. The main reason is the possibility of tagging the early activation, conduction system, and delineation of myocardial necrosis or scar as low-voltage areas. In addition, the authors have noticed that patients with ischemic cardiomyopathy often present with more than 1 ectopic focus. In the authors' experience, the risk of early recurrences of ES after successful ablation of 1 trigger supports the strategy to ablate all ectopic foci. Catheter ablation may address more Purkinje tissue along the margin of the affected tissue. In addition, this strategy could be used when no ectopy is present during the mapping or if catheter manipulation induces left bundle branch block, making an analysis of conduction system difficult. Finally, the electroanatomic system also can support modification of substrate for monomorphic VTs, should they occur at the same time.

SUMMARY

Currently, several strategies are being evaluated to improve the results of catheter ablation of unmappable VTs. They include both imaging techniques and novel mapping tools for assessment and modification of the arrhythmogenic substrate. Whether the use of MCS would change the outcome of the patients remains to be established. One of the most exciting areas seems to be the development of catheter ablation strategies in Brugada syndrome because it may correct the underlying pathology. Data on the results of catheter ablation in ES suggest that the prognosis is better when the patient is referred earlier than in ES. Finally, catheter ablation of focally triggered VF in early after acute myocardial infarction may be a life-saving procedure.

REFERENCES

1. Stevenson WG, Sager PT, Friedman PL. Entrainment techniques for mapping atrial and ventricular tachycardias. J Cardiovasc Electrophysiol 1995;6:201–16.
2. Killu AM, Mulpuru SK, Asirvatham SJ. Mapping and ablation procedures for the treatment of ventricular tachycardia. Expert Rev Cardiovasc Ther 2016;14:1071–87.
3. Marchlinski FE, Callans DJ, Gottlieb CD, et al. Linear ablation lesions for control of unmappable ventricular tachycardia in patients with ischemic and nonischemic cardiomyopathy. Circulation 2000;101:1288–96.
4. Dickfeld T, Tian J, Ahmad G, et al. MRI-Guided ventricular tachycardia ablation: integration of late gadolinium-enhanced 3D scar in patients with implantable cardioverter-defibrillators. Circ Arrhythm Electrophysiol 2011;4:172–84.
5. Perez-David, Arenal A, Rubio-Guivernau JL, et al. Noninvasive identification of ventricular tachycardia-related conducting channels using contrast-enhanced magnetic resonance imaging in patients with chronic myocardial infarction: comparison of signal intensity scar mapping and endocardial voltage mapping. J Am Coll Cardiol 2011;57:184–94.
6. Piers SR, Tao Q, van Huls van Taxis CF, et al. Contrast-enhanced MRI-derived scar patterns and associated ventricular tachycardias in nonischemic cardiomyopathy: implications for the ablation strategy. Circ Arrhythm Electrophysiol 2013;6:875–83.
7. Andreu D, Penela D, Acosta J, et al. Cardiac magnetic resonance-aided scar dechanneling: influence on acute and long-term outcomes. Heart Rhythm 2017;14:1121–8.
8. Sramko M, Hoogendoorn JC, Glashan CA, et al. Advancement in cardiac imaging for treatment of ventricular arrhythmias in structural heart disease. Europace 2019;21:383–403.
9. Cochet H, Komatsu Y, Sacher F, et al. Integration of merged delayed-enhanced magnetic resonance imaging and multidetector computed tomography for the guidance of ventricular tachycardia ablation: a pilot study. J Cardiovasc Electrophysiol 2013;24:419–26.
10. Komatsu Y, Cochet H, Jadidi A, et al. Regional myocardial wall thinning at multidetector computed tomography correlates to arrhythmogenic substrate in postinfarction ventricular tachycardia: assessment of structural and electrical substrate. Circ Arrhythm Electrophysiol 2013;6:342–50.
11. Esposito A, Palmisano A, Antunes S, et al. Cardiac CT with delayed enhancement in the characterization of ventricular tachycardia structural substrate: relationship between CT-segmented scar and electro-anatomic mapping. JACC Cardiovasc Imaging 2016;9:822–32.
12. Tian J, Jeudy J, Smith MF, et al. Three-dimensional contrast-enhanced multidetector CT for anatomic, dynamic, and perfusion characterization of abnormal myocardium to guide ventricular tachycardia ablations. Circ Arrhythm Electrophysiol 2010;3:496–504.
13. Tandri H, Calkins H. MR and CT imaging of arrhythmogenic cardiomyopathy. Card Electrophysiol Clin 2011;3:269–80.
14. Ashikaga H, Arevalo H, Vadakkumpadan F, et al. Feasibility of image-based simulation to estimate ablation target in human ventricular arrhythmia. Heart Rhythm 2013;10:1109–16.
15. Krahn PRP, Singh SM, Ramanan V, et al. Cardiovascular magnetic resonance guided ablation and intraprocedural visualization of evolving radiofrequency lesions in the left ventricle. J Cardiovasc Magn Reson 2018;20:20.
16. Peichl P, Wichterle D, Čihák R, et al. Catheter ablation of ventricular tachycardia in the presence of an old endocavitary thrombus guided by intracardiac echocardiography. Pacing Clin Electrophysiol 2016;39:581–7.
17. Hussein A, Jimenez A, Ahmad G, et al. Assessment of ventricular tachycardia scar substrate by

intracardiac echocardiography. Pacing Clin Electrophysiol 2014;37:412–21.

18. Bunch TJ, Weiss JP, Crandall BG, et al. Image integration using intracardiac ultrasound and 3D reconstruction for scar mapping and ablation of ventricular tachycardia. J Cardiovasc Electrophysiol 2010;21:678–84.

19. Bala R, Ren JF, Hutchinson MD, et al. Assessing epicardial substrate using intracardiac echocardiography during VT ablation. Circ Arrhythm Electrophysiol 2011;4:667–73.

20. Callans DJ, Ren JF, Michele J, et al. Electroanatomic left ventricular mapping in the porcine model of healed anterior myocardial infarction. Correlation with intracardiac echocardiography and pathological analysis. Circulation 1999;100:1744–50.

21. Arenal A, del Castillo S, Gonzalez-Torrecilla E, et al. Tachycardia-related channel in the scar tissue in patients with sustained monomorphic ventricular tachycardias: influence of the voltage scar definition. Circulation 2004;110:2568–74.

22. Mountantonakis SE, Park RE, Frankel DS, et al. Relationship between voltage map "channels" and the location of critical isthmus sites in patients with post-infarction cardiomyopathy and ventricular tachycardia. J Am Coll Cardiol 2013;61:2088–95.

23. Wijnmaalen AP, van der Geest RJ, van Huls van Taxis CF, et al. Head-to-head comparison of contrast-enhanced magnetic resonance imaging and electroanatomical voltage mapping to assess post-infarct scar characteristics in patients with ventricular tachycardias: real-time image integration and reversed registration. Eur Heart J 2011;32:104–14.

24. Vergara P, Trevisi N, Ricco A, et al. Late potentials abolition as an additional technique for reduction of arrhythmia recurrence in scar related ventricular tachycardia ablation. J Cardiovasc Electrophysiol 2012;23:621–7.

25. Della Bella P, Bisceglia C, Tung R. Multielectrode contact mapping to assess scar modification in post-myocardial infarction ventricular tachycardia patients. Europace 2012;14(Suppl 2):ii7–12.

26. Jaïs P, Maury P, Khairy P, et al. Elimination of local abnormal ventricular activities: a new end point for substrate modification in patients with scar-related ventricular tachycardia. Circulation 2012;125:2184–96.

27. Sacher F, Lim HS, Derval N, et al. Substrate mapping and ablation for ventricular tachycardia: the LAVA approach. J Cardiovasc Electrophysiol 2015;26:464–71.

28. Soejima K, Stevenson WG, Maisel WH, et al. Electrically unexcitable scar mapping based on pacing threshold for identification of the reentry circuit isthmus: feasibility for guiding ventricular tachycardia ablation. Circulation 2002;106:1678–783.

29. de Chillou C, Groben L, Magnin-Poull I, et al. Localizing the critical isthmus of postinfarct ventricular tachycardia: the value of pace-mapping during sinus rhythm. Heart Rhythm 2014;11:175–81.

30. Di Biase L, Burkhardt JD, Lakkireddy D, et al. Ablation of stable vts versus substrate ablation in ischemic cardiomyopathy: the VISTA Randomized Multicenter Trial. J Am Coll Cardiol 2015;66:2872–82.

31. Gökoğlan Y, Mohanty S, Gianni C, et al. Scar homogenization versus limited-substrate ablation in patients with nonischemic cardiomyopathy and ventricular tachycardia. J Am Coll Cardiol 2016;68:1990–8.

32. Nakahara S, Tung R, Ramirez RJ, et al. Distribution of late potentials within infarct scars assessed by ultra high-density mapping. Heart Rhythm 2010;7:1817–24.

33. Tung R, Nakahara S, Ramirez R, et al. Accuracy of combined endocardial and epi- cardial electroanatomic mapping of a reperfused porcine infarct model: a comparison of electrofield and magnetic systems with histopathologic correlation. Heart Rhythm 2011;8:439–47.

34. Tschabrunn CMRS, Dorman NC, Nezafat R, et al. High-resolution mapping of ventricular scar: comparison between single and multi-electrode catheters. Circ Arrhythm Electrophysiol 2016;9:e003841.

35. Berte B, Relan J, Sacher F, et al. Impact of electrode type on mapping of scar-related VT. J Cardiovasc Electrophysiol 2015;26:1213–23.

36. Anter E, Li J, Tschabrunn CM, et al. Mapping of a post-infarction left ventricular aneurysm-dependent macroreentrant ventricular tachycardia. HeartRhythm Case Rep 2015;1:472–6.

37. Viswanathan K, Mantziari L, Butcher C, et al. Evaluation of a novel high-resolution mapping system for catheter ablation of ventricular arrhythmias. Heart Rhythm 2017;14:176–83.

38. Tung R, Nakahara S, Maccabelli G, et al. Ultra high-density multipolar mapping with double ventricular access: a novel technique for ablation of ventricular tachycardia. J Cardiovasc Electrophysiol 2011;22:49–56.

39. Massé S, Magtibay K, Jackson N, et al. Resolving myocardial activation with novel omnipolar electrograms. Circ Arrhythm Electrophysiol 2016;9:e004107.

40. Magtibay K, Massé S, Asta J, et al. Physiological assessment of ventricular myocardial voltage using omnipolar electrograms. J Am Heart Assoc 2017;6 [pii:e006447].

41. Deno DC, Balachandran R, Morgan D, et al. Orientation-independent catheter- based characterization of myocardial activation. IEEE Trans Biomed Eng 2017;64:1067–77.

42. Jackson N, Gizurarson S, Viswanathan K, et al. Decrement evoked potential (DEEP) mapping: the

basis of a mechanistic strategy for ventricular tachy-car- dia ablation. Circ Arrhythm Electrophysiol 2015; 8:1433–42.

43. Porta-Sánchez A, Jackson N, Lukac P, et al. Multicenter study of ischemic ventricular tachycardia ablation h decrement-evoked potential(deep) mapping with extra stimulus. JACC Clin Electrophysiol 2018;4:307–15.

44. Jamil-Copley S, Vergara P, Carbucicchio C, et al. Application of ripple map- ping to visualise slow conduction channels within the infarct-related left ventricular scar. Circ Arrhythm Electrophysiol 2015; 8(1):76–86.

45. Luther V, Linton NW, Jamil-Copley S, et al. A prospective study of ripple mapping the postinfarct ventricular scar to guide sub- strate ablation for ventricular tachycardia. Circ Arrhythm Electrophysiol 2016;9(6) [pii:e004072].

46. Xie S, Kubala M, Liang JJ, et al. Utility of ripple mapping for identification of slow conduction channels during ventricular tachycardia ablation in the setting of arrhythmogenic right ventricular cardiomyopathy. J Cardiovasc Electrophysiol 2019;30:366–73.

47. Henz BD, do Nascimento TA, Dietrich Cde O, et al. Simultaneous epicardial and endocardial substrate mapping and radiofrequency catheter ablation as first-line treatment for ventricular tachycardia and frequent ICD shocks in chronic chagasic cardiomyopathy. J Interv Card Electrophysiol 2009;26: 195–205.

48. Sosa E, Scanavacca M, d'Avila A, et al. A new technique to perform epicardial mapping in the electrophysiology laboratory. J Cardiovasc Electrophysiol 1996;7:531–6.

49. Sacher F, Roberts-Thomson K, Maury P, et al. Epicardial ventricular tachycardia ablation a multicenter safety study. J Am Coll Cardiol 2010;55: 2366–72.

50. Nademanee K, Veerakul G, Chandanamattha P, et al. Prevention of ventricular fibrillation episodes in Brugada syndrome by catheter ablation over the anterior right ventricular outflow tract epicardium. Circulation 2011;123:1270–9.

51. Pappone C, Brugada J, Vicedomini G, et al. Electrical substrate elimination in 135 consecutive patients with brugada syndrome. Circ Arrhythm Electrophysiol 2017;10:e005053.

52. Patocskai B, Yoon N, Antzelevitch C. Mechanisms underlying epicardial radiofrequency ablation to suppress arrhythmogenesis in experimental models of brugada syndrome. JACC Clin Electrophysiol 2017;3:353–63.

53. Bunch TJ, Mahapatra S, Madhu Reddy Y, et al. The role of percutaneous left ventricular assist devices during ventricular tachycardia ablation. Europace 2012;14(Suppl 2):ii26–32.

54. Ostadal P, Mlcek M, Holy F, et al. Direct comparison of percutaneous circulatory support systems in specific hemodynamic conditions in a porcine model. Circ Arrhythm Electrophysiol 2012;5:1202–6.

55. Miller MA, Dukkipati SR, Mittnacht AJ, et al. Activation and entrainment mapping of hemodynamically unstable ventricular tachycardia using a percutaneous left ventricular assist device. J Am Coll Cardiol 2011;58:1363–71.

56. Bunch TJ, Darby A, May HT, et al. Efficacy and safety of ventricular tachycardia ablation with mechanical circulatory support compared with substrate-based ablation techniques. Europace 2012;14:709–14.

57. Reddy YM, Chinitz L, Mansour M, et al. Percutaneous left ventricular assist devices in ventricular tachycardia ablation: multicenter experience. Circ Arrhythm Electrophysiol 2014;7:244–50.

58. Turagam MK, Vuddanda V, Atkins D, et al. Hemodynamic support in ventricular tachycardia ablation: an international vt ablation center collaborative group study. JACC Clin Electrophysiol 2017;3(13): 1534–43.

59. Turagam MK, Vuddanda V, Koerber S, et al. Percutaneous ventricular assist device in ventricular tachycardia ablation: a systematic review and meta-analysis. J Interv Card Electrophysiol 2019;55(2): 197–205.

60. Enriquez A, Liang J, Gentile J, et al. Outcomes of rescue cardiopulmonary support for periprocedural acute hemodynamic decompensation in patients undergoing catheter ablation of electrical storm. Heart Rhythm 2018;15:75–80.

61. Noda T, Kurita T, Nitta T, et al. Significant impact of electrical storm on mortality in patients with structural heart disease and an implantable cardiac defibrillator. Int J Cardiol 2018;255:85–91.

62. Vergara P, Tung R, Vaseghi M, et al. Successful ventricular tachycardia ablation in patients with electrical storm reduces recurrences and improves survival. Heart Rhythm 2018;15:48–55.

63. Aldhoon B, Wichterle D, Peichl P, et al. Outcomes of ventricular tachycardia ablation in patients with structural heart disease: the impact of electrical storm. PLoS One 2017;12:e0171830.

64. Sacher F, Reichlin T, Zado ES, et al. Characteristics of ventricular tachycardia ablation in patients with continuous flow left ventricular assist devices. Circ Arrhythm Electrophysiol 2015;8:592–7.

65. Anderson RD, Lee G, Virk S, et al. Catheter ablation of ventricular tachycardia in patients with a ventricular assist device: a systematic review of procedural characteristics and outcomes. JACC Clin Electrophysiol 2019;5:39–51.

66. Haïssaguerre M, Shoda M, Jaïs P, et al. Mapping and ablation of idiopathic ventricular fibrillation. Circulation 2002;106:962–7.

67. Bänsch D, Oyang F, Antz M, et al. Successful catheter ablation of electrical storm after myocardial infarction. Circulation 2003;108:3011–6.

68. Enjoji Y, Mizobuchi M, Shibata K, et al. Catheter ablation for an incessant form of antiarrhythmic drug-resistant ventricular fibrillation after acute coronary syndrome. Pacing Clin Electrophysiol 2006;29: 102–5.

69. Peichl P, Cihák R, Kozeluhová M, et al. Catheter ablation of arrhythmic storm triggered by monomorphic ectopic beats in patients with coronary artery disease. J Interv Card Electrophysiol 2010;27:51–9.

70. Kautzner J, Peichl P. Catheter ablation of polymorphic ventricular tachycardia and ventricular fibrillation. Arrhythm Electrophysiol Rev 2013;2:135–40.

71. Friedman PL, Stewart JR, Fenoglio JJ Jr, et al. Survival of subendocardial Purkinje fibers after extensive myocardial infarction in dogs. Circ Res 1973; 33:597–611.

72. Friedman PL, Stewart JR, Wit AL. Spontaneous and induced cardiac arrhythmias in subendocardial Purkinje fibers surviving extensive myocardial infarction in dogs. Circ Res 1973;33: 612–26.

Mapping and Ablation of Ventricle Arrhythmia in Patients with Left Ventricular Assist Devices

Subodh R. Devabhaktuni, MD, Jonathan T. Shirazi, MD, John M. Miller, MD*

KEYWORDS

- Ventricular arrhythmias • Ventricular tachycardia • Mapping • Ablation • LVAD • Assist devices

KEY POINTS

- Ventricular arrhythmia (VA) is a common comorbidity in patients with left ventricular assist devices (LVADs).
- In contrast to what is expected, VA typically arise from areas of preexisting scar far from inflow cannula sites.
- Periprocedural planning is key to successful outcomes.
- Ablation appears to be a promising intervention in significantly reducing drug-refractory VA in LVAD patients.

INTRODUCTION

Ventricular arrhythmias (VAs), including ventricular tachycardia (VT) and ventricular fibrillation (VF), are well-known occurrences in patients with left ventricular assist devices (LVADs), with reported incidence ranging from 18% to as high as 52% (although there is some evidence of a recent decrease in incidence[1–3]). Although the use of implantable cardioverter-defibrillators (ICDs) in patients with LVADs has been shown to improve survival,[4] VT and VF events have been shown to adversely affect morbidity with recurrent ICD shocks, recurrent hospitalizations, and mortality from progressive right ventricular failure or by the arrhythmia itself (incessant or frequently recurrent VT/VF[5–7]). Antiarrhythmic drugs are commonly used to treat the VA as the first-line therapy; unfortunately, VA may become drug refractory.

Catheter ablation for VA in LVAD patients was initially reported by Dandamudi and colleagues[8] in a case series of 3 patients. Thereafter, catheter ablation has become common therapeutic intervention to address this problem, particularly with the increase and more widespread use of durable LVADs to bridge patients to transplantation or as destination therapy. In this article, we focus on etiology, mechanisms, periprocedural management, and mapping and ablation techniques for treatment of VA in patients with implanted, durable, LVADs.

PATHOGENESIS

Risk Factors

VA incidence has been traditionally categorized as early (<30 days) versus late (>30 days), with the prevalence of early occurrence being relatively

Conflicts of Interest: S.R. Devabhaktuni- None; J.T. Shirazi – None; J.M. Miller - Medtronic, Inc.; Boston Scientific Corp. (Training support; Lecturer); Biosense-Webster, Inc.; (Training support; Lecturer; Consultant); Abbott Electrophysiology (Advisor Board); Biotronik, Inc. (Lecturer).
Indiana University, Indianapolis, IN, USA
* Corresponding author. Krannert Institute of Cardiology, 1800 North Capitol Avenue, E-488, Indianapolis, IN 46202.
E-mail address: jmiller6@iu.edu

Card Electrophysiol Clin 11 (2019) 689–697
https://doi.org/10.1016/j.ccep.2019.07.001
1877-9182/19/© 2019 Elsevier Inc. All rights reserved.

higher.[1,9-11] Several risk factors have been shown to be predictors of VA incidence in post-LVAD patients, although these were not reconfirmed in other studies. **Box 1** shows reported risk factors.

Mechanisms of Ventricular Arrhythmia

Several mechanisms have been proposed to explain the VA occurrence in LVAD patients. **Table 1** lists these potential mechanisms. The primary mechanism of VT is scar-based reentry; additional factors may augment the likelihood of VA occurrence. In a study by Ziv and colleagues,[6] serum electrolyte abnormality was an independent predictor of post-LVAD VAs; use of inotropic agents to manage cardiogenic shock also increases the likelihood of VAs.[6,12] Molecular analysis has shown upregulation and downregulation of several ion channels possibly leading to VA. Upregulation of sodium–calcium exchanger (NCX) can lead to delayed after depolarizations resulting in triggered VA.[15,16] In addition, downregulation of the voltage-gated potassium channel (Kv4.3) as well as the sodium/potassium ATP pump results in an increased action potential duration.[15,17] In a study by Rodrigue-Way and colleagues,[18] upregulation in calcium handling and sarcomeric genes, including calcium ATPase and ryanodine receptor 2, and an increase in cardiofibroblast genes were noted. Downregulation of connexin 43 (Cx43) can result in VA in animal studies.[15] New scar formation in the apical region along the suture lines, changes in autonomic tone, significant reduction in volume from left ventricular (LV) unloading and hemodynamic alteration from inotropic support can result in the milieu for arrhythmogenesis in the peri-implantation period. New or preexisting scar areas at or near the inflow cannula site can be a substrate for reentrant

Table 1
Mechanism and distribution of VAD-related VT

Mechanism of VT	Distribution, %
Scar-based reentry	90
Focal	5
Cannula adjacent VT	19
BBR VT	4

Abbreviations: BBR, bundle-branch reentry; VAD, ventricular assist device; VT, ventricular tachycardia.

From Anderson RD, Lee G, Virk S, et al. Catheter ablation of ventricular tachycardia in patients with a ventricular assist device: a systematic review of procedural characteristics and outcomes. *JACC Clin Electrophysiol.* 2019;5(1):39-51. https://doi.org/10.1016/j.jacep.2018.08.009; with permission.

VT.[6,12,19] Another mechanism is that of suction events, wherein from offset between the excessive LV unloading and preload volume. LV anteroseptum contacts the inflow cannula and can lead to sudden onset of monomorphic VT; these events can be resolved by decreasing LVAD speed and flows and thereby decreasing the degree of LV volume unloading.[20,21] The occurrence of VT in this setting may be due to mechanical irritation alone, or mechanical irritation as the initiator for sustained scar-based reentry.

Prolongation of the QT interval also can be seen following LVAD placement and this may increase the increase the risk of premature ventricular complex (PVC)-induced polymorphic VT. Electrocardiograms (ECGs) taken within 6 hours post-LVAD implant demonstrated statistically significant shortening of QRS duration and increase in QT and QTc duration (379 ± 10 to 504 ± 11 ms).[22] Mechanistic possibilities include inactivation of the swelling-activated chloride channel and an increase in the NCX.[14] PVC triggered VT or VF was observed in approximately 2.5% of the LVAD patients.[19,23] Bundle-branch reentry (BBR) was illustrated as another mechanism for VT in a study by Moss and colleagues.[24] In this study, 3 (14%) of 21 patients (14%) had BBR VT. **Table 1** summarizes the mechanisms of VT and their distribution from a systematic review of studies published to date.

Our experience with VT ablation in LVAD patients echoes the same results (**Table 2**).

MAPPING AND ABLATION
Preprocedural Planning

Preprocedural assessment is crucial for the treatment of VAs in all patients, and especially so for patients with LVAD. The clinical context of VA

Box 1
Risk factors

Elderly patients[5]

History of ischemic heart disease[12]

History of nonischemic heart disease[13]

History of ventricular tachycardia (VT) or ventricular fibrillation (VF) before left ventricular assist device (LVAD)[13]

Destination therapy[5]

Postoperative electrolyte abnormalities[6]

Increase in QT_c[14]

Low LVAD flows[6]

Nonuse of beta blockers[15]

Table 2
Indiana University experience

Pt. Profile	Pt. 1	Pt. 2	Pt. 3	Pt. 4	Pt. 5	Pt. 6	Pt. 7	Pt. 8	Pt. 9	Pt. 10
Age, y	43	70	53	76	74	70	42	66	59	41
Gender	M	M	M	M	M	F	M	F	M	M
Disease	ICM	NICM	NICM	ICM	NICM	ICM	NICM	ICM	NICM	NICM
LVAD indication	Shock and refract. VT	Recurrent VT	Advanced HF	Advanced HF	Advanced HF	Advanced HF	Refractory shock and VT	Advanced HF	Advanced HF	Advanced HF
LVAD model	Thoratec	HM 1	HM II	HM II	HM II	HM II	HM II	HeartWare	HeartWare	HM II
LVAD connection	LA to aorta	LV to aorta	LV to aorta	LV to aorta	LV to aorta	LV to aorta	LV to aorta	LV to aorta	LV to aorta	LV to aorta
VT morphology	RBRS	RBRI and RBLI	LBLS	LBLS and LBLS	LBRI and RBRS	RBLS	Multiple morphologies	No VT inducible	No VT inducible	RBRI
Mapping technique	Act/Entr	Act/Entr	Pace mapping	Act/Entr	Pace mapping	Act/Entr	Pace mapping	Substrate, pace mapping	Pace mapping	Pace mapping
VT mechanism	Reentry	Reentry	Focal	Reentry	Focal and reentry	Reentry	Focal + Purkinje related	n/a	n/a	Focal
Ablation sites	Basal inferior LV	Basal inferolateral LV	Inferoseptal, inferoapical RV	Apical LV septal near cannula	LSOV and apical inferior near cannula	Basal inferolateral LV	Mid anterior, anteroseptal, inferoseptal	Apical anterior and apical septal near cannula	Apical inferior LV near cannula	Basal anterolateral LV and CS epicardially
Ablation results	Success	Apparent success	Success	Success	Possible success	Success	Partial success; ablation limited to avoid heart block	Failure	Success	Success
Follow-up	No VT at 1 y	No VT; sepsis, died after 2 mo	No VT, transplant 9 mo later	No VT; died 4 y later from failure to thrive	Recurrent VT after 2 mo, died from stroke, seizures	No follow-up in EMR	Continued VT; died after 10 d from multiorgan failure	Complicated by pericardial hematoma; patient died	No VT	No VT

Abbreviations: Act/Ent, activation and entrainment mapping; CS, coronary sinus; EMR, electronic medical record; F, Female; HF, heart failure; HM, HeartMate; ICM, ischemic cardiomyopathy; LA, left atrium; LB R/L/S/I, left bundle right/left/superior/inferior; LV, left ventricle; LVAD, left ventricular assist device; M, male; n/a, not applicable; NICM, non-ischemic cardiomyopathy; Pt., patient; RB R/L/S/I, right bundle right/left superior/inferior; RV, right ventricle; SOV, sinus of Valsalva; VT, ventricular tachycardia.

occurrence is particularly relevant; for instance, VT due to suction events requires markedly different therapy from ablation. **Box 2** lists the periprocedural tools and techniques.

Role of 12-Lead Electrocardiogram

In traditional VT ablation planning, the 12-lead ECG of the clinical arrhythmia, as well as ICD electrograms, are useful tools to examine before any VA ablation procedures. However, in one study, ECG VT morphology correlated with the ablation sites in just 45% of patients with LVAD support.[9] Possible explanations for poor correlation could be due to development of progressive diffuse myopathy in the setting of intrinsic scar, distortion of LV from LVAD placement, hemodynamic effects of the LVAD, and LV decompression.

Preprocedural and Periprocedural Imaging

Consideration of a preprocedural computed tomography (CT) scans can be useful in defining the inflow cannula projection into the ventricle and aid with expeditious mapping during the procedure. Transesophageal echocardiography or intracardiac echocardiography (ICE) also may be helpful in assessing LV volume as well monitoring for pericardial effusion. Vigilance to keep the mapping catheter out of the inflow cannula is paramount; ICE also may be useful in incorporation of inflow cannula into the 3-dimensional (3D) LV electroanatomic "shell" constructed during electroanatomic mapping.

Multidisciplinary Involvement

Although there are multiple reports of patients with sustained, rapid VAs being hemodynamically stable with LVAD support, this may not be true when patients receive procedural anesthesia. Cardiovascular anesthesia, and extracorporeal membrane oxygenation/LVAD-trained personnel should be present for the ablation procedure not only for troubleshooting unforeseen developments during the procedure but also to change LVAD flow rates allowing for augmentation of LV volume and hemodynamic support.

Hemodynamic Monitoring

Hemodynamic monitoring to maintain adequate organ perfusion may be different in LVAD patients during ablation. Some investigators suggest additionally monitoring arterial lactate levels, as well as pulmonary capillary wedge pressure and central venous pressure (CVP) in addition to standard blood pressure, oxygen saturation, and urine output. Use of the cerebral oximetry device (FORE-SIGHT; CASMED, Branford, CT) noninvasively and continuously measures regional cerebral tissue oxygen saturation at the microvascular level in the watershed area of the frontal cortex[25] and it is used in some centers routinely during VT ablation.[26] In general, preload and afterload should be managed such that pump flow provides an acceptable cardiac output and by maintaining mean arterial blood pressure in the normal range. Right ventricular failure indicators, such as increasing CVP, should be monitored. Negative inotropic agents should be avoided. Positive inotropic agents, such as milrinone and dobutamine, are recommended, with dobutamine preferred because of its lesser tendency to hypotensive and vasodilatory effects compared with milrinone.

Periprocedural Anticoagulation

Patients with LVADs are both prone to bleeding and thrombogenesis. Von Willebrand factor multimers can be broken down and inactivated with continuous flow VADs leading to a propensity for bleeding. On the contrary, the coagulation cascade also may be activated in patients with ventricular support devices. VT ablations have been performed on warfarin with full therapeutic international normalized ratio of 2 to 3.[24] Anticoagulation with heparin with an ACT goal greater than 300 seconds should be standard procedural practice to reduce the risk of thromboembolic events. Extra caution should be exercised during vascular access, transseptal puncture, and during mapping and ablation; ultrasound guidance for vascular access may be helpful due to reduced or absent pulses that would ordinarily indicate entry sites. Some operators do not prefer retrograde

---

Box 2
Periprocedural considerations

Computed tomography imaging for inflow cannula and left ventricular (LV) anatomy

Toleration of periprocedural anticoagulation: Activated clotting time (ACT) greater than 300 seconds

Intraprocedural monitoring during the procedure: central venous pressure, cerebral oxygenation

Intraprocedural intracardiac echocardiography (ICE)

Left ventricular assist device (LVAD) adjustments during the procedure for left atrium/LV volume augmentation

Hemodynamic support with dobutamine and LVAD settings

aortic approach for this reason and also due to difficulty in crossing a minimally or nonopening aortic valve. Decreasing LVAD flow temporarily may allow LV ejection to open the aortic valve enough to allow catheter entry. In addition, some operators use a long sheath (deployed in the LV over a guidewire) to preserve LV access and prevent catheter dislodgement into the aortic root. LA volume is reduced due to the suction effect from the LVAD and adjustments of the LVAD settings may be needed before atrial septal puncture for accessing the LV.

Left Ventricular Assist Device Interactions with Electrocardiogram and Mapping Systems

It is important to be aware of specific LVAD interactions with electrophysiology recording and mapping systems. One common occurrence is high-frequency noise on the 12-lead ECG tracings (**Fig. 1**); this can be typically mitigated by reducing the low-pass filter of the surface ECG from 100 or 150 Hz to 40 to 50 Hz. More egregious, however, is electromagnetic interference (EMI) that can occur between electroanatomic mapping systems and partially or fully magnetic LVADs, such as the HeartWare and the HeartMate III, respectively. Specifically, mapping systems that are reliant on magnetic fields to create precise 3D shells encounter multiple LVAD interactions including loss of catheter visualization, electroanatomical point acquisition inhibition, loss of vector orientation, and loss of contact force readings, and thus inhibit accurate 3D mapping when the patient is being supported with a partially or fully magnetic LVAD.[9] These effects are most prominent when

the catheter is within approximately 4 cm of the apical inflow cannula. The current available solutions to these interactions include either reliance on fluoroscopy or ICE as the means of monitoring catheter tip location, or using a mapping system that is not dependent on magnetic fields for mapping.[27] Placement of patches on the lower back or reducing the speed of the LVAD also can provide improvement with EMI. Vaidya and colleagues[28] have shown that reducing the flow rate of the percutaneous VAD resulted in elimination of EMI and this can be applied in LVAD patients during ablation. Optimal settings for LVAD flow/rotational speed are yet to be defined.

Mapping

Catheters should be placed for recording the His bundle deflection (for diagnosing or excluding bundle-branch reentrant VT), coronary sinus (as an anatomic reference that also records basal LV activation), right ventricle (for stimulation and fiducial reference during activation mapping), and a mapping/ablation catheter, typically placed to the LV (**Fig. 2**). Following integration of an electro-anatomical shell with preprocedural cardiac CT (if available) or ICE, with special attention to represent the inflow cannula onto the LV shell (**Figs. 3 and 4**), substrate mapping of the LV may commence. Transseptal access may be slightly favored given the avoidance of the outflow cannula and output graft in the aorta. However, retrograde aortic access may be used if transseptal access cannot provide adequate reach, despite use of deflectable sheaths, to areas of importance, often the basal septum and basal inferior LV segments.

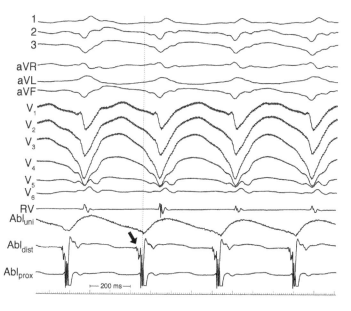

Fig. 1. ECG and intracardiac recordings during VT in an LVAD patient with a prior large inferoposterior infarction. Note high-frequency interference on ECG leads (especially V1–V3) due to interference from the LVAD. This patient had a focal VT from the right ventricular aspect of the interventricular septum; earliest site of activation showed a large but fragmented electrogram (*blue arrow*) 37 ms before QRS onset (*dashed line*). Ablation here accelerated then terminated VT. Abl, ablation catheter.

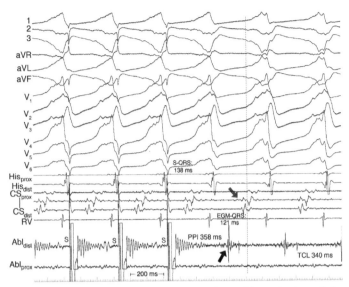

Fig. 2. ECG and intracardiac recordings during VT in an LVAD patient with a prior large inferoposterior infarction. Dashed line indicates QRS onset. At left, overdrive pacing is performed from the ablation catheter (Abl) located in the posterobasal LV where an early diastolic electrogram is recorded (*blue arrow*) when VT resumes after pacing concludes. Pacing from this site produces a QRS complex identical to that of VT in all 12 ECG leads, with a stimulus-QRS (S-QRS) interval 138, compared with the electrogram-QRS (EGM-QRS) interval 121 ms; the post-pacing interval at this site (358 ms) is 18 ms more than the tachycardia cycle length (TCL). These features indicate a good target site for ablation; radiofrequency energy delivery at this site terminated VT in 14 seconds after which VT was no longer inducible. Note also that ventricular electrograms (*red arrow*) in the coronary sinus (CS) recordings occur in late diastole.

It also should be noted that there have been cases wherein the aortic valve cannot be crossed because of low forward flow.[27] Augmentation of the LVAD pump speed may be beneficial in changing the LV volume to assist with mapping and ablation. For example, lowering the LVAD pump speed can yield an increased LA and LV volume that may be beneficial in transseptal puncture and aid in easier maneuverability with the LV during mapping. Despite large LV volumes before LVAD placement, chamber sizes are often markedly decreased during LVAD operation (and more

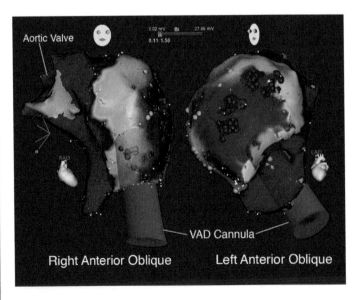

Fig. 3. Electroanatomic voltage map of LV. Right and left anterior oblique views are shown of bipolar voltage obtained from more than 400 points sampled during sinus rhythm in an LVAD patient undergoing VT ablation. Note the approximate location of the LVAD cannula. Extensive anterior wall and septal scarring in present (*red region*), with gray dots representing dense scar (no recordable voltage). Extensive substrate ablation was performed in the region of abnormal voltage and surrounding border zones (into *yellow and green colors*). Blue and Purple colors represents normal voltage. LAO, left aortic valve; RAO, right aortic valve.

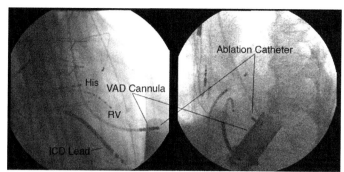

Right Anterior Oblique   Left Anterior Oblique

Fig. 4. Fluoroscopic views of VT ablation in an LVAD patient. Right and left anterior oblique views are shown, demonstrating intracardiac catheters at His bundle region, RV and the ablation catheter, in the LV from a retrograde aortic approach. The ablation catheter tip is near the LVAD inflow cannula.

tubular than spherical). Due to the ongoing suction from the LVAD intake cannula, the mapping catheter may be drawn toward the cannula or even into it; fortunately, this is more of a nuisance than a danger because moving elements of the LVAD are at least 3 cm beyond the open end of the inflow cannula. More problematic is the possibility that ablation targets are difficult or impossible to access due to the presence of the cannula where it contacts the apex or septum.

Detailed substrate mapping should include bipolar and unipolar voltage acquisition as well as notation of sites with abnormal electrograms, including sites with split, late, and fragmented signals that fall into the definition of LAVA (local abnormal ventricular activity). Substrate mapping should be performed with the same manner of ventricular activation; that is, the entire voltage map can be created with RV pacing or during sinus rhythm with acknowledgment that there can be variation in electrograms, including whether a site is a LAVA or not, based on the orientation of wave front propagation. **Fig. 3** shows an example of substrate mapping and ablation. Pace mapping may be used in concert with other mapping modalities as a means of narrowing in on possible exit sites of VT. When sites with reasonable matching to clinical VT are found, particularly when longer stimuli to QRS were noted, these sites should be tagged and further investigated as sites that may be important to the VT circuits.[29] These tools may provide a useful start in establishing areas of interest for activation and entrainment mapping of the patient's clinical arrhythmia. **Figs. 1** and **2** show case examples of good sites based on activation mapping and entrainment mapping.

Epicardial mapping and ablation, which may be necessary in some cases, can be problematic in LVAD patients due to obliteration of the pericardial space following LVAD placement, as well as the potential hazard of damaging mechanical components of the system (cannulae, motor housing) or causing infection. Mapping and ablation at the time of initial LVAD placement can be helpful in these situations.

Induction and study of the clinical arrhythmia remain important in successful ablation. For example, substrate modification, including the elimination of all LAVAs within an LV, would still result in ablation failure in a patient with bundle-branch reentrant VT. Furthermore, establishing the location of the critical diastolic corridor of a clinical macroreentrant VT through entrainment maneuvers provides strong evidence for the electrophysiologist that this specific region (diastolic corridor) is a prime target for ablation. Elimination of this corridor with ablation, rendering the macroreentrant arrhythmia noninducible, is a desirable endpoint. However, this approach is rarely without numerous obstacles. Eliminating a dominant inner loop and allowing the tachycardia to persist with identical exit sites at a longer tachycardia cycle length is not uncommon. A common scenario is elimination of one diastolic corridor, but a different circuit path involving the same entrance with a different diastolic corridor and different exit remains, allowing other VTs to be inducible in spite of successful ablation for the initial VT. Secondary and tertiary VT circuits are more commonly the rule than the exception; this may be in part facilitated by antiarrhythmic drugs such as amiodarone (used in many of these patients before ablation). Entrainment mapping is a versatile tool that can help differentiate excellent ablation sites from bystanders and other poor ablation targets (see **Fig. 2**). In addition, entrainment mapping is more feasible in LVAD patients than those without LVADs, as VTs in the former group are well tolerated. Acceptable procedural endpoints, as with other VT ablations, include termination and noninducibility of the clinical VT; whenever possible, additional substrate modification and targeting of nonclinical VT can be done.

Table 3
Complication rate noted in various case series studies

	Complication Rates, %
Minor	
Groin hematomas	2.9–4.7[24,31]
Pseudoaneurysm	4.7[30]
Atrioventricular fistula	0
Retroperitoneal bleed	0
Major	
Pericardial effusion	0
Catheter entrapment	0
Transient ischemic attack/stroke	5.8[31]
Cardiogenic shock	2.9[31]
Procedural death	0

Ablation Outcomes

Catheter ablation appears to be reasonable treatment option. According to the latest metanalysis, the acute procedural endpoint of noninducible clinical VT was achieved in 78%; noninducibility of any VT was achieved in 67%. Termination of VT storm was achievable in 18 (90%) of 20 cases.

Complications

Minor and major complications occur at rates similar to patients undergoing VT ablation without durable LVAD support. However, it should be noted that the reported complication rates are from centers with high volumes of VT ablations. **Table 3** lists complications from the 3 largest case series reported in the literature.[24,30,31] A specific complication noted in the case series by Moss and colleagues[24] was LVAD thrombosis post ablation. The earliest diagnosis of thrombosis was 148 days after the ablation procedure, and median time to diagnosis was 273 days, casting uncertainty on any causal relationship.

SUMMARY

VAs are frequent in patients with LVADs. Although medical therapy may control VT and VF, catheter ablation is also available to address these problems and has been shown to be effective in decreasing morbidity and mortality from VA. VAs arise from preexisting scar areas away from LVAD inflow cannula sites more commonly than from the cannula sites or mechanical irritation. Ablation outcomes have been good with excellent results, especially in LVAD patients with VT storm, although the evidence is from small studies. Further research is needed to overcome some of the challenges in successful mapping and ablation of VA in this increasing patient population.

REFERENCES

1. Kirklin JK, Naftel DC, Stevenson LW, et al. INTERMACS database for durable devices for circulatory support: first annual report. J Heart Lung Transplant 2008;27(10):1065–72.
2. Shirazi JT, Lopshire JC, Gradus-Pizlo I, et al. Ventricular arrhythmias in patients with implanted ventricular assist devices: a contemporary review. Europace 2013;15(1):11–7.
3. Greet BD, Pujara D, Burkland D, et al. Incidence, predictors, and significance of ventricular arrhythmias in patients with continuous-flow left ventricular assist devices: a 15-year institutional experience. JACC Clin Electrophysiol 2018;4(2):257–64.
4. Cantillon DJ, Tarakji KG, Kumbhani DJ, et al. Improved survival among ventricular assist device recipients with a concomitant implantable cardioverter-defibrillator. Heart Rhythm 2010;7(4):466–71.
5. Ambardekar AV, Allen LA, Lindenfeld J, et al. Implantable cardioverter-defibrillator shocks in patients with a left ventricular assist device. J Heart Lung Transplant 2010;29(7):771–6.
6. Ziv O, Dizon J, Thosani A, et al. Effects of left ventricular assist device therapy on ventricular arrhythmias. J Am Coll Cardiol 2005;45(9):1428–34.
7. Yoruk A, Sherazi S, Massey HT, et al. Predictors and clinical relevance of ventricular tachyarrhythmias in ambulatory patients with a continuous flow left ventricular assist device. Heart Rhythm 2016;13(5):1052–6.
8. Dandamudi G, Ghumman WS, Das MK, et al. Endocardial catheter ablation of ventricular tachycardia in patients with ventricular assist devices. Heart Rhythm 2007;4(9):1165–9.
9. Andersen M, Videbaek R, Boesgaard S, et al. Incidence of ventricular arrhythmias in patients on long-term support with a continuous-flow assist device (HeartMate II). J Heart Lung Transplant 2009;28(7):733–5.
10. Miller LW, Pagani FD, Russell SD, et al. Use of a continuous-flow device in patients awaiting heart transplantation. N Engl J Med 2007;357(9):885–96.
11. Pagani FD, Miller LW, Russell SD, et al. Extended mechanical circulatory support with a continuous-flow rotary left ventricular assist device. J Am Coll Cardiol 2009;54(4):312–21.
12. Bedi M, Kormos R, Winowich S, et al. Ventricular arrhythmias during left ventricular assist device support. Am J Cardiol 2007;99(8):1151–3.

13. Oswald H, Schultz-Wildelau C, Gardiwal A, et al. Implantable defibrillator therapy for ventricular tachyarrhythmia in left ventricular assist device patients. Eur J Heart Fail 2010;12(6):593–9.

14. Harding JD, Piacentino V, Rothman S, et al. Prolonged repolarization after ventricular assist device support is associated with arrhythmias in humans with congestive heart failure. J Card Fail 2005; 11(3):227–32.

15. Refaat M, Chemaly E, Lebeche D, et al. Ventricular arrhythmias after left ventricular assist device implantation. Pacing Clin Electrophysiol 2008;31(10): 1246–52.

16. Chaudhary KW, Rossman EI, Piacentino V, et al. Altered myocardial Ca2+ cycling after left ventricular assist device support in the failing human heart. J Am Coll Cardiol 2004;44(4):837–45.

17. Depre C, Shipley GL, Chen W, et al. Unloaded heart in vivo replicates fetal gene expression of cardiac hypertrophy. Nat Med 1998;4(11):1269–75.

18. Rodrigue-Way A, Burkhoff D, Geesaman BJ, et al. Sarcomeric genes involved in reverse remodeling of the heart during left ventricular assist device support. J Heart Lung Transplant 2005;24(1):73–80.

19. Anderson RD, Lee G, Virk S, et al. Catheter ablation of ventricular tachycardia in patients with a ventricular assist device: a systematic review of procedural characteristics and outcomes. JACC Clin Electrophysiol 2019;5(1):39–51.

20. Vollkron M, Voitl P, Ta J, et al. Suction events during left ventricular support and ventricular arrhythmias. J Heart Lung Transplant 2007;26(8):819–25.

21. Kassi M, Schettle S, Toeg H, et al. Suction event demonstrated by Valsalva maneuver in a patient with HM II LVAD. J Am Coll Cardiol 2018;71(11 Supplement):A2387.

22. Harding JD, Piacentino V, Gaughan JP, et al. Electrophysiological alterations after mechanical circulatory support in patients with advanced cardiac failure. Circulation 2001;104(11):1241–7.

23. Drakos SG, Terrovitis JV, Nanas JN, et al. Reverse electrophysiologic remodeling after cardiac mechanical unloading for end-stage nonischemic cardiomyopathy. Ann Thorac Surg 2011;91(3): 764–9.

24. Moss JD, Flatley EE, Beaser AD, et al. Characterization of ventricular tachycardia after left ventricular assist device implantation as destination therapy: a single-center ablation experience. JACC Clin Electrophysiol 2017;3(12):1412–24.

25. Fischer GW. Recent advances in application of cerebral oximetry in adult cardiovascular surgery. Semin Cardiothorac Vasc Anesth 2008;12(1): 60–9.

26. Miller MA, Dukkipati SR, Koruth JS, et al. How to perform ventricular tachycardia ablation with a percutaneous left ventricular assist device. Heart Rhythm 2012;9(7):1168–76.

27. Higgins SL, Haghani K, Meyer D, et al. Minimizing magnetic interaction between an electroanatomic navigation system and a left ventricular assist device. J Innov Card Rhythm Manag 2013;4:1440–6. Available at: http://www.innovationsincrm.com/cardiac-rhythm-management/2013/november/518-minimizing-magnetic-interaction. Accessed February 19, 2019.

28. Vaidya VR, Desimone CV, Madhavan M, et al. Compatibility of electroanatomical mapping systems with a concurrent percutaneous axial flow ventricular assist device. J Cardiovasc Electrophysiol 2014;25: 781–6.

29. Stevenson WG, Sager PT, Natterson PD, et al. Relation of pace mapping QRS configuration and conduction delay to ventricular tachycardia reentry circuits in human infarct scars. J Am Coll Cardiol 1995;26(2):481–8.

30. Cantillon DJ, Bianco C, Wazni OM, et al. Electrophysiologic characteristics and catheter ablation of ventricular tachyarrhythmias among patients with heart failure on ventricular assist device support. Heart Rhythm 2012;9(6):859–64.

31. Sacher F, Reichlin T, Zado ES, et al. Characteristics of ventricular tachycardia ablation in patients with continuous flow left ventricular assist devices. Circ Arrhythm Electrophysiol 2015;8(3):592–7.

The Spectrum of Idiopathic Ventricular Fibrillation and J-Wave Syndromes
Novel Mapping Insights

Michel Haïssaguerre, MD[a,b,c],*, Wee Nademanee, MD[d],
Mélèze Hocini, MD[a,b,c], Josselin Duchateau, PhD, MD[a,b],
Clementine André, MD[a,b], Thomas Lavergne, MD[b], Masa Takigawa, MD[a],
Frederic Sacher, MD[a,b], Nicolas Derval, MD[a,b], Thomas Pambrun, MD[a,b],
Pierre Jais, MD[a,b], Rick Walton, PhD[b], Mark Potse, PhD[b], Ed Vigmond, PhD[b],
Remi Dubois, PhD[b], Olivier Bernus, PhD[b,c]

KEYWORDS

- Sudden cardiac death • Ventricular fibrillation • Early repolarization syndromes
- J-wave syndromes • Purkinje system

KEY POINTS

- Idiopathic ventricular fibrillation (IVF) is defined as unexplained sudden cardiac death due to ventricular fibrillation (VF) without any identifiable structural or electrical cause after extensive investigations (no phenotype).
- Recent data show that the use of high-density electrophysiologic mapping may ultimately offer subclinical diagnoses of cardiac disease in about 90% of individuals with IVF. Two major conditions underlie the occurrence of VF: the presence of either depolarization abnormalities due to microstructural myocardial alteration or Purkinje abnormalities manifesting as triggering ectopy or reentry in the peripheral network.
- J-wave syndromes are defined as a distinct electrocardiographic phenotype (slurring/notch) affecting the junction between the QRS complex and the ST segment in inferolateral leads. Recent data provide evidence for heterogeneous substrates, related to either delayed depolarization due to microstructural alterations or early repolarization abnormalities.
- IVF and J-wave syndromes are the result of a wide spectrum of pathophysiologic processes. The individual phenotypic characterization is essential given its implications in therapy, genetic testing, and risk stratification.

Disclosure Statement: The authors have nothing to disclose.
This work was supported by the National Research Agency (ANR-10-IAHU04-LIRYC), the European Research Council (FP7/2007-2013 grant agreement number 322886–SYMPHONY), and the Leducq Foundation (RHYTHM network).
[a] Electrophysiology and Cardiac Stimulation, Bordeaux University Hospital, 311 President Wilson Boulevard, Bordeaux 33200, France; [b] IHU LIRYC, Electrophysiology and Heart Modeling Institute, Avenue du Haut Leveque, Bordeaux 33604, Passes Cedex, France; [c] Univ Bordeaux, CRCTB, U1045, Bordeaux, France; [d] Bumrungrad Hospital, Bangkok 10110, Thailand
* Corresponding author. Institute of Rythmology and Heart Modelling, Hopital Cardiologique Haut-Leveque, Avenue de Magellan, Bordeaux-Pessac, France.
E-mail address: michel.haissaguerre@chu-bordeaux.fr

cardiacEP.theclinics.com

Sudden cardiac death (SCD) remains a major health problem in all continents. Estimates vary around 350,000 victims per year in the United States or in Europe and are even higher in Southeast Asia. Coronary artery disease and cardiomyopathies are the main causes in older persons.[1–4] However, in victims younger than 35 years, a common finding is the absence of structural heart disease (SHD) at autopsy, reported in 29% to 40% of cases particularly in young men.[5–9] In the patients surviving after resuscitation maneuvers, ventricular fibrillation (VF) is consistently the lethal heart rhythm identified at the time of event.[10,11] Over the last 20 years considerable efforts have been devoted to the search for discrete electrocardiographic or imaging signs and genetic markers in survivors.[1,4,12] Despite this progress, unexplained SCD remains frequent in young adults.

The authors report here novel insights based on recent mapping data on 2 subsets: *idiopathic VF* defined as an idiopathic ventricular fibrillation (IVF) with no apparent structural or electrical heart disease after extensive investigations (eg, no phenotype) and *J-wave syndromes* defined as an electrocardiographic phenotype affecting the junction (J-wave) between the QRS complex and the ST segment in inferolateral leads.

IDIOPATHIC VENTRICULAR FIBRILLATION

SCD is commonly defined as death from an unexpected circulatory arrest, occurring within an hour of the onset of symptoms. Unexplained SCD is defined as no apparent structural or electrical heart disease after extensive investigations. When VF has been documented by electrocardiography during resuscitation maneuvers, unexplained SCD is termed as IVF.[5,13,14]

Criteria Defining Idiopathic Ventricular Fibrillation

Based on published guidelines, patients classified as having IVF have no clinical evidence for drug abuse/intoxication or electrolyte abnormality at the time of initial presentation, no identifiable SHD demonstrated by normal echocardiographic and delayed gadolinium-enhanced MRI, no detectable coronary artery disease on coronary angiography or exercise testing, and no known repolarization abnormalities associated with long or short QT interval or J-wave syndromes.[4,5,13] Pharmacologic testing with infusion of a sodium-channel blocker (ajmaline, flecainide, or procainamide) is performed to exclude Brugada syndrome. Catecholamine infusion (isoprenaline and adrenaline) is performed to exclude catecholaminergic polymorphic ventricular tachycardia or arrhythmogenic right ventricular cardiomyopathy and to confirm the absence of long QT syndrome. **Box 1** shows the flow diagram of diagnostic tests performed in patients referred for SCD.

According to the guidelines, genetic testing is recommended "for genetic arrhythmia syndromes in young patients (<40 years of age) with IVF." The yield of genetic testing is higher if a family history of SCD at a young age is present.[2,4] Familial screening is recommended in first-degree relatives and should include resting electrocardiogram (ECG), exercise testing, and echocardiography. In selected cases, Holter and signal-averaged ECGs, MRI, and pharmacologic testing may be performed.

International protocols using whole exome sequencing are currently performed for improving the diagnosis yield of inherited disorders.

The absence of clinical phenotype defining a VF as idiopathic obviously depends on the resolution of investigations performed in each patient. The same reasoning also applies to the autopsy's results concluding for the absence of SHD. The authors have previously reported the ability of noninvasive mapping to identify the location of drivers (focal or reentrant) responsible for VF in man.[9,15] This information has allowed to subsequently investigate the driver areas using high-density electrogram mapping and demonstrate the presence of microstructural cardiomyopathic alterations, which are a substrate of VF reentries.

The other chapters in this issue will emphasize the role of these microstructural myocardial alterations and that of Purkinje tissue in the pathophysiology of human IVF.

Pathology of the Purkinje System in Idiopathic Ventricular Fibrillation

The specialized Purkinje system constitutes a tiny part (about 2%) of the myocardial mass, but its pathologic role in arrhythmogenesis is disproportionally high and pleomorphic.[16,17] Purkinje pathology in IVF can manifest either as triggering ectopies or as arrhythmia maintenance via its complex network.

Purkinje cells triggering idiopathic ventricular fibrillation

When they can be identified in IVF (eg, in patients with frequent VF initiations), the great majority (85%) of triggering ectopy originates from the Purkinje system or muscular structures associated with the Purkinje system, such as the moderator band and the papillary muscles. VF is usually triggered by short-coupled premature ventricular

Box 1
Diagnostic tests performed in patients with sudden cardiac death

Structural imaging

   Including MRI (before ICD)

Electrocardiographic monitoring

   Careful 12-lead documentation of ectopy morphologies and couplings

   Repolarization during cycle length variations and dynamic maneuvers

   Signal-averaged ECG

Stress test and pharmacologic tests

   Na + blocker—adrenaline, isoprenaline

Electrophysiologic studies

   High-density endoepicardial mapping

   Programmed stimulation

   EP-guided biopsy (optional)

Genetic testing

Abbreviations: ECG, electrocardiogram; EP, electrophysiology; ICD, implantable cardioverter defibrillator; SCD, sudden cardiac death.

complexes (PVCs) but the authors have observed some patients with IVF in whom all documented Purkinje PVCs had long-coupling intervals greater than 360 ms (**Fig. 1**). The right ventricular outflow tract and less frequently the left ventricular outflow tract, or other myocardial locations are seen in 15% of cases, in the authors' current experience of 78 patients. The origin of ectopic trigger can be demonstrated by mapping the earliest origin (see **Fig. 1**) or by pace mapping if ectopies are rare. Many reports of successful ablation of triggering PVCs have been published, however, most of the time including only one or few cases.[16] In the cases where runs of polymorphic PVCs have been reported, not only the initial one but also subsequent beats can be associated with Purkinje activity, suggesting repetitive reentry or triggered activity (see **Fig. 1**). This suggests that in addition to Purkinje firing, there is a potential to sustain activity within the Purkinje network, explaining the observations of successful outcome after ablation despite the persistence of isolated short-coupled ectopy.

The ectopy morphology is essential to document on the 12-lead ECG as it guides mapping techniques by allowing focus on the area of interest. When originating from the left Purkinje fibers, the PVCs are narrow (<120 ms) with a right-bundle-branch block morphology. They demonstrate right or left axis deviation when originating from the anterior or the posterior Purkinje fibers, respectively. Morphology changes are frequently observed in the left Purkinje PVCs, indicating different exit sites or origins and thus a need for larger ablation. When originating from the right Purkinje arborization, the PVCs have a left-bundle-branch block morphology and left axis.[16] They display a rapid initial deflection but have a wider QRS duration than left Purkinje PVCs, as the right Purkinje has a more limited spatial arborization. More discrete PVC morphology changes are observed, as compared with left Purkinje PVC.

In sinus rhythm, distal Purkinje potentials precede the QRS complex by less than or equal to 15 ms. Longer intervals indicate a fascicular origin (with the risk of creating significant QRS changes if targeted for ablation). Special care should be taken during catheter manipulation to avoid inadvertent bumping of the right bundle, which will conceal Purkinje potentials within the local electrograms, the left-bundle-branch being much less vulnerable. When they are rare, PVCs can be inducible by creating postpacing (atrial or ventricular) pauses and/or drug infusion such as isoproterenol (1–2 mcg/kg/min) or class I drugs.

Repetitive reentry in the Purkinje network
Reentry in the proximal Purkinje system has been described in the form of monomorphic ventricular tachycardia, either as bundle branch reentry or as left fascicular reentry. Polymorphic ventricular tachycardia has also been reported, with all QRS complexes being associated with Purkinje activity (see **Fig. 1**). The authors have observed 5 patients, survivors of IVF, who had neither short-coupling Purkinje ectopy nor microstructural myocardial alteration. A distinct electrophysiologic response was however observed during programmed stimulation at the distal left fascicular system.

No VF or repetitive activity was induced by stimulation from the right ventricle (in 4 of 5 patients), while pacing (S2-S3 extrastimuli) from the left posterior fascicle, and could consistently induce repetitive polymorphic ventricular tachycardia within the distal Purkinje system. The polymorphic QRS complexes were associated with distal Purkinje potentials on a beat-to-beat basis, whereas the proximal Purkinje fascicle and bundle branch potentials were slower or absent (excluding a bundle branch reentry). The variations in ventricular cycles were preceded by a similar change in Purkinje cycles; and arrhythmia termination was

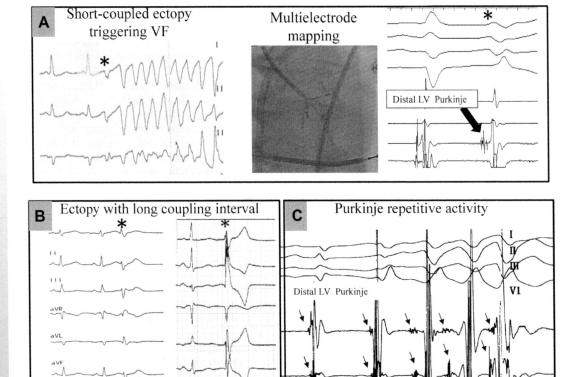

Fig. 1. Different patterns of Purkinje activity in 4 patients with IVF. (*A*) Typical short-coupled ectopy (*asterisk*) initiating VF. Multielectrode mapping with a multispline catheter (*center*) allows to record the earliest activity preceding ectopic beat in the distal left posterior fascicle (*right*). (*B*) Purkinje ectopy with long-coupling intervals (370 and 440 ms) in 2 patients with IVF. (*C*) Spontaneous polymorphic ventricular tachycardia associated with 1- to- 1 distal Purkinje activity. Note the varying Purkinje activation sequence between the distal and proximal bipoles that suggest changes in activation pathway. LV, left ventricle.

preceded by the disappearance of Purkinje activity (**Fig. 2**). Two of these cases have been published recently.[18]

These observations suggest that pacing performed near the distal left posterior Purkinje captures and invades retrogradely the Purkinje network. Although triggered activity cannot be ruled out, the repetitive responses are likely re-entries induced in peripheral Purkinje system, with a gradual shift in trajectory and ventricular exit as demonstrated by computer modeling studies. These responses have been considered as clinically abnormal by the authors, as they are uncommon in their experience and have not been reported in the unique study evaluating left ventricular pacing in control patients.[18] Further investigations are needed to confirm their pathologic significance and whether this electrophysiologic protocol may offer methods to reveal Purkinje abnormalities that can underlie VF susceptibility.

MICROSTRUCTURAL MYOCARDIAL SUBSTRATE IN IDIOPATHIC VENTRICULAR FIBRILLATION

In high-resolution experimental setups, VF requires the continuous formation of reentry for its maintenance, of which a critical determinant is the presence of normal (fiber arrangement) or abnormal (fibrosis) structural heterogeneities. In cardiomyopathic post-transplant human hearts, reentry has been shown to self-perpetuate for many cycles, as it can anchor to a myocardial scar.[10,19] The authors have used multielectrode body surface recordings (ECGi) in clinics to identify the reentries during ongoing VF. Because patients with IVF are free of SHD, VF reentries were expected to be distributed homogeneously across both ventricles. However, a clustering of reentries was observed, and mapping of these regions in sinus rhythm revealed, in some of them, abnormal electrogram characteristics, indicating the presence of "microstructural" cardiomyopathic alteration.

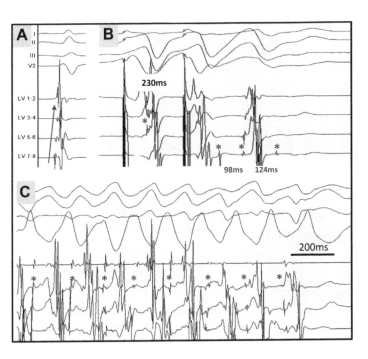

Fig. 2. Inducible repetitive activity in distal Purkinje. Recordings are performed along a decapolar catheter on the distal left posterior fascicle in sinus rhythm (*A*) and during programmed stimulation (*B, C*). Fig. 2B shows double extrastimulation (230–230 ms), producing splitting of Purkinje (*asterisks*) activity (98 ms) followed by a third Purkinje activity 124 ms later: note the different involvement of parts of peripheral Purkinje system (LV7-8 vs LV 5-6). Fig. 2C shows double extrastimulation producing a polymorphic ventricular tachycardia in which each ventricular beat preceded by Purkinje activity, with varying sequence between recording bipoles. Arrhythmia termination is preceded by the disappearance of Purkinje activity. Repetitive Purkinje reentry was consistently reproducible and was the only electrophysiologic abnormality observed in this young woman surviving an episode of IVF. VT, ventricular tachycardia.

Invasive Electrogram Mapping in Sinus Rhythm

High-density recordings of endocardial and epicardial electrograms were performed using multispline catheter (Lasso or PentaRay catheter with 2 mm interelectrode distances) in the epicardium and PentaRay or decapolar catheters in the right and left endocardium. A transseptal or retroaortic approach was performed to access the endocardial left ventricle and a subxyphosternal approach to access into the pericardial space. The objective was to analyze electrograms present at the main driver areas (with the maximal number of rotations) compared with nondriver regions. Electroanatomical mapping was performed using magnetic geolocalization (CARTO system, Biosense Webster, CA); in a prior study, the authors mapped a mean of 590 ± 403 (endocardial right ventricle), 547 ± 292 (endocardial left ventricle), and 2081 ± 1278 (epicardium) sites per patient. Electrogram criteria were identical to those defining fibrotic and cardiomyopathic tissue during mapping of ischemic or dilated cardiomyopathies. Areas of low-amplitude electrograms were delineated in bipolar (less than 1 mV) and unipolar modes (less than 8.3 and 5.5 mV in left and right ventricles respectively) on 3-dimensional ventricular reconstruction (CARTO system, BiosenseWebster,CA). Because low-amplitude electrograms can be due to normal fat tissue

on the epicardium, epicardial electrograms were only considered abnormal if they harbored fragmented signals with a duration superior to 70 ms with more than 3 components or split/late potentials.[20–22] Greater mapping density was acquired in cases of abnormality to delineate the abnormal surface area.

Results

In the authors' current experience, myocardial areas manifesting low-amplitude and prolonged fractionated signals were found in 32 of 48 (67%) patients. The abnormal tissue was clustered in 1 or 2 areas, whereas 4 patients had scattered abnormal areas. In a previous study the abnormal surface area covered a mean of 13±5 cm^2, ranging from 6 to 22, representing 3.9 ± 1.7% of the total ventricular surface. This finding is in keeping with prior experimental studies, which showed that even small ventricular lesions in the range of 4 cm^2 are sufficient to promote VF.[23,24]

The right ventricle was the structure preferentially harboring the abnormal area, whereas the left ventricle or the septum was less frequently affected (**Fig. 3**). The comparison of endocardial and epicardial recordings at the same location showed that the abnormal signals were recorded in one side, mostly epicardial, indicating that the pathology involved a part of the ventricular wall rather than being transmural.

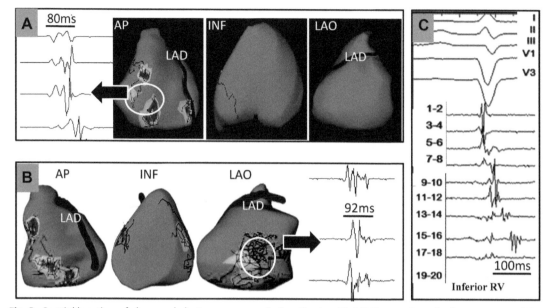

Fig. 3. Spatial location of abnormal electrogram areas in 3 patients with IVF. Two patients had spontaneous (*A*) or induced (*B*) sustained VF, with VF drivers mapped using body surface mapping. The trajectories of unstable and stable reentries are shown by the blue curves and red areas, respectively in 3 views, whereby the anterior view shows the right ventricle and the left anterior oblique view shows the left ventricle. The abnormal signals recorded in sinus rhythm during epicardial mapping are present within the white dotted contours, which collocated with a dominant area of VF reentries, in the epicardial right (*B*) or left (*C*) ventricle. All other ventricular regions show narrow signals indicating healthy underlying tissue. Case C had no VF inducible by electrical stimulation. An area of prolonged and late electrograms was detected in the epicardial inferior right ventricle. AP, anteroposterior; LAD, left anterior descending; LAO, left anterior oblique; RV, right ventricle.

This aspect may explain why the abnormalities were unperceived by MRI. The reexamination of imaging data or retesting with ajmaline failed to identify structural abnormality or Brugada syndrome.

Among all abnormal areas, 86% colocalized within or at the border of a main driver region (see **Fig. 3**). This finding indicates that the mechanism of VF is linked to microstructural alterations acting as a substrate maintaining reentry, in the same way as overt structural heterogeneities maintain VF in SHDs.

SPECTRUM OF IDIOPATHIC VENTRICULAR FIBRILLATION SUBSTRATES

The phenotypic screening performed in 48 consecutive patients referred for IVF concluded that 11 patients (23%) presented a Purkinje abnormality without microstructural myocardial abnormality, 32 patients (67%) presented microstructural myocardial abnormalities, and 5 of them also having Purkinje triggers. Five patients had no apparent Purkinje or microstructural abnormality. Therefore, only 10% of IVF remained unexplained after comprehensive

investigations. Unexplained SCD may result from an external ephemeris factor (as fever, vagal burst, hypokalemia, etc) necessary to reach a critical arrhythmogenic threshold and concealed causes such as long QT syndromes, Purkinje or microstructural abnormality etc., which may become detectable during follow-up or by genetic testing using genome wide sequencing (see **Box 1**).

The differentiation of IVF depending on Purkinje or myocardial dominant substrates has implications in terms of pathogenesis, diagnostic, genetics, and therapy. It is likely that both common and distinct diseases are involved in these different substrates and that a spectrum of different diseases such as genetic, inflammatory, or acquired cardiomyopathies can affect them. Improvements in imaging or electrophysiologic methods may be implemented in the future to identify the myocardial arrhythmogenic substrate before the occurrence of SCD. In terms of genetic predisposition, mutations in genes coding for specific Purkinje proteins versus genes coding for structural myocardial proteins may be differentiated as well as the interpretation of gene variants within the GWAS database, depending on the individual phenotype. Finally, in addition to Purkinje trigger ablation, the capability to identify localized structural alterations allows substrate ablation targeting the fragmented electrograms, such as in Brugada syndrome or SHDs.

Inferolateral J-Wave Syndromes

Early repolarization indicates a distinct electrocardiographic phenotype affecting the junction (J-wave) between the QRS complex and the ST segment in inferolateral leads. It was initially described as a benign ECG finding or in association with hypothermia.[24] Subsequently, many conditions producing this phenotype have been described such as hypercalcemia, acute ischemia, brain injury, and others.[25] The link with an increased risk of arrhythmic death was demonstrated in sporadic cases and in case-control studies of unexplained SCD then finally in association with various types of SHD.[26–32] The later section reviews most recent mapping data in humans, which provide evidence for heterogeneity of substrates, which underlie inferolateral J-wave syndromes. For a comprehensive review of risk stratification and clinical management of J-wave syndromes the readers are guided to other articles.[33–35]

Diagnosis of early repolarization and inferolateral J-wave syndromes

Expert consensus recommendations[33] defined the syndrome (the term indicating symptomatic patients) as follows: (1) the presence of J-point elevation greater than or equal to 1 mm in greater than or equal to 2 contiguous inferior and/or lateral leads of a standard 12-lead ECG in a patient resuscitated from otherwise unexplained VF; (2) an SCD victim with a negative autopsy and medical chart review with a previous ECG demonstrating J-point elevation greater than or equal to 1 mm in greater than or equal to 2 contiguous inferior and/or lateral leads of a standard 12-lead ECG. The ECG pattern (asymptomatic subjects) is defined by a distinct J-wave or J-point elevation greater than or equal to 1 mm that is a notch or a slur, with or without ST-segment elevation.

This definition may be sometimes ambiguous owing to the small amplitude and spontaneous changes of the J-wave. Strong inspiration or Valsalva maneuvers can amplify J-wave possibly by changing the heart shape and position relative to the chest. The dynamic changes in J-waves during cycle-length prolongation, either unchanged pattern or amplification, are an important sign to evaluate, as it relates to the individual substrate underlying the J-wave.

High-density mapping of the J-wave

In contrast to experimental wedge models focusing on repolarization abnormalities,[31] recent high-density electrogram mapping in humans both in vivo and ex vivo experimental conditions provide evidence that a spectrum of heterogeneous substrates, related either to delayed depolarization or to early repolarization abnormalities, underlie inferolateral J-wave syndromes.

Clinical mapping data have been collected from patients with inferolateral J-wave syndrome in 3 centers.[36] These patients had no apparent SHD on MRI, and most were referred for VF recurring despite antiarrhythmic drugs including quinidine. A J-wave syndrome combined with a Brugada syndrome was observed in a subset, either spontaneously or with sodium channel blocker. High-density endocardial and epicardial (2000–6000 recorded points) electrograms were performed during sinus rhythm in bipolar and unipolar mode. A specific attention was paid to the electrograms coincident with the timing of J-wave. The electrograms occurring within the J-wave were considered as belonging to depolarization if they were in temporal continuity of the surrounding depolarization field and sharp. They were considered as indicating ventricular repolarization if there was no continuity with surrounding depolarization electrograms and a slow pattern (hump) in unipolar mode.[37,38]

J-wave due to delayed depolarization abnormality In patients referred with an isolated inferolateral J-wave syndrome, the J-wave was the expression of an area of delayed depolarization in the inferior part of ventricles in 15% to 30% of cases (depending on the inclusion center), whereas an early repolarization was the cause of J-wave in the others (70%–85%). The true prevalence of depolarization versus repolarization abnormality varied between the inclusion centers and was also biased as the patients could be referred after quinidine failure, which may have selected more patients with delayed depolarization. Delayed-depolarization J-waves were recorded at the sites of terminal activation in the right ventricle or left ventricle. Most of the abnormal electrograms are found in epicardium, whereas 3 patients had abnormal electrograms recorded endocardially and epicardially. The terminology of early repolarization here is erroneous and "inferolateral J-wave" is more appropriate. An example of a late depolarization J-wave is shown in **Fig. 4.**

In contrast, in the patients with combined J-wave and Brugada syndrome, J-wave was consistently caused by a delayed depolarization.

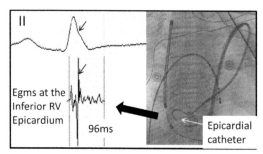

Fig. 4. A case of inferolateral J-wave syndrome due to abnormal depolarization. Epicardial depolarization in the inferobasal right ventricle occurs at the J-wave onset (*small arrow*) and is prolonged by low-voltage fragmented electrograms coincident with the J-wave body. Fluoroscopic anterior view shows the recording of circular 20-pole catheter in the epicardial infero-basal right ventricle and an endocardial decapolar catheter along the septum. ER, early repolarization.

The abnormal electrograms were recorded in infe-rior right ventricle and similar to those in the RVOT, suggesting structural alteration from the same pathogenesis. The absence of ST elevation in infe-rior leads, in contrast to V1-V2 leads, may be due to specific properties of the RVOT tissue, more prone to develop marked repolarization changes secondary to altered depolarization.[39–42]

Ajmaline testing was performed in all patients of the cohort and resulted in J-wave amplification or ST elevation in the inferior leads in only 5 patients. All 5 patients had a delayed depolarization, whereas no patient with early repolarization had J/ST wave amplification on Ajmaline.

The results mentioned earlier are in keeping with the high prevalence of J-waves described in various cardiomyopathies including noncom-paction or arrhythmogenic right ventricular cardiomyopathies. In this context, it is likely that most of the J-waves express delayed depolarization.

J-wave due to early repolarization In this subset of patients there was no depolarization electro-gram coincident with J-wave, but low-frequency signals (hump) were present particularly in unipolar recordings. Electrocardiographically, the increase of J-waves during cycle-length prolongation was likely the most specific sign associated with early repolarization syndrome (**Fig. 5**).

The early repolarization potentials were domi-nantly located epicardially in the inferior septum and adjacent left ventricle including the regions of papillary muscles.

The J-wave mechanism is likely here a voltage gradient across the ventricular wall during early phase of repolarization, as shown by Antzelevitch and Yan.[31] However, the current clinical mapping

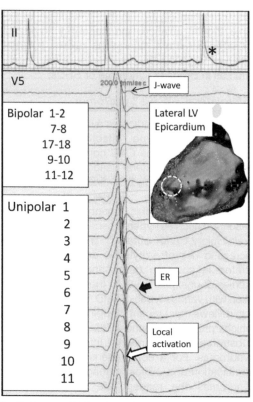

Fig. 5. A case of inferolateral J-wave syndrome due to early repolarization syndrome. The ECG shows J-wave amplification occurring in the third beat (*asterisk*) following a longer cycle length. Electrograms are re-corded during epicardial mapping within the white dotted contour. Bipolar and unipolar recordings show the sharp local depolarization coincident with the very onset of J-wave (*vertical line*). The electrocar-diographic J-wave is coincident with low-frequency ("ER") signals in unipolar recordings 1 to 11, which cover the entire half-inferior surface of left ventricle in this patient.

techniques do not allow to measure repolarization parameters precisely and to demonstrate a gradient of repolarization or a phase 2 reentry. In patients with spontaneous VF initiation, the au-thors found an important triggering role of the Pur-kinje system further confirmed by favorable outcome after ablation (**Fig. 6**).

J-wave in human optical mapping In order to elucidate the substrates underlying J-wave syndrome, the authors' team had the unique opportunity to investigate human hearts with electrocardiographic J-wave patterns obtained through an organ donor program at the Univer-sity Hospital. Epi- and endocardial optical mapping and microelectrode recordings were performed on either the left or the right ventricle. In one subject, the J-wave phenotype

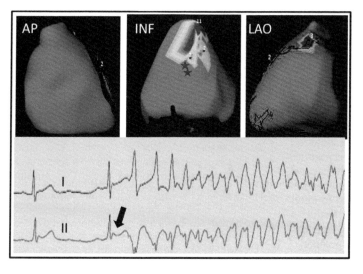

Fig. 6. Location of VF reentries in a 14-year-old patient with early repolarization (*arrow*). Noninvasive mapping is performed during the initial 2 seconds following spontaneous initiation of VF (ECG shown). The initial 2 beats seem as focal breakthroughs (2 *red stars*), whereas the subsequent 15 beats seem as reentries (in *red*) clustered in the inferior septal area (inferior view). The latter (epicardial) location is compatible with an exit from the (endocardial) left posterior Purkinje fascicle. INF, inferior.

was due to delayed conduction in the LV basal region with 80% activation time prolongation compared with control (*P*<.05) and was exacerbated with increasing pacing frequency. For the other 2 subjects (who were siblings), J-waves increased during bradycardia and were associated with a heterogeneous increase of the action potential notch (phase 1 repolarization) and

delayed action potential plateau on the right and/or left ventricular endocardium, but not epicardium, with no associated conduction abnormalities. These unique human heart data demonstrate that a variety of individual conduction and repolarization substrates, not limited to the epicardium, can underlie J-wave syndromes in humans.[15]

	Conduction Abnormality	Repolarization Abnormality	Excitation Abnormality
Primary VF substrate	Structural abnormality - Heterogeneity of depolarization	Electrical abnormality - heterogeneity of repolarization	Rapid or multifocal ectopic activity
Diagnostic	*Localized prolonged depolarization*	*Repolarization parameters*	*Consistent Ectopy at arrhythmia initiation and no myocardial abnormality*
Type	Brugada syndrome Inferolateral J wave IVF with localized structural abnormality	Long QT Early repolarization Short QT	IVF from Purkinje or myocardial foci Catecholaminergic Polymorphic VT Accidental : Commotio cordis, electrocution, drugs ..
Therapy	*Ablation*	*Drugs*	*Drugs or Ablation*

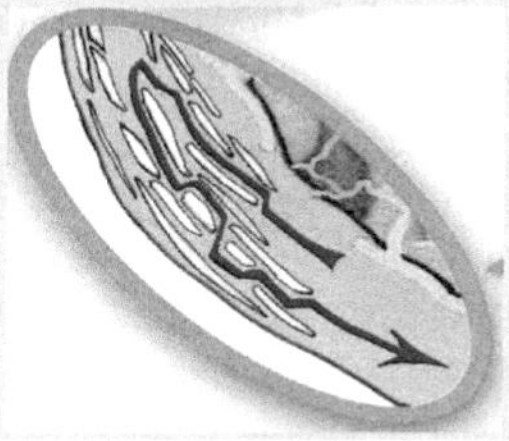

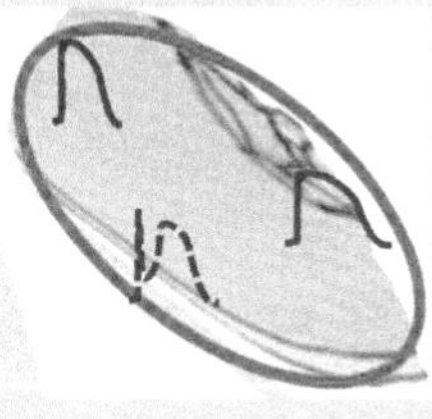

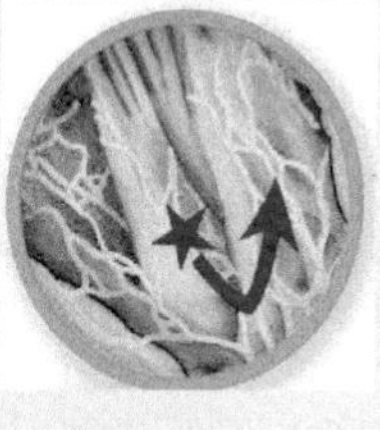

Fig. 7. The spectrum of arrhythmogenic diseases leading to SCD in apparently normal hearts, in 3 categories, based on the primary pathogenesis.

SUMMARY

The present review shows that arrhythmogenic diseases leading to SCD in apparently normal hearts may be underlined by fundamentally different substrates despite similar ECG phenotypes (such as J-wave) or the absence of phenotype (IVF).

An important category is emerging in which the primary substrates maintaining VF are localized depolarization abnormalities due to microstructural myocardial alterations. Their pathogenesis is potentially of multiple causes, altering myocardial cells or their connections or leading to intervening fibrotic, inflammatory, or fatty tissue. A common feature of these substrates is that they constitute a target for efficient catheter ablation.

In a second category of SCD with structurally normal hearts, the primary VF substrates are repolarization abnormalities (long/short or early repolarization) for which drugs are the most appropriate therapy. In a third category the arrhythmia, mechanism seems dominated by "focal" activities from Purkinje or myocardial origin, such as catecholaminergic polymorphic ventricular tachycardia or a subset of IVF. This simplified classification (**Fig. 7**) does not exclude overlapping mechanisms. It puts together arrhythmogenic diseases, which are clinically distinct but share similar modes of pathogenesis and therapy, and potentially common genetic variants.

REFERENCES

1. Fishman GI, Chugh SS, Dimarco JP, et al. Sudden cardiac death prediction and prevention: report from a National Heart, Lung, and Blood Institute and Heart Rhythm Society Workshop. Circulation 2010;122:2335–48.
2. Priori SG, Blomström-Lundqvist C, Mazzanti A. 2015 ESC Guidelines for the management of patients with ventricular arrhythmias and the prevention of sudden cardiac death. Eur.Heart J 2015;36:2793–867.
3. Murakoshi N, Aonuma K. Epidemiology of arrhythmias and sudden cardiac death in Asia. Circ J 2013;77:2419–31.
4. Al-Khatib SM, Stevenson WG, Ackerman MJ, et al. 2017 AHA/ACC/HRS guideline for management of patients with ventricular arrhythmias and the prevention of sudden cardiac death. Heart Rhythm 2018; 15(10):e190–252.
5. Visser M, van der Heijden JF, Doevendans PA, et al. Idiopathic ventricular fibrillation: the Struggle for definition, diagnosis, and follow-up. Circ Arrhythm Electrophysiol 2016;9:e003817.
6. Eckart R, Shry EA, Burke AP, et al. Sudden death in young adults. An autopsy-based series of a population undergoing active surveillance. J Am Coll Cardiol 2011;58:1254–61.
7. Winkel BG, Holst AG, Theilade J J, et al. Nationwide study of sudden cardiac death in persons aged 1-35 years. Eur Heart J 2011;32:983–90.
8. Bagnall RD, Weintraub RG, Ingles J J, et al. A prospective study of sudden cardiac death among children and young adults. N Engl J Med 2016;374:2441–52.
9. Haissaguerre M, Hocini M, Cheniti G, et al. Localized structural alterations underlying a subset of unexplained sudden cardiac death. Circ Arrhythm Electrophysiol 2018;11:e006120.
10. Gray RG, Pertsov AM, Jalife J. Spatial and temporal organization during cardiac fibrillation. Nature 1998; 392:75–8.
11. Nash MP, Mourad A, Clayton RH, et al. Evidence for multiple mechanisms in human ventricular fibrillation. Circulation 2016;114:536–42.
12. Torkamani A A, Muse ED, Spencer EG, et al. Molecular autopsy for sudden unexpected death. JAMA 2016;316:1492–4.
13. Krahn AD, Healey JS, Chauhan V. Systematic assessment of patients with unexplained cardiac arrest: cardiac arrest survivors with preserved ejection fraction registry (CASPER). Circulation 2009;120: 278–85.
14. Viskin S, Lesh MD, Eldar M, et al. Mode of onset of malignant ventricular arrhythmias in idiopathic ventricular fibrillation. J Cardiovasc Electrophysiol 1997;8(10):1115–20.
15. Haissaguerre M, Vigmond E, Stuyvers B, et al. Ventricular arrhythmias and the His-Purkinje system. Nat Rev Cardiol 2016;13:155–66.
16. Wilde AAM, Garan H, Boyden PA. Role of the Purkinje system in heritable arrhythmias. Heart Rhythm 2019;16:1121–6.
17. Haissaguerre M, Cheniti G, Escande W, et al. Idiopathic ventricular fibrillation associated with repetitive activity inducible within the distal Purkinje system. Heart Rhythm 2019. https://doi.org/10.1016/j.hrthm. 2019.04.012 [pii:S1547-5271(19)30312-1].
18. Nair K, Umapathy K, Farid T. Intramural activation during early human ventricular fibrillation. Circ Arrhythm Electrophysiol 2011;4:692–703.
19. Hsia H, Callans DJ, Marchlinski FE. Characterization of endocardial electrophysiological substrate in patients with nonischemic cardiomyopathy and monomorphic ventricular tachycardia. Circulation 2003; 108:704–10.
20. Soejima K, Stevenson WG, Sapp JL, et al. Endocardial and epicardial radiofrequency ablation of ventricular tachycardia associated with dilated cardiomyopathy: the importance of low-voltage scars. J Am Coll Cardiol 2004;43:1834–41.
21. Cano O, Hutchinson M, Lin D. Electroanatomic substrate and ablation outcome for suspected

epicardial left ventricular tachycardia in non-ischemic cardiomyopathy. J Am Coll Cardiol 2009; 54:799–808.

22. Janse MJ, Kléber AG. Electrophysiological changes and ventricular arrhythmias in the early phase of regional myocardial ischemia. Circ Res 1981;49: 1069–81.

23. Kubota I, Lux RL, Burgess MJ, et al. Activation sequence at the onset of arrhythmias induced by localized myocardial warming and programmed premature stimulation in dogs. J Electrocardiol 1988;21:345–54.

24. Tomaszewski W. Changements electrocardiographiques observes chez un homme mort de froid. Arch Mal Cœur 1938;31:525–8.

25. Gussak I, Antzelevitch C. Early repolarization syndrome: clinical characteristics and possible cellular and ionic mechanisms. J Electrocardiol 2000;33: 299–309.

26. Otto CM, Tauxe RV, Cobb LA, et al. Ventricular fibrillation causes sudden death in southeast Asian immigrants. Ann Intern Med 1984;101:45–7.

27. Aizawa Y, Tamura M, Chinushi M, et al. Idiopathic ventricular fibrillation and bradycardia-dependent intraventricular block. Am Heart J 1993;126:1473–4.

28. Haissaguerre M, Derval N, Sacher F, et al. Sudden cardiac arrest associated with early repolarization. N Engl J Med 2008;358:2016–23.

29. Tikkanen JT, Anttonen O, Junttila MJ, et al. Long-term outcome associated with early repolarization on electrocardiography. N Engl J Med 2009;361: 2529–37.

30. Rosso R, Kogan E, Belhassen B, et al. J-point elevation in survivors of primary ventricular fibrillation and matched control subjects: incidence and clinical significance. J Am Coll Cardiol 2008;52:1231–8.

31. Antzelevitch C, Yan GX. J-wave syndromes: Brugada and early repolarization syndromes. Heart Rhythm 2015;12:1852–66.

32. Macfarlane PW, Antzelevitch C, Haissaguerre M, et al. The early repolarization pattern: a consensus paper. J Am Coll Cardiol 2015;66:470–7.

33. Viskin S, Rosso R, Halkin A. Making sense of early repolarization. Heart Rhythm 2012;9:566–9.

34. Obeyesekere N, Krahn AD. Early repolarization – what should the clinician do? Arrhythm Electrophysiol Rev 2015;4:96–9.

35. Nademanee K, Haissaguerre M, Hocini M, et al. Ventricular Fibrillation substrates and Electrophysiological Abnormalities In Early Repolarization Syndrome: A Tale Of Two Phenotypes. HRS San francisco. Heart Rhythm Scientific Sessions S-PO01-131. 2019.

36. Haissaguerre M, Nademanee W, Hocini M, et al. Depolarization versus repolarization abnormality underlying inferolateral J wave syndromes–new concepts in sudden cardiac death with apparently normal hearts. Heart Rhythm 2018;16(5):781–90.

37. Boineau J. The early repolarization variant-an electrocardiographic enigma with both QRS and J-STT anomalies. J Electrocardiol 2007;40:3.e1-10.

38. Coronel R, Casini S, Koopmann TT, et al. Right ventricular fibrosis and conduction delay in a patient with clinical signs of Brugada syndrome: a combined electrophysiological, genetic, histopathologic, and computational study. Circulation 2005;112: 2769–77.

39. Martini M, Nava A, Thiene G, et al. Ventricular fibrillation without apparent structural heart disease. Am Heart J 1989;118:1203–9.

40. Hoogendijk MG, Potse M, Linnenbank AC, et al. Mechanism of right precordial ST-segment elevation in structural heart disease: excitation failure by current-to-load mismatch. Heart Rhythm 2010;7: 238–48.

41. Benoist D, Charron S, Dubes VN, et al. Arrhythmogenic Molecular Substrate In The Healthy Right Ventricular Outflow Tract Heart Rhythm Scientific Sessions C-PO01-04. 2017.

42. Bernus O, Walton RD, Hof T, et al. A Wide Spectrum Of Substrates Underlie J-wave Syndromes In Humans. HRS chicago. Heart Rhythm Scientific Sessions S-MP13-05. 2019.

Challenges in Ablation of Complex Congenital Heart Disease

George F. Van Hare, MD

KEYWORDS

- Ablation • Congenital heart disease • Intra-atrial reentry • Fontan • Senning • Mustard
- Ventricular tachycardia

KEY POINTS

- The field of congenital cardiac electrophysiology is growing rapidly due to the rapid growth in the population of survivors of childhood critical congenital heart disease surgery.
- Chronic arrhythmias pose one of the biggest challenges in this patient population, and catheter ablation, despite its challenges, is still the most desirable and acceptable approach when successful.
- Clinicians who propose catheter ablation in such patients need to understand the congenital anatomy, should carefully review the details of all prior cardiac surgery, and should be prepared to deal with the various challenges posed by lack of normal cardiac access and the possibility of poor hemodynamics.
- Still, experienced laboratories can achieve excellent results in this difficult patient population.

One of the major accomplishments of pediatric cardiac surgical programs is the increasing expectation that children born with complex critical congenital heart disease can now be managed in a way that allows them to survive into adulthood.[1] Surgical management involves closure of septal defects, relief of obstructions, placement of valves and conduits, and sometimes, palliative repair in situations of single ventricle or other severe and complex defects. For these children, generally the highest risk they face is at the time of initial repair, which now usually occurs in infancy. They are then managed throughout childhood, often requiring additional cardiac operations, particularly to manage the effects of growth on things like prosthetic valves and homograft conduits. In the modern era, aside from atrioventricular (AV) block and junctional tachycardia in the immediate postoperative period, arrhythmias tend not to be a large problem for the vast majority of these children. It is when they reach adulthood, however, that arrhythmias often become the most important problem that these patients face. This can be quite disappointing to families who may have come to believe that repair of the hemodynamic defects was the main hurdle they needed to overcome. Increasingly, the field of congenital cardiac electrophysiology has grown in prominence, along with the dramatic rise in patients living to adulthood, who then experience these late-developing arrhythmias. Many electrophysiology clinicians have found the conjunction of congenital anatomy, hemodynamic compromise, and unusual arrhythmias to be compelling and fascinating, and the number of practitioners in this field is growing rapidly.[2]

Disclosures: No pertinent disclosures.
Washington University School of Medicine, One Children's Place, Campus Box 8116, Saint Louis, MO 63110, USA
E-mail address: vanhare@wustl.edu

The management of these arrhythmias certainly may involve long-term antiarrhythmic medication, and for some patients, repair of residual hemodynamic abnormalities is important as well, because residual defects can exacerbate arrhythmias in patients with these substrates. Likewise, there is increasing interest in surgical management of these arrhythmias, particularly when such a surgical approach to arrhythmia management can be combined with correction of hemodynamic defects. For example, in the situation of a patient with an atriopulmonary connection Fontan for single ventricle, who is having surgical revision to a more hemodynamically favorable external conduit Fontan, arrhythmia surgery also can be accomplished via an atrial Maze procedure.[3] However, catheter ablation holds particular appeal as a method of definitively dealing with a chronic arrhythmia, without resorting to sternotomy or lifelong antiarrhythmic medications. Catheter ablation in this setting, however, poses a number of significant challenges, which this article reviews. These challenges can be subdivided into those related to congenital anatomy, the potential for preexisting substrates, along with the understanding the ways in which surgical repair creates the substrate for arrhythmia, difficulties with access to the heart, and finally the contribution of natural history to decision-making when managing such patients.

CHALLENGES RELATED TO CONGENITAL ANATOMY

Any proposed ablation procedure needs to proceed from a thorough understanding of the cardiac anatomy present. In complex congenital heart disease, there is a seeming endless variety of malformations that may be encountered. The most extreme of these arguably are the heterotaxy syndromes in which one may encounter dextrocardia, mesocardia, situs inversus, AV canal defects, single ventricles of either right or left ventricular morphology, and valve malformations, including Ebstein anomaly. In addition, the great majority of patients suffering from arrhythmias will have undergone some type of cardiac repair, and the details of those repairs are critically important in understanding both likely substrate for arrhythmia and the subsequent approach to ablation. Furthermore, critical structures are often not where they would normally be expected, and this includes locations and sidedness of great vessels and caval veins, coronary arteries, and notably, the AV conducting tissue. Avoiding the complication of inadvertent AV block is particularly important in these patients, as long-term pacing may not be available via the transvenous route, and

may not be well tolerated by whatever route pacing is accomplished.[4]

ATRIOVENTRICULAR CONDUCTION SYSTEM ANATOMY

There are several important details about AV conduction anatomy that must be remembered. First, for patients with so-called congenitally corrected transposition, also known as L-transposition or ventricular inversion, there is an increased rate of spontaneous development of complete AV block, thought to be due to fragility of the conduction system related to the long course it must take the ventricles due to AV malalignment. The conduction system arises more superiorly than in a normal heart and is more prone to injury. In patients with AV canal defects, the compact AV node is not in the usual septal location, as that portion of the septum never formed embryologically, and instead, is found in close proximity to the mouth of the coronary sinus. This poses the particular hazard of inadvertent AV block during procedures such as posterior septal accessory pathway ablation, slow pathway ablation in AV nodal reentry tachycardia (AVNRT), and cavotricuspid isthmus flutter ablation.[5]

Superimposed on these congenital structural cardiac abnormalities will be surgically created lines of block, as most such patients will have undergone surgical repair of some type. We now understand that the propensity for cardiac arrhythmias following cardiac surgical repair is largely the result of a macroreentry circuits, which use both preexisting anatomic obstacles and surgically created obstacles in long reentrant circuits. Although the tendency to develop sustained atrial or ventricular tachycardia is certainly influenced by adverse hemodynamics, it is the long incisions that most likely play the most important part in creating these large reentrant circuits.

Clearly any clinician who plans catheter ablation in a patient with complex congenital heart disease needs to understand both the preexisting congenital cardiac anatomy along with the details of prior surgery. It is often helpful to review original operative reports, if available, so that the details of cardiac incisions, suture lines, and baffle are understood before embarking on the procedure.

THE OCCURRENCE OF PREEXISTING SUBSTRATES

Although a large amount of the focus in arrhythmias in repaired congenital heart disease is related to the effects of prior surgery, it should not be forgotten that common tachyarrhythmias also can occur in this patient population. Arrhythmias such as AVNRT and accessory pathway tachycardia can certainly be seen, and when that happens, the congenital anatomy may present particular challenges related to access and avoidance of complications. An example is when AVNRT occurs in a patient following the Mustard or Senning procedure for d-transposition of the great arteries. In this circumstance, generally access to the pulmonary venous atrium is required to access the region of the slow pathway and this can be done either retrograde or by transseptal approach.

The Ebstein anomaly deserves special mention. Isolated Ebstein anomaly poses specific challenges that have been well reported. There is a high incidence of Wolff-Parkinson-Shite syndrome (WPW) and concealed accessory pathways in patients with this condition, which are often multiple, and the abnormal anatomy poses particular challenges in achieving stable catheter contact as well as interpretation of electrograms due to prominent fractionation related to the presence of atrialized right ventricle.[6] It should be remembered as well that there is a high incidence of Ebstein anomaly in patients with congenitally corrected transposition, and in that situation, because the tricuspid valve is the left-sided systemic AV valve, the Ebstein anomaly is on the left side of the heart. Ablation of pathways in that location will require access to the left atrium via a preexisting atrial septal defect or by a transseptal approach, or alternatively by a retrograde approach to the left-sided systemic right ventricle.

One completely unique arrhythmia substrate seen in complex congenital heart disease is so-called "duplicated AV conduction systems." This is seen in heterotaxy patients, typically those with AV discordance and AV canal defects, in whom there may be 2 separate AV nodes and His bundles.[7] Reentry can occur between the 2 conduction systems and appears as AV reciprocating tachycardia with a somewhat long ventriculoatrial (VA) time. Electrophysiologically, these act very much like Mahaim pathways, in that the QRS morphology changes depending on which conduction system is engaged.

CHALLENGES RELATED TO ACCESS

Preexisting venous anomalies that create challenges for access include such variations as interruption of the inferior vena cava with azygos continuation to the superior vena cava (SVC), or persistent left SVC to the coronary sinus connection. Surgically created access issues include, most importantly, the various forms of the Fontan procedure in which all systemic venous return is routed directly to the pulmonary arteries, preventing access to the ventricle as well as most of the atrial mass, depending on the type of repair. Finally, isolated venous obstructions can exist due to a history of indwelling lines, permanent pacing leads, and frequent cardiac catheterizations. These can be severe and may include complete obstruction of the inferior vena cava (IVC) or narrowing of the SVC. All of these variations present challenges when planning an ablation procedure and should be detected before a procedure, by echocardiography, MRI, or computed tomography angiography, or careful review of the surgical history. Novel and creative approaches may be needed. For example, in patients who have undergone the Fontan procedure, access to the heart via perforation of the baffle is commonly described,[8] but the ventricle may also be approached by a retrograde catheter course from the aorta to the ventricle, crossing the semilunar valve. Rarely, direct transthoracic access may be used. This approach has the advantage of delivering the catheter directly into the atrium from the chest and is notable for the easy maneuverability of the catheter via this approach. The use of this approach, of course, carries with it some risk of intrathoracic bleeding. Finally, for patients who have lost femoral venous access due to thrombosis, or occasionally in Fontan patients, access to the heart may be gained via transhepatic access.[9]

EFFECT OF NATURAL HISTORY

In the moderate era, most patients with significant congenital heart disease can now be expected to survive many decades, and so definitive treatment catheter ablation is attractive as an alternative to lifelong antiarrhythmic medication. In addition, the cardiologist needs to be aware that the development of serious arrhythmias is often delayed into adulthood, most likely due to the cumulative effect of suboptimal hemodynamics over years. For example, the incidence of ventricular tachycardia and sudden death after repair of tetralogy of Fallot is low in childhood but increases dramatically beyond 20 to 25 years after initial repair. Specific risk factors can be assessed in such patients, and include indices of right ventricular function and dilation, QRS duration, left ventricular systolic or diastolic dysfunction, and the occurrence of either spontaneous ventricular tachycardia or its inducibility in the electrophysiology laboratory.[10] Similarly, intra-atrial reentry is often diagnosed in adults who have undergone repair of more simple cardiac defects, such as atrial septal defect, in childhood. Finally, atrial fibrillation is increasingly being recognized and managed with ablation technology in adults with repaired congenital heart disease, and it appears earlier than in adults without a history of congenital heart disease surgery.[11]

SPECIFIC SURGICALLY-CREATED ARRHYTHMIA SUBSTRATES
Intra-atrial Reentry Tachycardia

One of the most common postoperative arrhythmias seen in patients following congenital heart disease (CHD) surgery is atrial flutter, also known as intra-atrial reentry tachycardia (IART). It is now well understood that in most cases, this is in fact a rhythm that uses both surgically created and preexisting anatomic obstacles that act to constrain atrial activation and that define the macroreentry pathway.[12] In many cases, the resulting arrhythmia is quite similar to common atrial flutter, in that it uses the cavotricuspid isthmus as a critical isthmus. In this situation, the atriotomy that was used to perform the repair (of atrial septal defect, ventricular septal defect [VSD], AV canal, or tetralogy of Fallot) substitutes for the crista terminalis as the long line of block supporting reentry. In this circumstance, approaching ablation using standard techniques for common atrial flutter

is reasonable. In other patients, with long atriotomies, the reentrant circuit is entirely incisional, as it in fact orbits the atriotomy and does not involve the cavotricuspid isthmus as a critical isthmus.[12] Finally, patients who have had left atriotomy can experience left atrial flutter that orbits the mitral annulus. In all these circumstances, the approach to ablation typically involves a combination of electroanatomic mapping to define possible target isthmus, combined with entrainment techniques to confirm the involvement of a proposed ablation target has a critical isthmus supporting tachycardia. In the case of incisional reentry, around the right atrial incision, this critical isthmus often is between the inferior end of the atriotomy and either the IVC or the tricuspid annulus depending on the placement of the atriotomy. Standard techniques should be used to document the achievement of bidirectional block in such patients following ablation. It is well known of that simple termination of tachycardia during application of energy is an insufficient criterion, to minimize the chances of clinical recurrence. Finally, as atrial tissue is sometimes quite thick, the use of irrigated tip radiofrequency ablation is advisable in these patients.[13]

A particular special case that deserves mention is IART occurring in patients following either the Senning or the Mustard procedure for

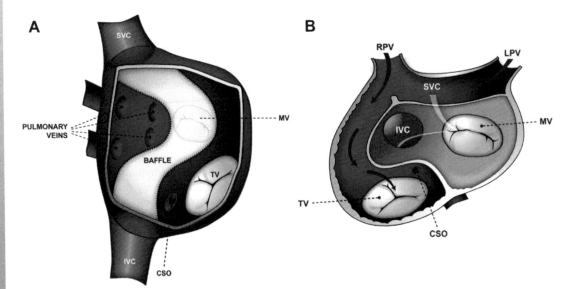

Fig. 1. Cavotricuspid isthmus in D-TGA with Mustard (*A*) or Senning (*B*) baffles. (*A, B*) A right anterior oblique view of a Mustard baffle and axial view of a Senning baffle are schematically depicted, respectively. Systemic venous return via the superior (SVC) and inferior (IVC) vena cavae are directed toward the mitral valve (MV), whereas pulmonary venous return is oriented toward the tricuspid valve (TV). Note that the cavotricuspid isthmus is divided in 2, with the IVC portion on the systemic and TV portion on the pulmonary venous side of the circulation. CSO, coronary sinus ostium; D-TGA, complete transposition of the great arteries; LPV, left pulmonary vein; RPV, right pulmonary vein. (*From* Khairy P, Van Hare GF. Catheter ablation in transposition of the great arteries with Mustard or Senning baffles. Heart Rhythm. 2009 Feb;6(2):283-9, with permission.)

A

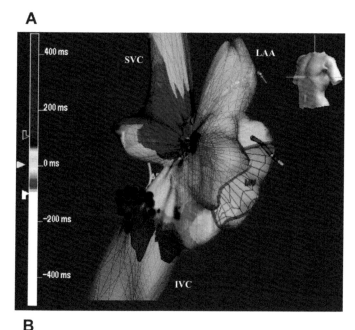

B

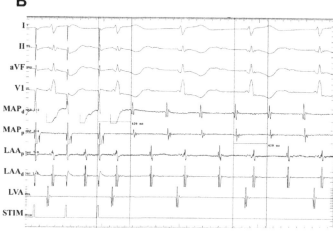

Fig. 2. Electroanatomic and entrainment mapping of IART in a patient with D-TGA and a Mustard baffle. (*A*) A left anterior oblique view of an electroanatomic map of the systemic venous atrium. Local activation times are color-coded, from white to red, orange, yellow, green, light blue, dark blue, and purple. Along the septal portion of the baffle, the wavefront propagates from a superior to inferior direction. The systemic venous atrium contained approximately half of the 428-m tachycardia cycle length, as estimated by subtracting the earliest from the latest activation times on the scale shown on the left. This activation sequence and incomplete circuit within the systemic venous atrium was compatible with the patient's clockwise circuit around the left-sided tricuspid valve. Brown circles indicate ablation lesions in the pulmonary venous portion of the cavotricuspid isthmus. (*B*) Recordings from surface electrocardiograph leads I, II, aVF, and V1; distal (MAP$_d$) and proximal (MAP$_p$) ablation catheter on the systemic venous portion of the cavotricuspid isthmus; proximal (LAA$_p$) and distal (LAA$_d$) left atrial appendage; and left ventricular apex (LVA). A stimulation (STIM) channel is also shown. Entrainment with concealed fusion occurs by pacing from the ablation catheter at 410 ms at a site in the IART circuit associated with a post-pacing interval of 420 ms, equivalent to the tachycardia cycle length. D-TGA, complete transposition of the great arteries; MV, mitral valve. (*From* Khairy P, Van Hare GF. Catheter ablation in transposition of the great arteries with Mustard or Senning baffles. Heart Rhythm. 2009 Feb;6(2):283-9, with permission.)

d-transposition of the great arteries (**Figs. 1** and **2**). Although that operation is no longer performed, there are many adults living with this surgical repair and atrial arrhythmias may be life-threatening in them. Because of the details of surgical anatomy, both the cavotricuspid isthmus and the long right atriotomy are in the pulmonary venous portion of the baffle, and access to these areas is not straightforward. One may approach the pulmonary venous atrium either with a retrograde catheter course to the systemic right ventricle retroflexing across the tricuspid valve into the pulmonary venous atrium, or alternatively via puncture of the baffle by a modified transseptal technique.[14]

In general, success rates are high for all but the most complex forms of atrial surgery, but success rates have been fairly disappointing for the atriopulmonary connection form of the Fontan procedure. This is most likely due to the thickness of the atrial wall in such patients, along with multiple tachycardia circuits mediated by atrial scarring.

Ventricular Tachycardia in Tetralogy of Fallot and Related Defects

It is now well understood that the problem of sudden death in tetralogy patients late after repair is mainly related to the occurrence of macroreentrant ventricular tachycardia. As is the case with atrial arrhythmias, macroreentrant ventricular tachycardia is made possible through a combination of surgically created and naturally occurring barriers to impulse propagation that define the reentrant circuit. As in atrial arrhythmias, hemodynamic changes tend to encourage the development of these arrhythmias, and in tetralogy, this is mainly related to chronic pulmonary insufficiency with resulting right ventricular dilation and, presumably, conduction delay. Zeppenfeld and colleagues[15] have defined 4 critical isthmuses (**Fig. 3**) that are created surgically in most tetralogy patients and those with related conditions such as double outlet right ventricle and transposition with pulmonary stenosis. Induced arrhythmias can be shown to use these isthmuses, and catheter ablation directed to the sites is effective. Similar to the situation in atrial tachycardia, electroanatomic mapping is quite useful. However, in many cases, induced ventricular arrhythmias may not be well enough tolerated to allow entrainment mapping, and so clinicians usually rely on substrate mapping provided by electroanatomic mapping systems, paying particular attention to voltage mapping as a method of defining areas of scar or incision. Kapel, Zeppenfeld and colleagues[16] also

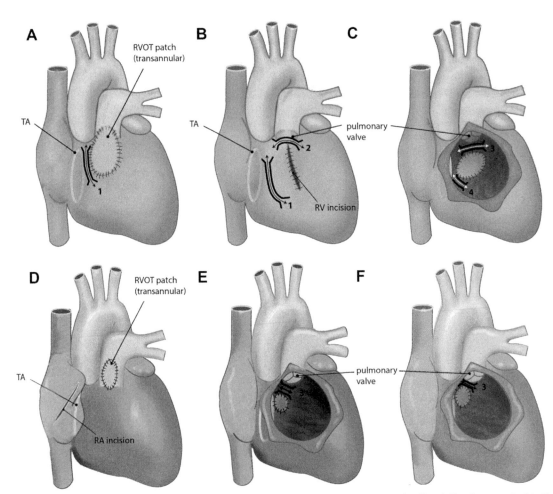

Fig. 3. Schematic overview of the 4 potential anatomic isthmuses in tetralogy of Fallot following repair. (*A–C*) Transventricular approach. Isthmus 1 bordered by tricuspid annulus (TA) and right ventricular outflow tract (RVOT) patch or RV incision, isthmus 2 by RV incision and pulmonary valve, and isthmus 3 by pulmonary valve and VSD patch. Isthmus 4 is bordered by VSD patch and TA but is only present in case of a subaortic VSD with muscular posteroinferior rim. (*D–F*) Transatrial-transpulmonary approach with small TA patch and VSD patch, preventing isthmuses 1 and 2. Isthmus 4 not shown. Anatomic isthmuses are labeled using black brackets. RA, right atrium. (*From* Brouwer C, Kapel GFL, Jongbloed MRM, Schalij MJ, de Riva Silva M, Zeppenfeld K. Noninvasive Identification of Ventricular Tachycardia-Related Anatomical Isthmuses in Repaired Tetralogy of Fallot: What Is the Role of the 12-Lead Ventricular Tachycardia Electrocardiogram. JACC Clin Electrophysiol. 2018: Oct;4(10):1308-1318, with permission.)

emphasized the importance of the outlet septum and the occurrence of slow conduction through this region as the final common pathway for most sustained ventricular tachycardia in these patients. They also drew attention to the occasional need to approach this part of the heart via a combined retrograde and antegrade approach given the thickness of the structure. Finally, the increasing use of transcatheter pulmonary valves (Melody, Sapien) particularly in native right ventricular outflow tracts raises a concern that obtaining access to this region in the future for ablation will be difficult.

Given the propensity for sudden death in adults following tetralogy of Fallot repair, the ability to successfully ablate a ventricular tachycardia substrate may not free the patient from a need for an implantable cardioverter defibrillator (ICD), particularly if other risk factors are present, such as left ventricular dysfunction. Indeed, most reported ablation procedures for ventricular tachycardia in tetralogy patients have been done following implantation of an ICD, after the occurrence of appropriate defibrillator therapy.

Approach to More Common Substrates

Supraventricular tachycardia is rather common in the adolescent and adult population, and so it may very well occur randomly in patients who have undergone repair of complex congenital heart disease. It is important that a careful diagnosis is made in such cases before moving to electroanatomic mapping and ablation attempts. For example, the most common form of supraventricular tachycardia (SVT), AVNRT, when seen in patients with the Mustard or the Senning procedure for transposition can masquerade as atrial tachycardia or flutter. It may well be necessary to establish a diagnosis with fewer than the usual complement of 4 intracardiac catheters in these situations. In addition, the typical location for slow pathway ablation in AVNRT will actually be on the pulmonary venous atrial side of the baffle in such patients, requiring either a retrograde or transseptal approach.[17]

Also of note is that patients with preexisting bundle branch block, such as those who have undergone successful repair of tetralogy, when presenting with supraventricular arrhythmias, will of course have a wide QRS. It is important not to be misled into thinking that the patient has ventricular tachycardia when in fact they simply have SVT or, commonly, IART in the presence of preexisting bundle branch block.

Atrial Fibrillation

Increasingly, as repaired patients with congenital heart disease age, atrial fibrillation begins to become a problem. A number of large adult congenital electrophysiology centers have begun to attack this problem, with some success, although success rates are not as high as in the noncongenital population. The congenital and surgical anatomy, of course, presents specific challenges and barriers to approaching the left atrium for the purpose of pulmonary vein isolation.[18]

Atrioventricular Junction Ablation

Although less frequently used in the noncongenital population, AV junction ablation for rate control in chronic atrial fibrillation with placement of a pacemaker is still a reasonable approach for specific patients, and is also a possibility for selected congenital patients experiencing refractory atrial arrhythmias who have failed, or are not candidates for, attempted catheter ablation of the substrate. One example may be persistent or poorly tolerated paroxysmal atrial fibrillation or atrial flutter. In such patients, placement of a pacemaker with ablation of the AV junction may be the most reasonable option, but carries with it some difficulties and hazards. First, as noted previously, the AV conduction system may not be located in its expected location because of the congenital anatomy. Second, transvenous pacing may not be reasonable due to access issues or intracardiac shunting, mandating an epicardial approach that of course will require a sternotomy or thoracotomy. These may be risky implantation procedures. Also of concern is the predictable decline in ventricular function that occurs when pacing is initiated in a patient who previously had narrow QRS complexes, due to dyssynchrony, and pacing may be very poorly tolerated. Before embarking on AV junction ablation for such patients, it would be important to assess their tolerance for chronic pacing, with consideration for multisite ventricular pacing to minimize dyssynchrony.

SUMMARY

The field of congenital cardiac electrophysiology is growing rapidly due to the rapid growth in the population of survivors of childhood critical congenital heart disease surgery. Chronic arrhythmias pose one of the biggest challenges in this patient population, and catheter ablation, despite its challenges, is still the most desirable and acceptable approach when successful. Clinicians who propose catheter ablation in such patients need to understand the congenital anatomy, should carefully review the details of all prior cardiac surgery, and should be prepared to deal with the various challenges posed by lack of normal cardiac access and the possibility of poor hemodynamics. Still, experienced laboratories can achieve excellent results in this difficult patient population.

REFERENCES

1. Stout KK, Daniels CJ, Aboulhosn JA, et al. 2018. AHA/ACC Guideline for the Management of Adults With Congenital Heart Disease: Executive Summary: A Report of the American College of Cardiology/ American Heart Association Task Force on Clinical Practice Guidelines. J Am Coll Cardiol 2019 Apr 2; 73(12):1494–563.

2. Khairy P, Van Hare GF, Balaji S, et al. PACES/HRS expert consensus statement on the recognition and management of arrhythmias in adult congenital heart disease: developed in partnership between the pediatric and congenital electrophysiology Society (PACES) and the Heart Rhythm Society (HRS). Endorsed by the governing bodies of PACES, HRS, the American College of Cardiology (ACC), the American Heart Association (AHA), the European Heart Rhythm Association (EHRA), the Canadian Heart Rhythm Society (CHRS), and the International Society for Adult Congenital Heart Disease (ISACHD). Heart Rhythm 2014;11(10):e102–65.

3. Mavroudis C, Stulak JM, Ad N, et al. Prophylactic atrial arrhythmia surgical procedures with congenital heart operations: review and recommendations. Ann Thorac Surg 2015;99(1):352–90.

4. Idriss SF. Ventricular pacing in single-ventricle complex congenital heart disease: how hard it is to achieve the ideal. JACC Clin Electrophysiol 2018; 4(10):1298–9.

5. Ávila P, Bessière F, Mondésert B, et al. Cryoablation for perinodal arrhythmia substrates in patients with congenital heart disease and displaced atrioventricular conduction systems. JACC Clin Electrophysiol 2018;4(10):1328–37.

6. Sherwin ED, Abrams DJ. Ebstein anomaly. Card Electrophysiol Clin 2017;9(2):245–54.

7. Epstein MR, Saul JP, Weindling SN, et al. Atrioventricular reciprocating tachycardia involving twin atrioventricular nodes in patients with complex congenital heart disease. J Cardiovasc Electrophysiol 2001;12(6):671–9.

8. Correa R, Walsh EP, Alexander ME, et al. Transbaffle mapping and ablation for atrial tachycardias after Mustard, Senning, or Fontan operations. J Am Heart Assoc 2013;2(5):e000325.

9. Shim D, Lloyd TR, Cho KJ, et al. Transhepatic cardiac catheterization in children. Evaluation of efficacy and safety. Circulation 1995;92(6): 1526–30.

10. Khairy P, Dore A, Poirier N, et al. Risk stratification in surgically repaired tetralogy of Fallot. Expert Rev Cardiovasc Ther 2009;7(7):755–62.

11. Labombarda F, Hamilton R, Shohoudi A, et al. Increasing prevalence of atrial fibrillation and permanent atrial arrhythmias in congenital heart disease. J Am Coll Cardiol 2017;70(7):857–65.

12. Kalman JM, Van Hare GF, Olgin JE, et al. Ablation of 'incisional' reentrant atrial tachycardia complicating surgery for congenital heart disease. Use of entrainment to define a critical isthmus of conduction. Circulation 1996;93(3):502–12.

13. Triedman JK, DeLucca JM, Alexander ME, et al. Prospective trial of electroanatomically guided, irrigated catheter ablation of atrial tachycardia in patients with congenital heart disease. Heart Rhythm 2005;2(7): 700–5.

14. Baysa SJ, Olen M, Kanter RJ. Arrhythmias following the Mustard and Senning operations for dextro-transposition of the great arteries: clinical aspects and catheter ablation. Card Electrophysiol Clin 2017;9(2):255–71.

15. Zeppenfeld K, Schalij MJ, Bartelings MM, et al. Catheter ablation of ventricular tachycardia after repair of congenital heart disease: electroanatomic identification of the critical right ventricular isthmus. Circulation 2007;116(20):2241–52.

16. Kapel GFL, Brouwer C, Jalal Z, et al. Slow conducting electroanatomic isthmuses: an important link between QRS duration and ventricular tachycardia in tetralogy of Fallot. JACC Clin Electrophysiol 2018;4(6):781–93.

17. Upadhyay S, Marie Valente A, Triedman JK, et al. Catheter ablation for atrioventricular nodal reentrant tachycardia in patients with congenital heart disease. Heart Rhythm 2016;13(6):1228–37.

18. Liang JJ, Frankel DS, Parikh V, et al. Safety and outcomes of catheter ablation for atrial fibrillation in adults with congenital heart disease: a multicenter registry study. Heart Rhythm 2019;16(6): 846–52.

Fluoroless Catheter Ablation of Cardiac Arrhythmias

Hany Demo, MD, FACC, FHRS[a], Cameron Willoughby, DO[b],
Mohammad-Ali Jazayeri, MD[c], Mansour Razminia, MD[d],*

KEYWORDS

• Fluoroless • Fluoroless ablation • Atrial fibrillation • Cryoablation • Intracardiac echo (ICE)

KEY POINTS

• Steps to perform fluoroless catheter ablation of cardiac arrhythmia.
• The role of intracardiac echocardiogram in fluoroless catheter ablation.
• Fluoroless transseptal access.
• Fluoroless cryoballoon ablation of atrial fibrillation.
• Esophageal temperature monitoring during cardiac ablation without the use of fluoroscopy.

INTRODUCTION

Catheter ablations of cardiac arrhythmias are traditionally performed using fluoroscopic guidance for catheter placement. It is well-established that radiation exposure increases the lifetime risk of malignancies, genetic defects, skin injuries, and cataracts.[1–6] In addition, long-term use of heavy protective lead aprons and other apparel is known to contribute to adverse orthopedic effects.[7] The duration of ablation procedures is variable depending on a number of factors, but on average the effective radiation dose was approximately 15 mSv, or the equivalent of 150 chest radiographs, in 1 study.[8] Other studies have estimated the cumulative radiation burden from 53 to 60 minutes of fluoroscopy during ablation procedures results in 0.7 to 1.4 fatal malignancies per 1000 women and 1.0 to 2.6 per 1000 men.[9,10] Although total fluoroscopy time is less accurate as a predictor of radiation-related malignancies when compared with the total radiation dose; nonetheless, strategies to decrease fluoroscopy time should be pursued in any laboratory seeking optimal safety for its users, including patients, physicians, and laboratory staff.

Newer imaging and mapping techniques have proven important to accomplishing this aim. Pulse fluoroscopy and optimization of fluoroscopy exposure parameters have also resulted in reduced radiation burden.[9] Recently, several studies have illustrated that nonfluoroscopic or "fluoroless" catheter ablation can be safely and effectively performed in adults with a variety of arrhythmias by relying only on intracardiac electrograms, electro-anatomic mapping (EAM), and, in most instances, intracardiac echocardiography (ICE) for catheter guidance.[11,12]

MAPPING SYSTEM

Fluoroless endocardial ablation is possible using most currently available EAM systems, rendering it feasible for a variety of operators. The mapping

[a] Swedish Covenant Hospital, 5140 North California Avenue Suite 780, Chicago, IL 60625, USA; [b] McLaren Health-Macomb Campus, 21550 Harrington Boulevard, Suite C, Clinton Township, MI 48036, USA; [c] Department of Cardiovascular Medicine, University of Kansas Medical Center, 3901 Rainbow Boulevard, MS 3006, Kansas City, KS 66160, USA; [d] Amita Health-Elign Campus, 1975 Lin Lor Lane, Suite 155, Elgin, IL 60123, USA
* Corresponding author.
E-mail address: raz1@hotmail.com

Card Electrophysiol Clin 11 (2019) 719–729
https://doi.org/10.1016/j.ccep.2019.08.013
1877-9182/19/© 2019 Elsevier Inc. All rights reserved.

system enables reliable visualization of catheter placement and produces geometry representing the heart and vascular system within which the catheters can then be manipulated (**Fig. 1**).

INTRACARDIAC ECHOCARDIOGRAPHY

ICE is an essential tool to reduce and even eliminate reliance on fluoroscopy during catheter ablation procedures. It permits real-time visualization of catheters and cardiac structures, monitoring for procedural complication(s) (eg, pericardial effusion), and direct visualization of structures that are not identifiable on fluoroscopy or the 3-dimensional EAM map. ICE also allows operators to monitor ablation progression by edema formation and tissue–catheter contact, although it cannot measure contact force.

Developing comfort with ICE generally features an unencumbered learning curve. If one is new to it or has limited experience, it is recommended to integrate ICE during simple ablation procedures at first: manipulating the catheter and identifying structures during downtime in procedures, such as after anticoagulation reversal, while allowing tissue edema to subside, or at the conclusion of the case.

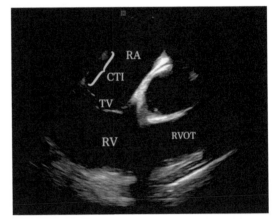

Fig. 2. Home view in ICE. CTI, cavotricuspid isthmus; RV, right ventricle; RVOT, right ventricular outflow tract; TV, tricuspid valve.

The most basic view with ICE is the home view, which can be found by advancing the ICE catheter in a neutral position, that is, ICE catheter ridge pointing to patient nose or 12 o'clock, into the mid right atrium (RA; **Fig. 2**). Visible structures in this view are the RA, cavotricuspid isthmus, tricuspid valve anterior and posterior leaflets, and the right ventricle (RV) and right ventricular outflow tract (RVOT).

INTRACARDIAC ECHOCARDIOGRAPHY MANEUVERS TO VISUALIZE LEFT ATRIAL STRUCTURES

Generally speaking, rotation of the ICE catheter clockwise (CW) allows visualization of anterior to posterior structures until the posterior wall and esophagus are in view. Afterward, continued application of CW rotation permits visualization

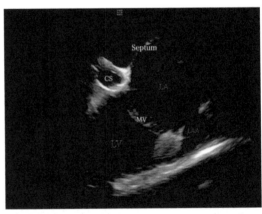

Fig. 3. CCW rotation of the ICE catheter to the 2 o'clock to 3 o'clock position allows visualization of the CS ostium, septum, left atrium (LA), left atrial appendage (LAA), mitral valve (MV), and the left ventricle (LV).

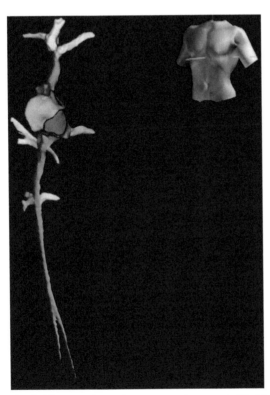

Fig. 1. The mapping system can create a geometry of the heart and the vascular system.

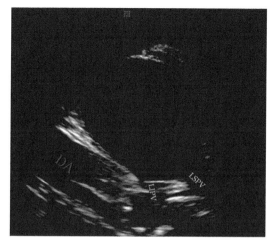

Fig. 4. CCW rotation of the ICE catheter to the 4 o'clock to 5 o'clock position allows visualization of the LSPV, left inferior pulmonary vein (LIPV), part of the left atrial roof, and the descending aorta (DA).

of intracardiac structures in a posterior to anterior sequence.

- Starting from home view, left atrial structures can be brought into the field of view by applying CW rotation of the ICE catheter.
- CW rotation to the 2 o'clock to 3 o'clock position allows visualization of the coronary sinus (CS) ostium, as well as the mitral valve and left atrial appendage (**Fig. 3**).
- Additional CW rotation to the 4 o'clock to 5 o'clock position typically reveals the left superior pulmonary vein (LSPV), left inferior pulmonary vein, and the descending aorta (**Fig. 4**).

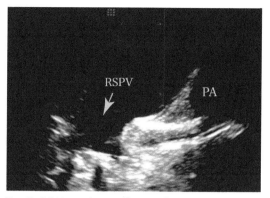

Fig. 6. CCW rotation to the 7 o'clock to 8 o'clock position allows visualization of the right superior pulmonary vein (RSPV), as well as the pulmonary artery (PA).

- CW rotation to the 6 o'clock position allows the operator to bring the right inferior pulmonary vein and esophagus into view (**Fig. 5**).
- Further CW rotation to the 7 o'clock to 8 o'clock position will allow visualization of the right superior pulmonary vein as well as the pulmonary artery (**Fig. 6**).

ADVANCING THE INTRACARDIAC ECHOCARDIOGRAPHY CATHETER INTO THE LEFT ATRIUM

For enhanced visualization of the pulmonary veins during catheter ablation, the ICE catheter can be

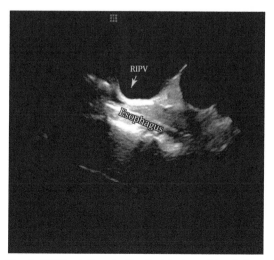

Fig. 5. CCW rotation to the 6 o'clock position brings into view the right inferior pulmonary vein (RIPV) and the esophagus.

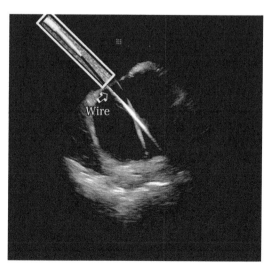

Fig. 7. After successful transseptal access, the transseptal needle is removed and the J-wire is advanced into the LSPV. The transseptal dilator assembly is pulled back into the RA, maintaining the J-wire in the LSPV. While applying an anterior curve to the ICE catheter, the entry point of the J-wire through the transseptal puncture is visualized on ICE.

advanced into the left atrium (LA). To do so, the ICE catheter may be introduced via a previously performed transseptal puncture, that is, for positioning of LA ablation catheter(s). Once successful transseptal access is obtained, the transseptal needle is withdrawn, and the J-wire is advanced into the LSPV. Next, the transseptal dilator assembly is pulled back into the RA while maintaining the J-wire in the LSPV. While applying an anterior curve to the ICE catheter, the entry point of the J-wire through the transseptal puncture is visualized on ICE (**Fig. 7**). The ICE catheter is advanced parallel to the J-wire through the same transseptal puncture. Afterward, the transseptal sheath–dilator assembly is then readvanced into the LA over the wire and both dilator and wire are then removed. Once the ICE catheter is in the LA, adding a posterior tilt facilitates visualization of the left-sided pulmonary veins, and CW rotation permits visualization of the right-sided pulmonary veins.

INTRACARDIAC ECHOCARDIOGRAPHY VIEWS FROM THE RIGHT VENTRICLE

ICE catheter placement in the RV allows for evaluation of pericardial effusion, as well as visualization of left ventricular structures. From the home view, the ICE catheter can be maneuvered into the RV by applying anterior tilt to visualize the tricuspid valve and advancing the catheter through the valve, after which the anterior tilt is released.

CW rotation of the ICE catheter in the RV allows visualization of the left ventricular structures posterior to anterior, beginning with the interventricular septum, followed by the posteromedial papillary muscle (**Fig. 8**), and the anterolateral papillary muscle (**Fig. 9**).

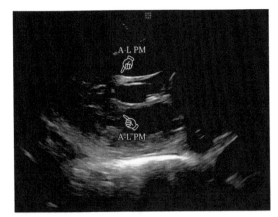

Fig. 9. Anterolateral papillary muscle (A-L PM), viewed from the RV.

Minimal withdrawal while maintaining slight CW rotation of the ICE catheter, after viewing the left ventricular outflow tract, positions the ICE catheter adjacent to the proximal septum and the base of the RVOT. Structures that can be seen in this position include the aortic valve cusps, the LA and left atrial appendage, the Coumadin ridge, and the LSPV (**Fig. 10**). Further CW rotation reveals the ascending aorta (**Fig. 11**). Further advancement of the ICE catheter, in contrast, allows visualization of the RVOT and pulmonic valve (**Fig. 12**).

Back-up ventricular pacing should be considered and preparations made before ICE catheter manipulation in this region in patients with left bundle branch block.

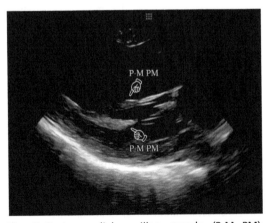

Fig. 8. Posteromedial papillary muscle (P-M PM), viewed from the RV.

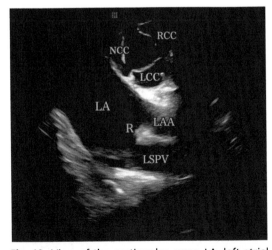

Fig. 10. View of the aortic valve cusps, LA, left atrial appendage (LAA), Coumadin ridge, and LSPV from the RVOT. LCC, left coronary cusp; NCC, noncoronary cusp; RCC, right coronary cusp.

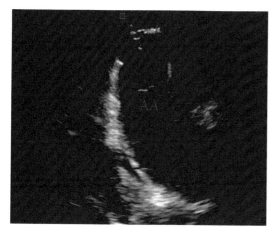

Fig. 11. View of the ascending aorta (AA) from the RVOT.

INTRACARDIAC ECHOCARDIOGRAPHY VIEW FROM THE PULMONARY ARTERY

Once the pulmonary valve is in view, applying anterior tilt and advancing the ICE catheter through the pulmonary valve places the catheter in the pulmonary artery. The left atrial appendage can then be visualized via counterclockwise (CCW) rotation of the ICE catheter (**Fig. 13**).

STEPS TO PERFORM FLUOROLESS CATHETER ABLATION
Vascular Access

Percutaneous femoral venous access is obtained via the modified Seldinger technique, using vascular ultrasound guidance, for placement of the introducer sheaths. This same technique is used for femoral arterial access when ablating left ventricular tachycardias using a retrograde approach.

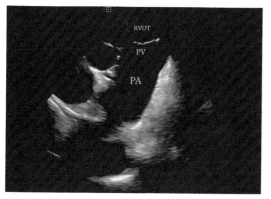

Fig. 12. Visualization of the pulmonary valve from the RVOT. PA, pulmonary artery; PV, pulmonary valve.

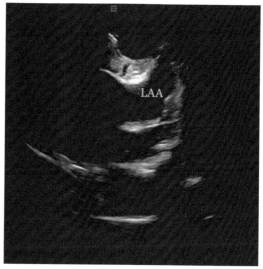

Fig. 13. The ICE catheter in the pulmonary artery; the left atrial appendage (LAA) can be visualized from this position.

Catheter Placement

For cases involving intracardiac ultrasound guidance, a phased-array ICE catheter is advanced through a sheath in the left femoral vein. The ICE catheter is advanced through the femoral vein and into the external iliac vein. An echo clear space is maintained at the transducer's tip during advancement of the ICE catheter toward the RA (**Fig. 14**).

For most cases, a deflectable decapolar catheter is advanced through the femoral vein and into the inferior vena cava with EAM guidance. The geometry of the inferior vena cava is collected throughout this time. When electrograms are first noted on the distal bipoles of the catheter, the catheter tip has traversed the border of the inferior vena cava and inferior RA (**Fig. 15**). It is then advanced superiorly into the RA until loss of electrogram signals noted on all but the very proximal poles of the decapolar catheter signifies that the catheter is approximating the border of the superior RA and the superior vena cava (SVC)

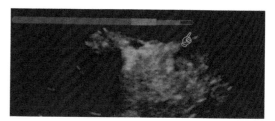

Fig. 14. An echo clear space is maintained at the transducer tip during advancement of the ICE catheter.

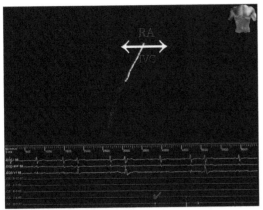

Fig. 15. Electrograms are first noted on the distal bipoles of the catheter which indicates the catheter tip has traversed the border of the inferior vena cava (IVC) and inferior RA.

(**Fig. 16**). The geometry of the SVC is then collected, and the decapolar catheter is withdrawn into the RA and manipulated under EAM guidance to collect the geometry of the RA. The right atrial appendage and CS ostia are delineated. If ICE is used, it serves as an additional tool to ensure the accuracy of the EAM geometry model. The decapolar catheter is usually advanced last into the CS. The CS is cannulated by manipulating the catheter such that its tip is in the posteroseptal region of the RA under EAM guidance. When Electrograms compatible with the CS ostium are noted in this region, the catheter tip is placed into the CS.

The geometry created with the deflectable decapolar catheter serves as a "shell" in which the remaining diagnostic and ablation catheters can be positioned and tracked appropriately.

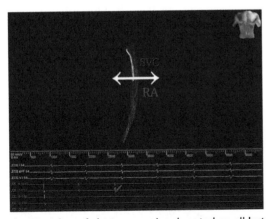

Fig. 16. A loss of electrogram signals noted on all but the very proximal poles of the decapolar catheter signifies the catheter is approximating the border of the superior RA and SVC.

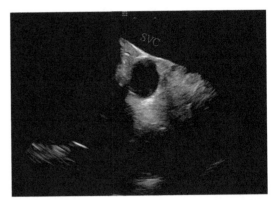

Fig. 17. View of the SVC for transseptal puncture. From the home view on ICE, CCW rotation is added to visualize the interatrial septum and the LA. A posterior tilt is added, and minimal CCW rotation is applied to visualize the SVC.

Transseptal Access

From the ICE home view, CW rotation is performed to bring into view the interatrial septum and LA. After a posterior tilt, minimal CCW rotation allows visualization of the SVC (**Fig. 17**).

Through a short, 8F sheath in the right femoral vein, a 180-cm 0.032-inch J-wire (Fixed-core J-tip guidewire, Medtronic, Mounds View, MN) is advanced into the SVC under direct ICE visualization. The short sheath is then removed and the transseptal sheath–dilator assembly (SL0, Abbott Laboratories, Abbott Park, IL) is inserted and carefully advanced over the wire into the SVC under direct ICE visualization (**Fig. 18**). The wire is withdrawn from the body, and the transseptal needle (NRG RF Transseptal Needle, Baylis Medical Company Inc., Montreal, Canada) is placed in the sheath–dilator and advanced such that its distal end aligns with the very distal

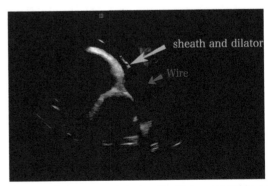

Fig. 18. The transseptal sheath–dilator assembly is advanced over the wire into the SVC.

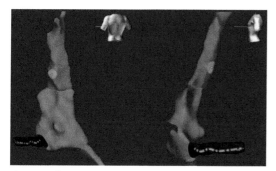

Fig. 19. The transseptal assembly is withdrawn into the RA, while tracking on the EAM system (*green circle*).

end of the dilator. The sheath–dilator assembly is withdrawn minimally to expose the blunt tip of the NRG transseptal needle. The transseptal assembly is then withdrawn into the RA, while being tracked via the EAM system (**Fig. 19**) and ICE, until tenting of the interatrial septum is seen observed on ICE (**Fig. 20**). Successful radiofrequency transseptal access requires the left pulmonary vein to be visualized on ICE while performing the puncture. Hemodynamic pressure monitoring is used to confirm entry into the LA, in addition to direct visualization by ICE.

If a standard (ie, non-radiofrequency) transseptal needle is used, the operator must rely solely on ICE to track the sheath–dilator assembly position as it is withdrawn from the SVC down to the interatrial septum. Care must be taken to avoid prematurely exposing the needle tip.

LEFT ATRIAL CATHETER PLACEMENT

For radiofrequency ablation of atrial fibrillation and other left-sided arrhythmias, such as atrial tachycardias and supraventricular tachycardias using a left-sided accessory pathway, once transseptal access has been obtained, the geometry of the LA is collected by manipulating the ablation catheter or circular mapping catheter under EAM and ICE guidance. The geometries for the pulmonary veins and the left atrial appendage can be constructed in the same fashion.

VENTRICULAR AND OUTFLOW TRACT CATHETER PLACEMENT

For RVOT tachycardias, the RV and RVOT geometries are constructed with EAM using a deflectable decapolar catheter under ICE guidance.

For left ventricular tachycardias, using a retrograde approach, femoral arterial access is obtained under ultrasound guidance using the modified Seldinger technique. An ablation catheter is advanced retrograde via the femoral artery into the iliac system and subsequently into the aorta, all of which is performed with EAM guidance. The geometry of the arterial system is collected as the ablation catheter traverses the abdominal and thoracic portions of the aorta in retrograde fashion (**Fig. 21**). The catheter tip is deflected to produce a distal U-curve, which is confirmed by reversal in the sequence of distal electrode numbering on the EAM (**Fig. 22**). This U-curve facilitates advancement of the ablation catheter along the aortic arch and across the aortic valve. The aortic valve is crossed by prolapsing the catheter across the valve under ICE guidance. Once the catheter has successfully crossed the aortic valve, the geometry of the left ventricular outflow

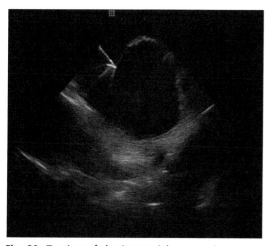

Fig. 20. Tenting of the interatrial septum is seen on ICE.

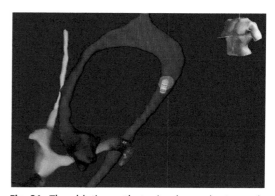

Fig. 21. The ablation catheter is advanced retrograde through the abdominal aorta, descending thoracic aorta, aortic arch, and ascending aorta to the level of the aortic valve.

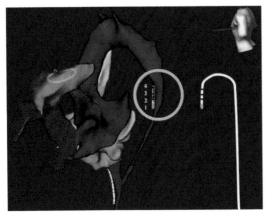

Fig. 22. The catheter tip is deflected to produce a U-curve, which is confirmed by reversal in the sequence of distal electrode numbering on the EAM.

tract and left ventricle can be created with ICE guidance.

For some cases of left ventricular tachycardia, a transseptal approach is used to access the LA. The ablation catheter can then be advanced from the LA into the left ventricle under ICE guidance (**Fig. 23**).

RADIOFREQUENCY CATHETER ABLATION

A stable catheter position and contact during ablation can be confirmed on EAM and ICE. ICE allows for monitoring lesion formation, in addition to safe maneuvering of the ablation and mapping

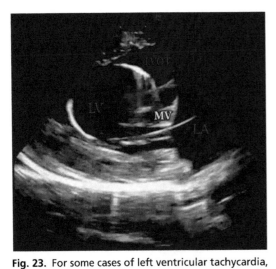

Fig. 23. For some cases of left ventricular tachycardia, a transseptal approach is used to access the LA. The ablation catheter can then be advanced from the LA into the left ventricle with ICE guidance. LV, left ventricle; LVOT, left ventricular outflow tract; MV, mitral valve.

catheters. Critical structures, such as the coronary artery ostia, can be clearly delineated on ICE and marked on the EAM.

CRYOBALLOON CATHETER ABLATION

When performing cryoballoon ablation, the transseptal sheath is exchanged for a 15F steerable sheath (FlexCath Advance, Medtronic) under direct ICE visualization. The 10.5F, 28-mm cryoballoon (Arctic Front Advance, Medtronic) and a 10-pole circular mapping catheter (Achieve, Medtronic) are placed through the FlexCath into the LA.

The ostia of the PVs, as visualized by ICE, are delineated on EAM using the mapping catheter. The Achieve catheter is advanced into the target PV, after which the cryoballoon is inflated and positioned in the antrum of the vein. ICE can confirm the alignment of the transseptal sheath and the balloon before cryoenergy application (**Fig. 24**). Achievement of a pulmonary capillary wedge pressure waveform on hemodynamic pressure monitoring signifies complete occlusion of the vein (**Fig. 25**). A lack of color flow Doppler imaging within the targeted PV serves as an additional indicator of adequate PV occlusion. A thorough search for leaks around the cryoballoon's circumference on color flow Doppler imaging should be performed by applying small degrees of CW and CCW rotation to ICE catheter to evaluate for leaks. It is also imperative to ensure that the sheath, balloon, and vein are coaxial in the same view. If the balloon seems to be coaxial to the vein, but the sheath is not clearly seen in the same view, slight CW or CCW rotation applied to the ICE catheter can help to determine the relative location of the sheath. From there, a counter maneuver is applied to the sheath to achieve coaxiality. For

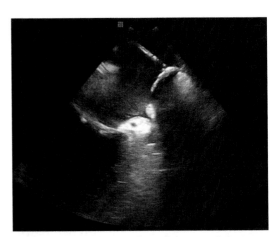

Fig. 24. ICE is used to confirm alignment of the transseptal sheath and the balloon before cryoenergy application.

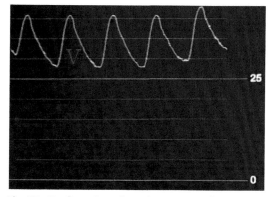

Fig. 25. Confirmation of a pulmonary capillary wedge pressure waveform on hemodynamic pressure monitoring signifies complete occlusion of the pulmonary vein.

example, if the ICE catheter is rotated slightly CW to find the sheath relative to the balloon and vein, then the sheath should be rotated slightly CCW to make it coaxial to the balloon and vein. Finally, to ensure the antral position of the balloon is optimized during ablation, the majority of the equator of the balloon should be seen on ICE like a golf ball on a tee (Fig. 26). Cryotherapy is then applied with a goal temperature of −40°C to −50°C to ideally achieve PV conduction block within the first 60 seconds of the application.

Before cryoballoon ablation of the right-sided PVs, a 6F decapolar catheter is advanced to the SVC with ICE and EAM guidance. It is used to pace the SVC at high output to monitor the integrity of the phrenic nerve during cryoenergy applications.

ESOPHAGEAL TEMPERATURE MONITORING

Esophageal temperature monitoring is important during atrial fibrillation ablation. Traditionally, assessment of the location of the esophageal temperature probe was performed under fluoroscopy. A nonfluoroscopic approach to esophageal temperature monitoring can be achieved using ICE.

A multisensor probe, CIRCA S-Cath MSP (CIRCA Scientific, LLC, Englewood, CO) is used to monitor the esophageal temperature. When the probe is advanced into the esophagus under ICE guidance, the thermistors on the probe can be seen on ICE, with the most distal thermistor designated as 1 and the most proximal as 12 (Fig. 27).

From the home view, CW rotation is applied to the ICE catheter to visualized the left PVs. To better visualize the esophagus, the ICE catheter is withdrawn slightly, and minimal left steer is applied. A slight CW rotation is then applied to bring the right inferior pulmonary vein into view. Because the level of the right inferior pulmonary vein often indicates the posterior aspect of the LA, this position is ideal for visualization of the esophagus. In this view, the esophagus should be seen in a longitudinal view (Fig. 28). At this point, the temperature probe is advanced into the esophagus. Once the sixth thermistor is seen at the level of the right inferior pulmonary vein, the stylet for the probe is withdrawn and the serpentine shape of the temperature probe is seen under ICE (Fig. 29). With the sixth thermistor at the level of the right inferior pulmonary vein, the first thermistor is typically distal to the inferior border of the LA, and this method has been validated using fluoroscopy in our laboratory (Fig. 30). The benefits of the multipolar temperature probe include increased sensitivity to temperature

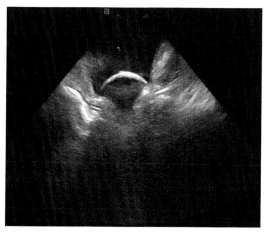

Fig. 26. To ensure a relatively antral location of the balloon during ablation, the majority of the equator of the balloon should be seen on ICE, producing a golf ball on a tee appearance.

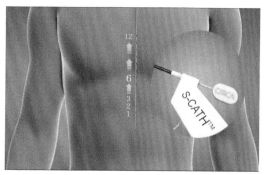

Fig. 27. The CIRCA catheter is used to monitor the esophageal temperature. It is advanced into the esophagus under ICE guidance. The thermistors on the probe can be seen on ICE, with the most distal thermistor designated as 1 and the most proximal as 12. (CIRCA S-Cath MSP courtesy of CIRCA Scientific, Englewood, CO; with permission.)

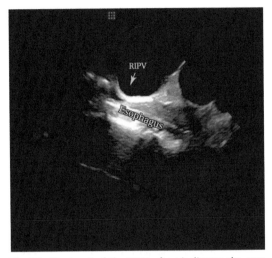

Fig. 28. The level of the RIPV often indicates the posterior aspect of the LA. This location is favored for visualizing the esophagus. In this view, the esophagus is seen in a longitudinal orientation.

increased and reduced temperature probe adjustments in the esophagus as ablation is being performed.

ADVANTAGES AND LIMITATIONS OF INTRACARDIAC ECHOCARDIOGRAPHY

Fluoroless catheter ablation carries the advantages of eliminating harmful radiation to patients, electrophysiology laboratory staff, and physicians. The avoidance of heavy lead garments may result

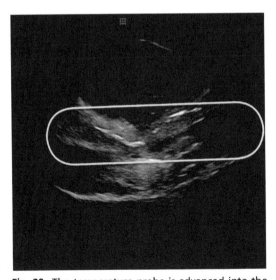

Fig. 29. The temperature probe is advanced into the esophagus. Once the sixth thermistor is positioned at the level of the RIPV with ICE guidance, the stylet for the probe is withdrawn, and the serpentine shape of the temperature probe is seen on ICE.

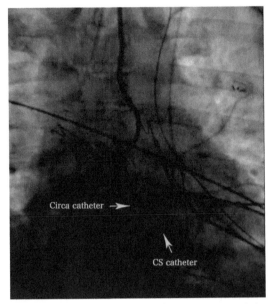

Fig. 30. With the sixth thermistor at the level of the RIPV, the first thermistor is typically distal to the inferior border of the LA as seen on fluoroscopy.

in fewer orthopedic injuries and downstream disability for electrophysiology laboratory staff and physicians. Also, members of the anesthesia team and other special populations, such as pediatric and adolescent patients and pregnant patients or colleagues, can more safely participate in fluoroscopy-free ablation procedures.

The extensive use of ICE in nonfluoroscopic techniques often results in a better understanding of anatomic variations and potential obstacles, such as left common and right middle PVs, accessory PVs with unusual takeoffs (**Fig. 31**), and cor triatriatum sinister (**Fig. 32**), during cryoballoon

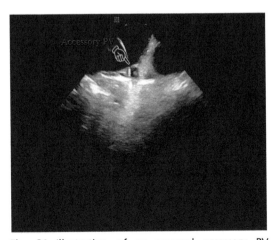

Fig. 31. Illustration of an unusual accessory PV takeoff.

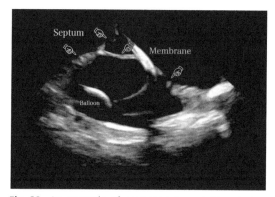

Fig. 32. An example of cor triatriatum sinister during cryoablation for atrial fibrillation. As seen on ICE, the cryoballoon sheath and catheter cross the intra-atrial septum, as well as atrial membrane via its extant perforation. The cryoballoon is in the RIPV.

ablation of the pulmonary veins. Proficient use of ICE may decrease or even eliminate the need for routine preprocedural imaging, including computed tomography scans and cardiac MRI for the purposes of identifying anatomic variations.

A potential disadvantage of nonfluoroscopic endocardial catheter ablation is the cost associated with ICE. However, in many laboratories ICE is routinely used during left-sided ablation procedures regardless of whether or not fluoroscopy is also being used. Thus, accessibility should not be an insurmountable barrier. Finally, if routine preprocedural computed tomography scans and cardiac MRI can be avoided before catheter ablation, then potentially significant cost savings may be achieved by intraprocedural ICE rather than these respective modalities. Broader societal impact and long-term cost effectiveness may result from avoidance of employment disability owing to orthopedic injury, and the downstream effects of reduced radiation exposure for patients, physicians, and allied health professionals participating in catheter ablation procedures.

REFERENCES

1. Vano E, Arranz L, Sastre JM, et al. Dosimetric and radiation protection considerations based on some cases of patient skin injuries in interventional cardiology. Br J Radiol 1998;71:510–6.

2. Kovoor P, Ricciardello M, Collins L, et al. Risk to patients from radiation associated with radiofrequency ablation for supraventricular tachycardia. Circulation 1998;98:1534–40.

3. Calkins H, Niklason L, Sousa J, et al. Radiation exposure during radiofrequency catheter ablation of accessory atrioventricular connections. Circulation 1991;84:2376–82.

4. Rehani MM, Ortiz-Lopez P. Radiation effects in fluoroscopically guided cardiac interventions: keeping them under control. Int J Cardiol 2006; 109:147–51.

5. Park TH, Eichling JO, Schechtman KB, et al. Risk of radiation induced skin injuries from arrhythmia ablation procedures. Pacing Clin Electrophysiol 1996;19: 1363–9.

6. McFadden SL, Mooney RB, Shepherd PH. X-ray dose and associated risks from radiofrequency catheter ablation procedures. Br J Radiol 2002;75: 253–65.

7. Klein LW, Miller DL, Balter S, et al. Occupational health hazards in the interventional laboratory: time for a safer environment. Radiology 2009;250: 538–44.

8. Picano E, Vañó E, Rehani MM, et al. The appropriate and justified use of medical radiation in cardiovascular imaging. A position document of the ESC associations of cardiovascular imaging, percutaneous cardiovascular interventions and electrophysiology. Eur Heart J 2014;35:665–72.

9. Lickfett L, Mahesh M, Vasamreddy C, et al. Radiation exposure during catheter ablation of atrial fibrillation. Circulation 2004;110:3003–10.

10. Rosenthal LS, Mahesh M, Beck TJ, et al. Predictors of fluoroscopy time and estimated radiation exposure during radiofrequency catheter ablation procedures. Am J Cardiol 1998;82: 451–8.

11. Razminia M, Willoughby MC, Demo H, et al. Fluoroless catheter ablation of cardiac arrhythmias: a 5-year experience. Pacing Clin Electrophysiol 2017; 40:425–33.

12. Razminia M, Manankil MF, Eryazici PL, et al. Nonfluoroscopic catheter ablation of cardiac arrhythmias in adults: feasibility, safety, and efficacy. J Cardiovasc Electrophysiol 2012;23: 1078–86.

Toward a Uniform Ablation Protocol for Paroxysmal, Persistent, and Permanent Atrial Fibrillation

Domenico Giovanni Della Rocca, MD[a],*, Carlo Lavalle, MD[b],
Carola Gianni, MD, PhD[a], Marco Valerio Mariani, MD[b],
Sanghamitra Mohanty, MD[a], Chintan Trivedi, MD, MPH[a],
Ugur Canpolat, MD[a,c], Bryan MacDonald, MD[a], Huseyin Ayhan, MD[a,d],
Agostino Piro, MD[b], Mohamed Bassiouny, MD[a], Amin Al-Ahmad, MD[a],
John David Burkhardt, MD[a], Joseph G. Gallinghouse, MD[a],
Rodney P. Horton, MD[a], Javier Sanchez, MD[a], Nicola Tarantino, MD[f],
Luigi Di Biase, MD, PhD[a,e,f,g], Andrea Natale, MD[a,e,h,i,j]

KEYWORDS

- Atrial fibrillation • Catheter ablation • Outcome • Trigger • Substrate • Anticoagulation • Stroke

KEY POINTS

- Atrial fibrillation is the most widely recognized arrhythmia and is associated with increased relative risk of cardiovascular and all-cause mortality, stroke, heart failure, and chronic cognitive impairment.
- Atrial fibrillation catheter ablation has emerged as the most effective strategy to restore and maintain sinus rhythm.
- A lack of agreement exists regarding other targets to seek for ablation, as well as how to identify them.

Disclosures: Dr A. Al-Ahmad has received honoraria from Medtronic and St. Jude Medical. Dr L. Di Biase is a consultant for Biosense Webster, Boston Scientific, Stereotaxis, and St. Jude Medical; and has received speaker honoraria from Medtronic, Atricure, EPiEP, and Biotronik. Dr A. Natale has received speaker honoraria from Boston Scientific, Biosense Webster, St. Jude Medical, Biotronik, and Medtronic; and is a consultant for Biosense Webster, St. Jude Medical, and Janssen. All other authors have reported that they have no relationships relevant to the contents of this article to disclose.

[a] Texas Cardiac Arrhythmia Institute, St. David's Medical Center, Austin, TX, USA; [b] Department of Cardiovascular, Respiratory, Nephrological, Anesthesiological and Geriatric Sciences, "Sapienza" University of Rome, Policlinico Umberto I, Rome, Italy; [c] Arrhythmia and Electrophysiology Unit, Department of Cardiology, Hacettepe University, Sihhiye, Ankara 06532, Turkey; [d] Department of Cardiology, Ankara Yildirim Beyazit, Ankara, Turkey; [e] Department of Biomedical Engineering, University of Texas, 107 West Dean Keeton Street, Austin, TX 78712, USA; [f] Montefiore Medical Center, Albert Einstein College of Medicine, 1300 Morris Park Avenue, Bronx, NY 10461, USA; [g] Department of Clinical and Experimental Medicine, University of Foggia, Via A. Gramsci, Foggia, Italy; [h] Interventional Electrophysiology, Scripps Clinic, 9898 Genesee Avenue, La Jolla, CA 92037, USA; [i] MetroHealth Medical Center, Case Western Reserve University School of Medicine, 10900 Euclid Avenue, Cleveland, OH 44106, USA; [j] Division of Cardiology, Stanford University, 291 Campus Drive, Stanford, CA 94305, USA
* Corresponding author. Texas Cardiac Arrhythmia Institute, St. David's Medical Center, 3000 North I-35, Suite 720, Austin, TX 78705.
E-mail address: domenicodellarocca@hotmail.it

Card Electrophysiol Clin 11 (2019) 731–738
https://doi.org/10.1016/j.ccep.2019.08.014
1877-9182/19/© 2019 Elsevier Inc. All rights reserved.

cardiacEP.theclinics.com

INTRODUCTION

Atrial fibrillation (AF) is the most widely recognized arrhythmia and is associated with increased relative risk of cardiovascular and all-cause mortality, as well as stroke, heart failure (HF), and chronic cognitive impairment. Additionally, a significant impact on exercise tolerance and quality of life has been widely documented in AF patients regardless of symptoms. Over the last decades, the total cost of AF care has steadily risen, amounting to $6.65 billion only in the United States in 2005.[1]

Nearly two-thirds of the total economic burden of AF is represented by direct and indirect costs associated with hospitalization, as well as the monitoring of pharmacologic treatment and its adverse events.[1] Considering the important socioeconomic and health burden carried by AF, several studies have been conducted aiming at identifying the optimal therapeutic strategies to contain the predicted epidemic of AF, its associated events, and the estimated increase in health care costs.

Among available therapies, catheter ablation (CA) has emerged as the most effective strategy to restore and maintain sinus rhythm.[2–4] Its benefits in terms of arrhythmia burden and clinical event reduction, symptoms relief, and quality of life improvement have been consistently demonstrated in large randomized clinical trials[2,4] and confirmed in subpopulations with specific clinical conditions (eg, HF, hypertrophic cardiomyopathy, elderly).[5–7] Nowadays, the cornerstone of AF ablation is elimination of triggers from the pulmonary veins (PVs) by means of PV antral isolation (PVAI).[8] Nevertheless, a variable number of patients may experience atrial tachyarrhythmia recurrences even in the presence of permanent PVAI.[9] Whether and in which patients PVAI should be considered as the only ablation strategy remains a matter of debate. Similarly, a lack of agreement exists regarding other targets to seek for ablation, as well as how to identify them.

In this review, we aimed at summarizing the rationale and effectiveness of different ablation approaches and identifying some key points for a uniform AF ablation strategy.

INDICATIONS AND GENERAL CONSIDERATIONS

AF CA is indicated for symptomatic AF patients refractory or intolerant to at least 1 class I or III antiarrhythmic medication.[8] More specifically, as reported in the 2017 HRS/EHRA/ECAS/APHRS/SOLAECE expert consensus statement on catheter and surgical ablation of AF,[8] CA is recommended for patients with symptomatic paroxysmal AF who have failed antiarrhythmic drug (AAD) therapy (Class I, level of evidence [LOE] A). CA in symptomatic patients who have failed AAD therapy has a Class IIa, LOE B-NR indication if AF is persistent and a Class IIb, LOE C-LD indication if AF is long-standing persistent.

CA is considered reasonable before initiation of antiarrhythmic therapy with a Class I or III antiarrhythmic medication in symptomatic patients with paroxysmal (Class IIa, LOE B-R) or persistent (Class IIa, LOE C-EO) AF and may be considered in those with long-standing persistent AF (Class IIb, LOE C-EO).

All procedures should be conducted under general anesthesia, to control respiration and patient movements. This point is of pivotal importance to improve catheter and mapping stability and achieve more effective lesions, as well as decrease the risk of complications. A few studies have assessed the safety and effectiveness of different anesthesia settings during CA. Among them, a prospective randomized clinical trial reported higher success rates, lower incidence of PV reconnection, and shorter procedure and fluoroscopy times with general anesthesia compared with conscious sedation.[10]

To minimize procedural embolic risk, patients taking vitamin K antagonists (VKAs) should be prescribed with at least 4 weeks of therapeutic oral anticoagulation before the procedure. In the occurrence of subtherapeutic international normalized ratio, transesophageal echocardiography should be performed to exclude the presence of left atrial appendage (LAA) thrombosis. Novel oral anticoagulants (NOACs) have a faster onset of action and their management is easier compared with VKAs. A recent study on a large series of AF patients showed that performing CA in patients on uninterrupted NOACs without preprocedural transesophageal echocardiography is feasible and safe.[11]

All procedures should be performed on uninterrupted VKAs or NOACs. Recent studies in patients on NOACs suggest that a truly uninterrupted anticoagulation strategy does not increase the risk of procedural bleeding events and significantly decrease the risk of silent strokes compared with procedure day single-dose skipped and 24-hour skipped strategies.[12,13]

Real-time ultrasound examination is highly effective in minimizing the risk of vascular complications when venous accesses are obtained.

A heparin bolus (usually up to 10,000 U in patients taking VKAs and 12,000–15,000 U with NOACs) should be given before transseptal puncture is achieved. The bolus should be sufficient to target an activated clotting time (ACT) of more than 350 seconds and small boluses administered if needed based on ACT values. It is suggested to check ACT level every 10 to 15 minutes if therapeutic anticoagulation is not achieved, and every 15 to 30 minutes thereafter.

Access sheaths can be removed immediately at the end of the procedure once the ACT is less than 200 seconds. Ambulation should be avoided for 4 to 6 hours. Vascular closure devices may provide effective hemostasis and at the same time shorten ambulation time (2 hours) and the need for bladder catheterization, thereby decreasing the risk of access site and urinary complications.[14]

Oral anticoagulation should be restarted 3 to 5 hours after ablation, unless ongoing bleeding is documented. Similarly, it has to be continued for at least 2 months (Class I, LOE C-EO), regardless of individual thromboembolic risk, owing to the ablation-induced prothrombotic status resulting from reduced atrial contraction and endothelial damage.

The decision to discontinue oral anticoagulation is then made on an individual basis, with thromboembolic risk, bleeding risk, and procedural success (assessed via intense electrocardiographic monitoring) being the main factors to be considered.[15]

In patients who underwent LAA isolation, transesophageal echocardiography is required, usually between 3 to 6 months after the ablation to evaluate the residual LAA mechanical function. If low late systolic velocities (<0.4 m/s) are documented, oral anticoagulation should be continued indefinitely. Another alternative is LAA occlusion.

AAD therapy is generally continued for 2 to 3 months after the ablation. Further antiarrhythmic treatment depends on the results of an intense electrocardiographic monitoring with arrhythmia burden assessment.

PULMONARY VEIN TRIGGERS, ATRIAL SUBSTRATE, AND BEYOND: MAIN CONCEPTS

As discussed elsewhere in this article, PVAI is the cornerstone of every AF procedure. However, its effectiveness varies based on the type of AF, as well as the presence of unmodifiable and modifiable risk factors. These factors may promote electrophysiologic and structural changes that are involved in the development of AF triggers from PV and extra-PV sites, together with making the atria a vulnerable substrate to sustain AF.[16] As such, AF ablation aims at modifying the substrate that sustains AF and/or localizing and eliminating triggers promoting arrhythmia relapse.

Substrate-Based Ablation Strategies

Several substrate-based ablation strategies have been proposed over the years and some of them have found a widespread use in clinical practice. Specifically, substrate-based ablation can be achieved with linear lesions compartmentalizing the left atrium,[17,18] by targeting areas of complex electrograms (eg, complex fractionated atrial electrograms) or autonomic ganglionated plexi,[19,20] or with atrial scar homogenization.[21,22]

However, none of these modalities seem to confer a significant benefit over PVAI alone. Specifically, The Substrate and Trigger Ablation for Reduction of Atrial Fibrillation Trial Part II (STAR-AF II) did not find a decrease in the rate of AF recurrences when either linear ablation or ablation of complex fractionated atrial electrograms was performed in addition to PVAI in patients with persistent AF.[23] Similarly, in the prospective and randomized Alster-Lost-AF trial (Ablation at St. Georg Hospital for Long-Standing Persistent Atrial Fibrillation), no significant difference was observed between PVAI and a stepwise approach of PVAI plus complex fractionated atrial electrograms and linear ablation.[24]

On the basis of the hypothesis that AF could be sustained by discrete sources, recent research has focused on the impact of mapping and ablation of localized organized reentrant activity, such as rotors and high-frequency areas.

Results from a recent metanalysis evaluating the outcomes of PVAI with and without focal impulse and rotor modulation ablation did not show any therapeutic benefit of the focal impulse and rotor modulation approach over PVAI alone.[25] Similar results were reported in the recent Randomized Evaluation of Atrial Fibrillation Treatment With Focal Impulse and Rotor Modulation Guided Procedures (REAFFIRM) trial.[26]

Trigger Ablation

In patients with paroxysmal AF, achieving permanent PVAI is highly effective and associated with a high success rate. In this cohort, PVs are frequently the only source of triggers initiating AF. Conversely, the success rate of an ablation strategy exclusively targeting the PVs is significantly lower in patients with persistent and long-standing persistent AF, as well as in presence of specific unmodifiable and modifiable risk factors (eg, female gender, older age, obesity, HF, sleep-related breathing disorders, and hypertrophic cardiomyopathy). These subsets of patients share a higher prevalence of triggers from extra-PV sites; because PVs are unlikely to be the only source of triggers initiating paroxysms of atrial tachyarrhythmias, PVAI alone is not enough by itself to maintain sinus rhythm in these patients. A common pathophysiologic mechanism can be described. Specifically, as arrhythmia persists, as well as if these risk factors are present, structural and electrophysiologic changes occur in the atria, which predispose to the development of triggers from non-PV sites, together with making the atria a more vulnerable substrate to sustain AF.[16] As such, despite extensive substrate modification, the CA success rate does not improve without elimination of those triggers contributing to atrial tachyarrhythmia initiation. Non-PV triggers are ectopic beats initiating atrial tachyarrhythmias. They are harbored in specific areas outside the PVs,[27–29] the most frequent locations being left atrial posterior wall (PW), LAA, crista terminalis, interatrial septum, and other thoracic veins, such as coronary sinus (CS), superior vena cava (SVC), and vein of Marshall. When AF persists, or in the presence of other cardiac and extracardiac comorbidities, extracellular matrix remodeling, cell-to-cell coupling abnormalities, and myocyte density heterogenicity may occur. The result is the development of areas of slow conduction with abnormal electrical properties. However, some discrete atrial sites (non-PV sites) may maintain a preserved rapid conduction and become prone to abnormal automaticity, triggered activity, and/or microreentry. As a result, these sites may act as a cluster of ectopic beats, which may potentially initiate sustained arrhythmias. Similar findings can be reproduced in animal models via rapid pacing.[30] Rapid pacing promotes prolonged action potential duration and reduced resting potentials and delayed afterdepolarizations. Histologically, enlargement of atrial mitochondria, which show internal cristae disorganization, is observed. The resulting intracellular calcium overload promotes delayed afterdepolarizations-induced triggered activity and development of ectopic beats responsible for the initiation of sustained arrhythmias.

The prevalence of non-PV triggers widely varies among studies and several factors may explain these differences. First, AAD therapy may influence the electrophysiologic properties of atrial cells and may hinder trigger inducibility. Therefore, it is strongly recommended to stop any AADs at least 5 half-lives before ablation.

Second, the threshold of arrhythmia inducibility significantly changes based on the type of anesthesia. As an example, a high-dose isoproterenol infusion is necessary to induce triggers when ablation is performed under general anesthesia and not only ectopic beats triggering sustained runs of atrial tachycardia, but also nonsustained focal

tachycardias and frequent premature atrial contractions (PACs) should be considered significant and targeted for ablation.[31]

Third, the prevalence of non-PV triggers depends on the protocol adopted to induce them. Specifically, the prevalence of non-PV triggers is significantly lower if low-dose (<10 μg/min) or stepwise increasing doses of isoproterenol are used.[29,32–35]

Fourth, different definitions for significant non-PV triggers have been adopted by different groups.[33,35] Some investigators consider significant only non-PV triggers initiating reproducible sustained (>30 seconds) atrial tachyarrhythmias, whereas some others consider also those initiating runs of nonsustained (<30 seconds) focal atrial tachycardia or leading to repetitive PACs. In our center, procedures are conducted under general anesthesia and the protocol adopted to induce non-PV triggers is based on high-dose isoproterenol infusion (20–30 μg/min) for 10 to 15 minutes. Significant triggers targeted for ablation are those initiating either sustained and nonsustained atrial tachyarrhythmias, as well as repetitive (>10 minutes) isolated PACs.

The prevalence of non-PV ectopic beats triggering sustained runs of atrial tachyarrhythmias ranges between 8% to 15%[29,32,33]; however, extra-PV triggers can be induced in up to 80% of patients if nonsustained triggers and PACs are considered. Their prevalence is higher in nonparoxysmal AF, female, obese, and elderly patients, as well as in those with HF with reduced ejection fraction, sleep-related breathing disorders, hypertrophic cardiomyopathy, severe atrial scarring, and previous cardiac surgery.

CATHETER ABLATION OF ATRIAL FIBRILLATION: OUR APPROACH

The following protocol reflects the standard approach adopted at our center, a tertiary care hospital where approximately 2000 AF ablation procedures are performed every year. At our institution, all procedures are conducted under general anesthesia and uninterrupted oral anticoagulation. AADs, including amiodarone, are discontinued for at least 5 half-lives before the procedure to decrease the likelihood of noninducibility. Intracardiac echocardiography is used in all cases to guide ablation. Using an open irrigated tip ablation catheter, a power of 40 to 45 W is typically used with the goal of local potential abatement. Under circular mapping catheter (CMC) guidance, lesions are delivered throughout the antral surface of the PVs, including the areas between and around the PVs and the roof of the LAA. After completing

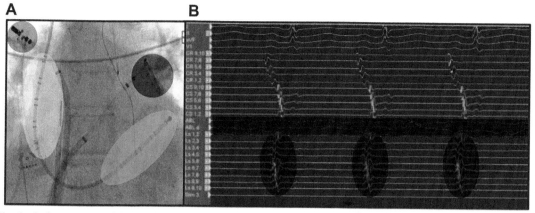

A   **B**

Fig. 1. Catheter setting (A) and intracardiac recordings (B) during high-dose isoproterenol challenge test. During the challenge test, catheters are positioned with the following setup: a 20-pole catheter with electrodes spanning from the SVC (*yellow*), right atrium/crista terminalis (*yellow*) to the CS (*blue*), the ablation catheter in the right superior PV recording the far-field interatrial septum (*violet*), the 10-pole CMC in the left superior PV recording the far-field LAA activity (*red*).

PVAI, PW isolation is achieved by targeting all potentials identified via a CMC moved along the PW. While ablating the PW, it is of pivotal importance to use real-time temperature monitoring, move the ablation catheter quickly along the PW, and titrate contact force and/or power to avoid significant esophageal damage and prevent the development of fistulas.

Subsequently, a pharmacologic challenge test with high-dose isoproterenol (starting at 20 μg/min and up to 30 μg/min for 10–15 minutes) is performed in sinus rhythm to elicit non-PV triggers and confirm persistent PVAI.

During the challenge test, catheters are positioned with the following setup (**Fig. 1**).

a. A 20-pole catheter with electrodes spanning from the SVC, right atrium/crista terminalis to the CS,
b. The ablation catheter in the right superior PV recording the far-field interatrial septum,
c. The 10-pole CMC in the left superior PV recording the far-field LAA activity.

Localization of non-PV triggers can be easily performed as follows.

d. Earliest activation in the proximal duo-decapolar catheter for ectopic beats originating from the right atrium,
e. Earliest activation in the distal duo-decapolar catheter for ectopic beats originating from the CS (**Fig. 2**);
f. Earliest far-field activity recorded from the CMC before the distal CS for beats originating from the LAA; and
g. Earliest far-field activity recorded from the ablation catheter, usually preceding the early

activation of both the CS and the proximal duo-decapolar catheter for beats originating from the interatrial septum.

If needed, a detailed activation mapping is performed to better localize the site of origin of non-PV triggers. Our definition for significant non-PV triggers includes those initiating AF, atrial flutter, sustained and nonsustained atrial tachycardia, as well as frequent PACs of 10 per minute or more.

At the end of the procedure, SVC isolation is performed in all patients, even if triggers from this site were not elicited.

As mentioned, the prevalence of non-PV triggers is higher in nonparoxysmal AF, female, obese, and elderly patients, as well as in those with HF with reduced ejection fraction, sleep-related breathing disorders, hypertrophic cardiomyopathy, severe atrial scarring, and previous cardiac surgery. Among them, non-PV triggers should be carefully documented and targeted for ablation at the time of the first procedure. In patients with recurrences and evidence of persistent PV isolation, non-PV triggers should be sought and targeted for ablation at the time of the repeat procedure, regardless of the type of AF (paroxysmal vs nonparoxysmal AF).

CS and LAA are the most common sources of triggers. The ablation strategy of choice for these sites, as well as for the SVC, should be complete isolation rather than focal ablation. In combination with PVAI and ablation/isolation of inducible triggers, PW should be empirically isolated in all patients, because it embryologically and electrophysiologically represents an extension of the PVs.[36] There is also strong evidence suggesting that empirical LAA isolation should be performed

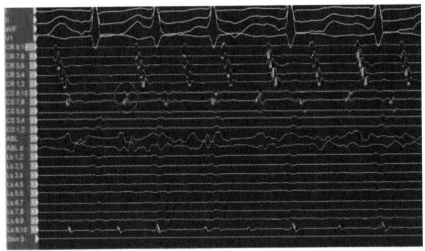

Fig. 2. Example of CS trigger (sustained atrial tachycardia). The earliest activation is recorded by the proximal electrodes of the distal segment of the duo-decapolar catheter inside the CS.

in long-standing persistent AF at the time of the first procedure to significantly improve outcomes.[33,37] Additionally, empirical isolation of the LAA and CS should be considered in patients presenting risk factors indicative of high non-PV trigger prevalence.

CS isolation is performed by ablating this structure both endocardially (from the left atrium) and epicardially (inside the CS). The ablation catheter has to be moved continuously while ablating inside the CS, making sure that the tip is not wedged in a branch to decrease the risk of steam pops. Given the proximity of the CS to the esophagus, esophageal temperature should be monitored and energy delivery stopped if the temperature significantly increases. The proximal CS is also close to the atrioventricular node; therefore, beat-to-beat PR monitoring is necessary while ablating close to the CS ostium to promptly recognize PR prolongation and prevent conduction system damage.

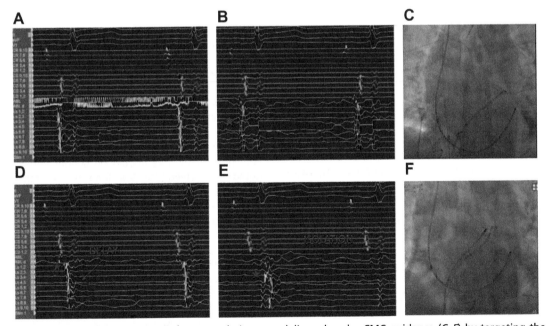

Fig. 3. Isolation of the LAA. Radiofrequency lesions are delivered under CMC guidance (C–F) by targeting the breakthrough (*red star*) recorded on the CMC positioned at the appendage ostium (A–E). LAA intracardiac recordings at baseline (A, B), showing delayed activation (D), and isolation (E).

The technique for LAA isolation is similar to that for PVAI. Briefly, lesions are delivered under CMC guidance by targeting the breakthrough recorded on the CMC (**Fig. 3**). Because the myocardium surrounding the LAA is thicker, longer RF application times and/or higher power are frequently necessary.

In our laboratory, SVC isolation is performed by targeting the septal segment of the SVC–right atrial junction and continues posteriorly and inferiorly with ablation of sites of early activation until electrical isolation is achieved.[36] This approach allows to eliminate any risk of sinus node injury or SVC stenosis; similarly, the chances of phrenic nerve injury are very limited and can be easily prevented by performing high-output pacing to localize the course of the nerve.

SUMMARY

The cornerstone of AF ablation is the elimination of triggers from the PVs. Nevertheless, a variable number of patients may experience atrial tachyarrhythmia recurrences even in the presence of permanent PVAI. Non-PV trigger ablation in combination to PVAI is the most effective approach to improve outcomes in AF ablation. Their localization can be easily achieved by means of multielectrode catheters positioned in specific areas of the right and left atrium during pharmacologic challenge test.

REFERENCES

1. Coyne KS, Paramore C, Grandy S, et al. Assessing the direct costs of treating nonvalvular atrial fibrillation in the United States. Value Health 2006;9: 348–56.
2. Packer DL, Mark DB, Robb RA, et al. Effect of catheter ablation vs antiarrhythmic drug therapy on mortality, stroke, bleeding, and cardiac arrest among patients with atrial fibrillation: the CABANA randomized clinical trial. JAMA 2019. https://doi.org/10.1001/jama.2019.0693.
3. Mark DB, Anstrom KJ, Sheng S, et al. Effect of catheter ablation vs medical therapy on quality of life among patients with atrial fibrillation: the CABANA randomized clinical trial. JAMA 2019. https://doi.org/10.1001/jama.2019.0692.
4. Blomstrom-Lundqvist C, Gizurarson S, Schwieler J, et al. Effect of catheter ablation vs antiarrhythmic medication on quality of life in patients with atrial fibrillation: the CAPTAF randomized clinical trial. JAMA 2019;321(11):1059–68.
5. Marrouche NF, Brachmann J, Andresen D, et al. Catheter ablation for atrial fibrillation with heart failure. N Engl J Med 2018;378:417–27.
6. Di Biase L, Mohanty P, Mohanty S, et al. Ablation versus amiodarone for treatment of persistent atrial fibrillation in patients with congestive heart failure and an implanted device: results from the AATAC multicenter randomized trial. Circulation 2016;133:1637–44.
7. Santangeli P, Di Biase L, Mohanty P, et al. Catheter ablation of atrial fibrillation in octogenarians: safety and outcomes. J Cardiovasc Electrophysiol 2012;23:687–93.
8. Calkins H, Hindricks G, Cappato R, et al. 2017 HRS/EHRA/ECAS/APHRS/SOLAECE expert consensus statement on catheter and surgical ablation of atrial fibrillation. Europace 2018;20(1):e1–160.
9. Mohanty S, Trivedi C, Gianni C, et al. Procedural findings and ablation outcome in patients with atrial fibrillation referred after two or more failed catheter ablations. J Cardiovasc Electrophysiol 2017;28:1379–86.
10. Di Biase L, Conti S, Mohanty P, et al. General anesthesia reduces the prevalence of pulmonary vein reconnection during repeat ablation when compared with conscious sedation: results from a randomized study. Heart Rhythm 2011;8:368–72.
11. Di Biase L, Briceno DF, Trivedi C, et al. Is transesophageal echocardiogram mandatory in patients undergoing ablation of atrial fibrillation with uninterrupted novel oral anticoagulants? Results from a prospective multicenter registry. Heart Rhythm 2016;13:1197–202.
12. Yu HT, Shim J, Park J, et al. When is it appropriate to stop non-vitamin K antagonist oral anticoagulants before catheter ablation of atrial fibrillation? A multicentre prospective randomized study. Eur Heart J 2019;40:1531–7.
13. Nagao T, Suzuki H, Matsunaga S, et al. Impact of periprocedural anticoagulation therapy on the incidence of silent stroke after atrial fibrillation ablation in patients receiving direct oral anticoagulants: uninterrupted vs. interrupted by one dose strategy. Europace 2019;21:590–7.
14. Mohanty S, Trivedi C, Beheiry S, et al. Venous access-site closure with vascular closure device vs. manual compression in patients undergoing catheter ablation or left atrial appendage occlusion under uninterrupted anticoagulation: a multicentre experience on efficacy and complications. Europace 2019. https://doi.org/10.1093/europace/euz004.
15. Themistoclakis S, Corrado A, Marchlinski FE, et al. The risk of thromboembolism and need for oral anticoagulation after successful atrial fibrillation ablation. J Am Coll Cardiol 2010;55:735–43.
16. Morton JB, Byrne MJ, Power JM, et al. Electrical remodeling of the atrium in an anatomic model of atrial flutter: relationship between substrate and triggers for conversion to atrial fibrillation. Circulation 2002;105:258–64.

17. Oral H, Chugh A, Lemola K, et al. Noninducibility of atrial fibrillation as an end point of left atrial circumferential ablation for paroxysmal atrial fibrillation: a randomized study. Circulation 2004;110:2797–801.

18. Jais P, Hocini M, Hsu LF, et al. Technique and results of linear ablation at the mitral isthmus. Circulation 2004;110:2996–3002.

19. Nademanee K, McKenzie J, Kosar E, et al. A new approach for catheter ablation of atrial fibrillation: mapping of the electrophysiologic substrate. J Am Coll Cardiol 2004;43:2044–53.

20. Pokushalov E, Romanov A, Artyomenko S, et al. Ganglionated plexi ablation for longstanding persistent atrial fibrillation. Europace 2010;12:342–6.

21. Rolf S, Kircher S, Arya A, et al. Tailored atrial substrate modification based on low-voltage areas in catheter ablation of atrial fibrillation. Circ Arrhythm Electrophysiol 2014;7:825–33.

22. Mohanty S, Mohanty P, Di Biase L, et al. Long-term follow-up of patients with paroxysmal atrial fibrillation and severe left atrial scarring: comparison between pulmonary vein antrum isolation only or pulmonary vein isolation combined with either scar homogenization or trigger ablation. Europace 2017;19:1790–7.

23. Verma A, Jiang CY, Betts TR, et al. Approaches to catheter ablation for persistent atrial fibrillation. N Engl J Med 2015;372(19):1812–22.

24. Fink T, Schlüter M, Heeger CH, et al. Stand-alone pulmonary vein isolation versus pulmonary vein isolation with additional substrate modification as index ablation procedures in patients with persistent and long-standing persistent atrial fibrillation: the randomized Alster-Lost-AF trial (ablation at St. Georg hospital for long-standing persistent atrial fibrillation). Circ Arrhythm Electrophysiol 2017;10(7). https://doi.org/10.1161/CIRCEP.117.005114.

25. Mohanty S, Mohanty P, Trivedi C, et al. Long-Term outcome of pulmonary vein isolation with and without focal impulse and rotor modulation mapping: insights from a meta-analysis. Circ Arrhythm Electrophysiol 2018;11(3):e005789.

26. ClinicalTrials.gov [Internet]. Bethesda (MD): National Library of Medicine (US). 2000 Feb 29. Identifier: NCT02274857. Randomized Evaluation of Atrial Fibrillation Treatment With Focal Impulse and Rotor Modulation Guided Procedures (REAFFIRM). 2014.

Available at: https://clinicaltrials.gov/ct2/show/NCT02274857. Accessed June 11, 2019.

27. Lin WS, Tai CT, Hsieh MH, et al. Catheter ablation of paroxysmal atrial fibrillation initiated by non-pulmonary vein ectopy. Circulation 2003;107:3176–83.

28. Tsai CF, Tai CT, Hsieh MH, et al. Initiation of atrial fibrillation by ectopic beats originating from the superior vena cava: electrophysiological characteristics and results of radiofrequency ablation. Circulation 2000;102:67–74.

29. Hung Y, Lo LW, Lin YJ, et al. Characteristics and long-term catheter ablation outcome in long-standing persistent atrial fibrillation patients with non-pulmonary vein triggers. Int J Cardiol 2017;241:205–11.

30. Stambler BS, Fenelon G, Shepard RK, et al. Characterization of sustained atrial tachycardia in dogs with rapid ventricular pacing-induced heart failure. J Cardiovasc Electrophysiol 2003;14:499–507.

31. Della Rocca DG, Mohanty S, Trivedi C, et al. Percutaneous treatment of non-paroxysmal atrial fibrillation: a paradigm shift from pulmonary vein to non-pulmonary vein trigger ablation? Arrhythm Electrophysiol Rev 2018;7:256–60.

32. Santangeli P, Zado ES, Hutchinson MD, et al. Prevalence and distribution of focal triggers in persistent and long-standing persistent atrial fibrillation. Heart Rhythm 2016;13:374–82.

33. Di Biase L, Burkhardt JD, Mohanty P, et al. Left atrial appendage isolation in patients with longstanding persistent AF undergoing catheter ablation: BELIEF trial. J Am Coll Cardiol 2016;68:1929–40.

34. Della Rocca DG, Mohanty S, Mohanty P, et al. Long-term outcomes of catheter ablation in patients with longstanding persistent atrial fibrillation lasting less than 2 years. J Cardiovasc Electrophysiol 2018;29:1607–15.

35. Santangeli P, Marchlinski FE. Techniques for provocation, localization and ablation of nonpulmonary vein triggers for atrial fibrillation. Heart Rhythm 2017;14:1087–96.

36. Gianni C, Sanchez JE, Mohanty S, et al. Isolation of the superior vena cava from the right atrial posterior wall: a novel ablation approach. Europace 2018;20:e124–32.

The Ideal Cardiac Mapping System

Mohammad Shenasa, MD, PhD, FHRS[a],*, Seyed-Mostafa Razavi, MD[a],
Hossein Shenasa, MD, FHRS[a], Amin Al-Ahmad, MD, FHRS[b]

KEYWORDS

• Arrhythmias • Imaging • Mapping • Cardiac magnetic resonance • CCT

KEY POINTS

The ideal mapping system in 2020 should have the following capabilities:

• To match patient anatomy and physiology at the same time.
• Completely noninvasive and radiation/fluoroscopy free.
• User friendly and safe in patients with cardiac implantable electronic devices, left ventricular assist devices, and other prosthesis. These issues are now being solved with MRI-safe machines.
• Real time, multimodality, affordable, widely available and capable of merging with other mapping/imaging technologies.
• Choice of mapping/imaging technique depends on several factors. Among important ones are operator preference, patient-specific substrate and arrhythmias, as well as associated structural heart disease and comorbidities.

INTRODUCTION

Milestones in Cardiac Mapping

Cardiac mapping has witnessed significant and unprecedented progress over more than a century. At present, several mapping/imaging technologies are commercially available, alone or in combination. This article briefly discusses the advantages and limitations (disadvantages) of each technique. The progress and milestones can be summarized as follows:

• Analog to digital conversion
• Multichannel computerized mapping
• Transcatheter mapping
• Cardiac activation mapping (isochronal mapping)
• Activation mapping
• Voltage mapping
• Electrical stimulation mapping (pace mapping, resetting, subthreshold mapping)
• Intraoperative mapping in humans
• Simultaneous intraoperative and computerized epicardial/endocardial mapping
• Electroanatomic and noncontact mapping
• Multimodality noninvasive mapping and imaging
• Optical mapping
• Molecular imaging
• Electrocardiogram imaging (ECGi)
• Fluoroless mapping

Fundamental to all maps is the ability to create an image. Modern cardiac mapping is analogous to a GPS (global positioning system) of the heart and can lead to unknown destinations.[1]

Current Technologies

Several technologies are currently available and are used in practice:

1. Nonfluoroscopic mapping systems
2. Noncontact mapping systems

Disclosures: None related to this article.
[a] Department of Cardiovascular Services, Heart and Rhythm Medical Group, O'Connor Hospital, San Jose, CA 95030, USA; [b] Texas Cardiac Arrhythmia Institute, 3000 North IH35, Suite 700, Austin, TX 78705, USA
* Corresponding author.
E-mail address: mohammad.shenasa@gmail.com

Card Electrophysiol Clin 11 (2019) 739–748
https://doi.org/10.1016/j.ccep.2019.08.015
1877-9182/19/© 2019 Elsevier Inc. All rights reserved.

3. Rotational angiography
4. Preprocedure computed tomography (CT)/MRI
5. Interventional cardiac MRI
6. Intracardiac echocardiography (ICE)
7. Intracardiac MRI
8. Real-time three-dimensional (3D) imaging/visualization
9. Navigation system
   - Remote magnetic navigation (stereotaxis)
   - Robotic navigation (Hansen system)
10. Fluoroless mapping[2]
11. CARTO
12. EnSite precision
13. NavX mapping system
14. Rhythmia Topera
15. Electrical stimulation mapping: pace mapping; resetting; subthreshold mapping

Some of these technologies are discussed in other articles in this issue or in the previous issue.

In general, any mapping and imaging technique should have the following capabilities:

1. Should be able to match each patient's anatomy, physiology, and arrhythmia substrate
2. Accurate mapping of specific arrhythmia and its substrate should be able to detect the mechanism, location of the arrhythmia focus, and determine the target for ablation without collateral damage
3. The mapping system should match the catheters and the energy source and be able to be integrated with other systems; for example, CARTO system with CT/MRI (CARTO-merge) or echocardiography (Cartosound) and other techniques (**Box 1** for details)
4. Completely noninvasive and radiation free
5. Real time
6. Multidimensional and multimodality
7. User friendly and safe
8. Affordable, widely available

SPECIFIC TECHNOLOGIES

Role, advantages and disadvantages of different mapping and imaging techniques are summarized in (**Tables 1** and **2**).

Electrocardiography

It is now more than a century since the invention of electrocardiograms (ECG) by Willem Einthoven in 1895[14] on the registration of cardiac electrical activity. It remains one of the most useful, widely available, and user friendly tests, and is capable

---

Box 1
Integrated technologies/systems (hybrid imaging)

- Electroanatomic mapping (EAM) + CT (Cartomerge)
- EAM + ICE (Cartosound), 3D phase array ICE with EAM
- EAM + echocardiography
- CT + fluoroscopy
- Noncontact mapping + MRI (Ensite NavX)
- EAM + MRI
- Echocardiography + contrast-enhanced cardiac CT (CCT)
- Echocardiography + cardiac MRI
- ICE + MRI
- PET + CT
- 3D CT + 3D ultrasonography (using ICE)
- Single-photon emission CT + CT
- CT + ICE
- PET + MRI
- CT + MRI
- Transesophageal echocardiography + MRI
- Magnetic navigation + EAM (CARTO RMT)
- Radiograph + MRI (referred to as coregistration or XFM)
- CT + MR + radiograph
- CT + Ensite NavX
- Rotational angiography + ICE
- Rotational angiography + MRI
- Cardiac C-arm CT + rotational angiography
- Navigation systems + EAM (CARTO RMT)
- PET + optical imaging
- All of the above

---

of providing information on many cardiac and noncardiac disorders as well as responses to specific pharmacologic and nonpharmacologic interventions.[4] Careful analysis of 12-lead ECG now provides useful and accurate information on the mechanism and location of specific arrhythmias. For example, 12-lead ECG has specific patterns of epicardial ventricular tachycardia (VT), VTs from unusual sites such as pulmonic of aortic valve cusps.[15]

Electrocardiogram imaging

This technique is well described by Yoram Rudi and Michel Heisseguerre and is based on

Table 1
Role of different imaging modalities in patients with atrial fibrillation

	TTE	TEE	CMRI	MDCT	Nuclear
Role					
Assessment of LA size and volume	++	++	+++	+++	—
Assessment of LV function	+++	+++	++	++	—
Evaluation of Underlying Heart Disease					
Valvular heart disease	+++	+++	++	++	—
Coronary heart disease	++	—	+++	+++	+++
Hypertensive heart disease	++	—	+	+	++
Congestive heart failure	+++	—	+++	+	++
Identification of LA thrombosis	—	+++	++	++	—
HCM	+++	=	+++	++	+
DCM	+++	++	+++	+++	++
RFCA Procedures					
Preablation	+	++	+++	+++	—
Intra-ablation periprocedure	—	+++	—	—	—
Postablation	++	—	++	—	—

Abbreviations: CMRI, cardiac MRI; DCM, dilated cardiomyopathy; HCM, hypertrophic cardiomyopathy; LA, left atrium; LV, left ventricle; MDCT, multidetector CT; RFCA, radiofrequency catheter ablation; TEE, transesophageal echocardiography; TTE, transthoracic echocardiography.

the registration of cardiac electrical activity on the torso, previously called body surface potential mapping. ECGi is capable of showing the mechanisms and location of arrhythmia, such as rotor activity on atrial or ventricular arrhythmias. It can also show the location of accessory pathways. Furthermore, it is useful to identify appropriate locations for cardiac resynchronization therapy implantation.[5,16,17]

Echocardiography

Transthoracic echocardiography

Like ECG, echocardiography is a useful noninvasive technique that provides both anatomic and physiologic information on the heart. It is usually used as first step in testing for cardiac and noncardiac disorders. Advanced modes of echocardiography, such as strain-rate imaging, provide useful information on wall motion abnormalities, as well as myocardial function.

Transesophageal echocardiography

This technique is useful for obtaining higher resolution of cardiac anatomy, such as congenital heart defects, presence of intracardiac thrombi, location of catheters during ablative procedures, and endocarditis.[18]

Intracardiac echocardiography

At present, intracardiac echocardiography (ICE) is being used as a first-line (or stand-alone) imaging technique to evaluate the anatomy and location of catheters during ablation procedures. ICE provides a two-dimensional image of cardiac anatomy without using fluoroscopy. The entire ablation procedure can be done with ICE only. ICE can also be integrated (merged) with virtually all the other mapping and imaging modalities.[19]

Cardiac Computed Tomography

CCT with or without contrast provides detailed multidimensional anatomic views of the heart. It can also detect intracardiac thrombus, shunts, cardiac mass, and valvular heart disease, such as mitral and aortic regurgitation. CCT is widely used to evaluate patients with chest pain, coronary artery disease, intracoronary stents, and bypass grafts. A major shortcoming of CCT is its radiation exposure and the need for contrast. For interventional electrophysiology procedures, CCT provides a shell for the cardiac chamber of interest for electroanatomic mapping and is often integrated with other imaging techniques.[20]

Cardiac MRI

Cardiac MRI (CMRI) is increasingly used as the imaging method of choice in evaluation and management of a variety of disorders, arrhythmia substrate, and response to catheter ablation of cardiac arrhythmias. CMRI is considered the gold standard technique for evaluation of

Table 2
Advantages and disadvantages of current and novel mapping and imaging techniques

Technique	Advantages	Disadvantages
ECG[3,4]	Readily available Widely used Can be used to localize arrhythmia focus	Low specificity and sensitivity in certain monogenic arrhythmias
ECGi[5]	Noninvasive mapping system Provides mechanisms of arrhythmias such as AF and VT	New and needs expert interpretation; patient needs to have a chest CT before the procedure; correlation between ECGi and invasive epicardial mapping reported to be poor in some cases
TTE	Readily available Real time Useful in cardiomyopathy risk stratification	Low resolution for small shunts and small thrombi
TEE	Real time Useful for intracardiac shunts, thrombi detection, electrophysiologic procedures	Invasive Rarely may cause esophageal rupture
ICE[6]	Real time, 3D–4D (excellent anatomic detail), shorter fluoroscopy times	Invasive Does not provide electrical data
CCT[7]	Fast, high sensitivity and specificity and predictive value	Radiation exposure, use of contrast in patients with impaired renal function, clinical significance of incidental findings is source of concern
CMRI[8]	Noninvasive, high resolution, 3D Expanded field of view Radiation free High reproducibility	Nephrogenic systemic fibrosis is associated with gadolinium in patients with impaired function High magnetic field limits Low SNR
MPI[9]	Extensively validated High reproducibility	Low resolution Radiation exposure
PET[10]	High resolution Allows molecular and metabolic imaging	High radiation exposure (an alternative approach is to use low-dose CT)
Optical mapping	Provides each cell's electrical activity with depolarization and repolarization mapping	In small experimental animals needs voltage-sensitive dye
CARTO[11]	Third generation of electroanatomic mapping Has been in use for a long time Provides catheter tracking and map visualization Can be integrated with MRI and CT	—
NavX/EnSite Precision[11]	Automatic high-resolution mapping Can be integrated with MRI and CT	Expensive Needs larger experience
Topera[11]	Rotor mapping system Mostly used for patients with AF	Complex workstation Used mostly in AF Electrode-tissue contact may be problematic
Rhythmia[11]	Rapid ultrahigh resolution, 3D, low noise, can register up to 200 intracardiac channels	Cost Larger experiments needed

(continued on next page)

Table 2
(continued)

Technique	Advantages	Disadvantages
Ripple[12]	Combines voltage and activation data conserving the signal; suboptimal window of interest does not harm the map; interpolated colors cannot deceive or distort the activation	—
High-density mapping[13]	Is a multielectrode mapping system with closely spaced electrodes Good SNR Has a basket electrode Provides high-resolution mapping in atrial and ventricular arrhythmias	

Abbreviations: AF, atrial fibrillation; CCT, cardiac CT; 4D, four-dimensional; ECG, electrocardiogram; ECGi, electrocardiogram imaging; MPI, myocardial perfusion imaging; SNR, signal/noise ratio; VT, ventricular tachycardia.

ventricular arrhythmias in most of the cardiomyopathies. For the role of CMRI in patients with atrial fibrillation, the readers are referred to Cardiac Electrophysiology Clinics (2019) Part I, Refs.[21,22] Furthermore, Late gadolinium enhancement (LGE) has been used as a diagnostic, prognostic (disease progression) and response to therapy method in patients with atrial and ventricular arrhythmias, and particularly in patients with a variety of cardiomyopathies, such as hypertrophic cardiomyopathy (HCM), dilated cardiomyopathy (DCM), and arrhythmogenic right ventricular dysplasia/cardiomyopathy.[22,23]

Furthermore, LGE-CMR is very useful for evaluation of catheter ablation in patients with coronary artery disease (scar-related VT) and non–ischemia-related VT.[24] Likewise, this technique is useful to detect intracardiac thrombus, such as detection of ventricular thrombus with LGE-CMR.[25] Several recent investigations have reported on the value of CMR and LGE-CMR in diagnosis and management of different disorders related to sudden cardiac death (SCD).[22,26–28] A comparison of CCT and MRI is shown in **Table 3**.

Multimodality Imaging

The unprecedented technological advances in cardiac mapping and imaging in the management of cardiac arrhythmias and ablation procedures allows clinicians to work in cardiac regions that 2 decades ago were considered inaccessible. Now it is possible to reach these areas either endocardially or epicardially. Integration of techniques that were once considered impossible, such as PET and MRI or CT and MRI, is now possible in 1 system and provides multimodality imaging. Accordingly, different disorders, such as HCM, DCM, other cardiomyopathies, scar-related VT, and VTs arising from uncommon sites, are currently amenable to precise localization and ablation.

Nonfluoroscopic Electroanatomic Mapping

Electroanatomic mapping is the cornerstone of cardiac mapping and imaging for a variety of complex anatomy and arrhythmia substrates. This technique was first developed in 1996. The system comprises a catheter that senses (detects) local electrical activity with simultaneous data acquisition. The mapping system creates a map of all collected data and constructs a 3D real-time image. For further details see Refs.[11,32]

Table 3
Comparison between cardiac MRI and cardiac computed tomography

Cardiac MRI	Cardiac CT
• Morphology • MRA • Function (increased stress) • Physiology • Myocardial perfusion • Viability assessment • Plaques characterization • Myocardial strain • Spectroscopy • DTI[29–31] • Valvular regurgitation	• Morphology • CTA) • Function • Myocardial infarction • Myocardial mass • Valvular regurgitation • Intracardiac mass and thrombus

Abbreviations: CTA, CT angiography; DTI, diffusion tensor imaging; MRA, magnetic resonance angiography.

Contact Mapping

Contact mapping is the most commonly used invasive technique in mapping arrhythmias. A catheter is manipulated in the chamber or chambers of interest and the local electrogram features are collected as the catheter is being manipulated. Both the voltage of the local electrogram, as well as the timing of the electrogram as compared with a reference. The reference used for timing is typically either a stable intracardiac signal such as the coronary sinus catheter for the mapping of atrial arrhythmias or the peak or nadir of an ECG lead when mapping ventricular arrhythmias. The location of the catheter in 3D space is accurately calculated by the mapping system using a magnetic field or an electrical field or a combination of the two.[33] Location accuracy within the chamber of interest is typically accurate to 1 mm range. As the catheter is manipulated in the chamber, it collects location data and a reconstruction of the chamber geometry is created. The electrical information is thus displayed on the geometry in a 3D map. Newer mapping systems also have features that can automatically tag signals that are fractionated for later review and potential ablation. Timing of the electrogram can also be at the onset or the end of the local electrogram, this allows for examination of late activation in areas such a ventricular scar. Multipolar catheter mapping is now a standard of all mapping systems. This allows for rapid geometry acquisition, as well as high density electrical mapping.[34] Ultrasound images can also be incorporated in one mapping system, thus allowing the delineation of some structures such as valves or papillary muscles (**Fig. 1**).

The major challenges of contact mapping are 1) lack of a stable or sustained arrhythmia 2) Poor contact in some regions of the chamber 3) Map distortion due to high catheter contact force 3) Electrical timing inaccuracy due to change or inconstancy of the timing refence 4) Map distortion or motion due to patient motion, or changes in impedance 5) Failure to annotate the correct signal (due to fractionation, noise, low voltage, far field signals).

Contact mapping can be extremely useful for substrate definition such as in VT (**Figs. 2 and 3**)[35], or timing such as in atrial arrhythmias (**Fig. 4**).

Further improvements with contact mapping will increase the accuracy and speed of mapping. In addition, the contact mapping may also provide important insight to arrhythmia mechanism and substrate.

Noncontact Mapping

Noncontact mapping is a 3D electroanatomic point-by-point (sequential) reconstruction acquired by a catheter in a cardiac chamber of interest, such as the left ventricle. This technique is limited by the time required to generate the chamber geometry and is also limited in cases of hemodynamically unstable or nonsustained arrhythmias.

This technique provides simultaneous data collection of the entire cardiac chamber, even in a single beat, in which direct contact with the cardiac chamber is not necessary.

FUTURE DIRECTIONS

With all these available technologies, it is important design prospective registries to evaluate proper indications, image quality, safety, and their effect on patient outcome. Large trials conducting prospective comparisons of imaging technologies and their impact on patients' survival and outcome are needed.

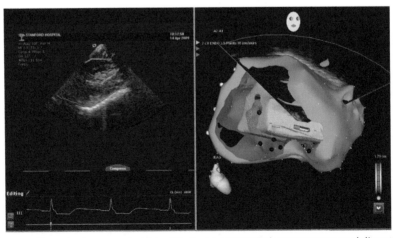

Fig. 1. Use of intracardiac echo incorporated in a 3D electroanatomical contact map to delineate the epicardial and endocardial borders of the left ventricle.

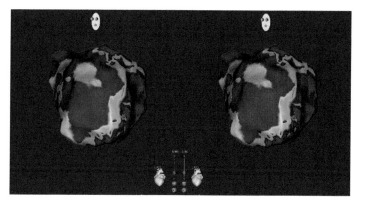

Fig. 2. Contact map of the left ventricle, the endocardial voltage is color coded such that voltage less than 0.5 mV is in red.

High diagnostic and prognostic performance and reliable assessment of complex anatomy and substrate are desirable. The use of cardiac imaging for screening in large populations needs to be validated in randomized trials.

Society guidelines have indicated the appropriate use of different mapping technologies such as CCT, MRI, CMRI, PET, and echocardiography.

Ideal Mapping System in the Twenty-first Century

The ideal mapping for the twenty-first century will have the following technical characteristics and capabilities (some of these are shown in **Fig. 5**):

- Matching patient anatomy, structure, function, and physiology
- Fully noninvasive or minimally invasive
- Matched with all other technologies and ablation catheters (integrable)
- Hybrid system approach (eg, PET/CT, PET/MRI)
- Real time (four-dimensional to six-dimensional)
- Multimodality
- Ionizing radiation free
- Appropriate use

- Fast, safe, affordable, and 100% effective
- Patient precision
- Multidisciplinary approach to SCD
- Improved and novel imaging methods, such as advanced CMRI, ECGi, electromechanical wave imaging, and diffusion MRI tractography
- Specific population studies (high-risk vs low-risk individuals)
- Reappraisal of SCD detection methods and epidemiology
- Focus more on inflammation, fibrosis, and biomarkers
- Better ECG markers for risk stratification of SCD in different substrates
- Better risk stratification models
- Multimarker approach
- Better design of future trials
- The heart-brain interaction and its relation to ventricular arrhythmias and SCD
- Heart-brain interactions, psychophysiologic coherence, and the emergence of system-wide order
- ECG as a mapping tool
- ECGi
- Noninvasive mapping and ablation (cyber ablation)

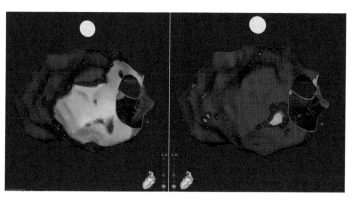

Fig. 3. Normal bipolar voltage on the right shown in purple. However, a unipolar voltage on the left map shows an area of low voltage accounting for epicardial or mid-myocardial scar.

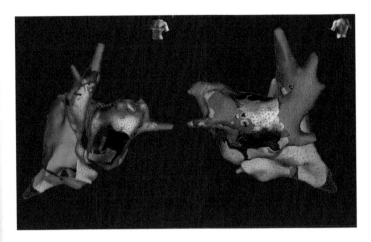

Fig. 4. Right and left atrial map of an atrial flutter showing the circuit in the posterior wall of the left atrium (color change from white to red going around the atrium).

- Hybrid technologies
- Hybrid suite and hybrid procedures
- Fluoroless mapping and ablation
- Computational systems
- Carbon beam
- Nuclear perfusion and functional scans
- Rotational angiography
- Structural, functional, coronary and perfusion MRI
- Ultrafast CT
- 3D to four-dimensional echocardiography

- 3D Biosense electromagnetic mapping
- Intracardiac/intravascular ultrasonography
- Optical coherence tomography
- One-stop shop with toolbox
- Remote navigation
- Real-time/virtual cardiac anatomy views
- Image-based guidance in ablation therapy
- Laser angiography
- 3D printing
- In vivo optical mapping
- Cardiac magnetic resonance spectroscopy

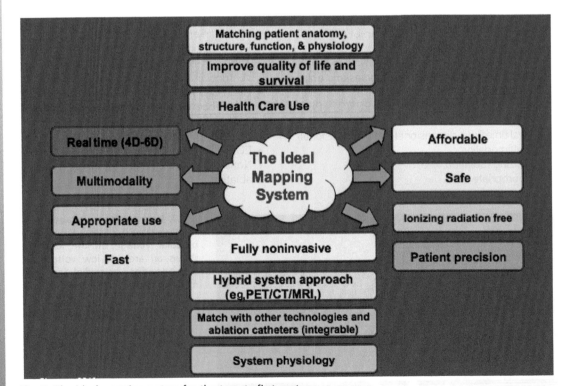

Fig. 5. The ideal mapping system for the twenty-first century.

- Laser optical spectroscopy
- Near-infrared spectroscopy
- Molecular imaging
- Fluorescence imaging
- Genetic engineering and drug delivery
- Biological pacemakers
- Stem cell imaging

SUMMARY

The ideal mapping and imaging systems should provide the most accurate localization of target sites of the arrhythmias with high success rate and no collateral damage.

The mapping and imaging technique should provide adequate information on the arrhythmia substrate as well as electrophysiologic characteristics of the mechanism of arrhythmias and the response to interventions.

The safety of the mapping and imaging techniques, such as their use in cardiac implantable electronic devices, left ventricular assist devices, and other prostheses, is being improved.

Better imaging agents to avoid contrast-induced nephropathy or neurogenic systemic fibrosis caused by MRI agents is of concern and needs to be resolved with newer imaging agents.[36,37]

A noninvasive, radiation-free (fluoroless) system is the way forward.

- Cardiovascular imaging is witnessing an rapid expansion of its armamentarium of non-invasive technologies capable of providing detailed information about the structure and function of the heart and vasculature.
- Many of these technologies are integration (ie, PET and CT, PET and MRI).
- The crucial role of imaging in early phenotyping of disease, risk definition, management guidance, and outcome assessment is expanding rapidly in ways previously thought unrealistic.
- Imaging options and their complexity will prompt the emergence of cardiovascular imaging specialists.
- In future there will be joint cardiology and radiology imaging departments.

REFERENCES

1. Zipes D. Foreword. In: Shenasa M, et al, editors. Cardiac mapping, fourth edition. Hoboken (NJ): Wiley-Blackwell; 2012.
2. Demo H, Willoughby C, Jazayeri M-A, et al. Fluoroless catheter ablation of cardiac arrhythmias. Card Electrophysiol Clin. 2019;11(4).
3. Wellens HJ, Gorgels AP. The electrocardiogram 102 years after Einthoven. Circulation 2004;109(5):562–4.
4. Stern S. Electrocardiogram: still the cardiologist's best friend. Circulation 2006;113(19):e753–6.
5. Cheniti G, Puyo S, Martin CA, et al. Noninvasive mapping and electrocardiographic imaging in atrial and ventricular arrhythmias (CardioInsight). Card Electrophysiol Clin 2019;11(3):459–71.
6. Kim SS, Hijazi ZM, Lang RM, et al. The use of intra-cardiac echocardiography and other intracardiac imaging tools to guide noncoronary cardiac interventions. J Am Coll Cardiol 2009;53:2117–28.
7. Motoyama S, Sarai M, Harigaya H, et al. Computed tomographic angiography characteristics of atherosclerotic plaques subsequently resulting in acute coronary syndrome. J Am Coll Cardiol 2009;54: 49–57.
8. Yang Q, Li K, Liu X, et al. Contrast-enhanced whole-heart coronary magnetic resonance angiography at 3.0-T: a comparative study with X-ray angiography in a single center. J Am Coll Cardiol 2009;54:69–76.
9. Hendel RC, Berman DC, Carli MFD, et al. ACCF/ASNC/ACR/AHA/ASE/SCCT/SCMR/SNM 2009 appropriate use criteria for cardiac radionuclide imaging: a report of the American College of Cardiology Foundation Appropriate Use Criteria Task Force, the American Society of Nuclear Cardiology, the American College of Radiology, the American Heart Association, the American Society of Echocardiography, the Society of Cardiovascular Computed Tomography, the Society for Cardiovascular Magnetic Resonance, and the Society of Nuclear Medicine. Circulation 2009;119: e561–87.
10. Bengel FM, Higuchi T, Javadi MS, et al. Cardiac positron emission tomography. J Am Coll Cardiol 2009;54:1–15.
11. Borlich M, Sommer P. Cardiac mapping systems: Rhythmia, Topera, EnSite precision, and CARTO. Card Electrophysiol Clin 2019;11(3):449–58.
12. Luther V, Linton NW, Koa-Wing M, et al. A prospective study of ripple mapping in atrial tachycardias: a novel approach to interpreting activation in low-voltage areas. Circ Arrhythm Electrophysiol 2016;9(1):e003582.
13. Laţcu DG, Saoudi N. High-resolution/density mapping in patients with atrial and ventricular arrhythmias. Card Electrophysiol Clin 2019;11(3):511–24.
14. Einthoven W. Le telecardiogtamme. Arch Int Physiol 1906;4:132–64.
15. Bazan VML, FE. Usefulness of the twelve lead ECG to identify epicardial substrate of ventricular tachycardia site of origin. In: Shenasa M, et al, editors. Cardiac mapping, fifth edition. Oxford (United Kingdom): Wiley; 2019. p. 1028–49.
16. Martin R, Hocini M, Dubois R, et al. Non-invasive body surface potential mapping of reentrant drivers in human atrial fibrillation. In: Shenasa M, et al, editors. Cardiac mapping, fifth edition. Oxford (United Kingdom): Wiley; 2019. p. 211–9.

17. Rudy Y. Electrophysiology of heart failure: non-invasive mapping of substrate and guidance of cardiac resynchronization therapy with Electrocardiographic imaging. In: Shenasa M, et al, editors. Cardiac mapping, fifth edition. Oxford (United Kingdom): Wiley; 2019. p. 220–35.

18. Sugeng L, Shernan SK, Salgo IS, et al. Live 3-dimensional transesophageal echocardiography: initial experience using the fully-sampled matrix array probe. J Am Coll Cardiol 2008;52(6):446–9.

19. Santangeli P, Hutchinson MD, Callans DJ. Intracardiac echocardiography. In: Shenasa M, et al, editors. Cardiac mapping, fifth edition. Oxford (United Kingdom): Wiley; 2019. p. 95–103.

20. Saremi F. Role of cardiac computed tomography imaging to guide catheter ablation of arrhythmias in complex cardiac morphologies. In: Shenasa M, editor. Cardiac mapping, fifth edition. Oxford (United Kingdom): Wiley; 2019. p. 104–22.

21. Kholmovski EG, Morris AK, Chelu MG. Cardiac MRI and fibrosis quantification. Card Electrophysiol Clin 2019;11(3):537–49.

22. Shenasa M. Fibrosis and ventricular arrhythmogenesis: role of cardiac MRI. Card Electrophysiol Clin 2019;11(3):551–62.

23. Lederman RJ. Cardiovascular interventional magnetic resonance imaging. Circulation 2005;112(19):3009–17.

24. Berruezo A, Fernandez-Armenta J, Penela D, et al. Scar-related ventricular tachycardia mapping and ablation using contrast-enhanced magnetic resonance imaging. In: Shenasa M, et al, editors. Cardiac mapping, fifth edition. Oxford (United Kingdom): Wiley; 2019. p. 1062–72.

25. Weinsaft JW, Kim HW, Shah DJ, et al. Detection of left ventricular thrombus by delayed-enhancement cardiovascular magnetic resonance: prevalence and markers in patients with systolic dysfunction. J Am Coll Cardiol 2008;52(2):148–57.

26. Kehat I, Molkentin JD. Molecular pathways underlying cardiac remodeling during pathophysiological stimulation. Circulation 2010;122(25):2727–35.

27. Markman TM, Nazarian S. Risk stratification for sudden cardiac death. Circulation 2017;135(22):2116–8.

28. Jackowski C, Schwendener N, Grabherr S, et al. Post-mortem cardiac 3-T magnetic resonance imaging: visualization of sudden cardiac death? J Am Coll Cardiol 2013;62(7):617–29.

29. Geerts L, Bovendeerd P, Nicolay K, et al. Characterization of the normal cardiac myofiber field in goat measured with MR-diffusion tensor imaging. Am J Physiol Heart Circ Physiol 2002;283(1):H139–45.

30. Mekkaoui C, Sosnovik DE. Diffusion magnetic resonance imaging tractography of the heart. In: Shenasa M, et al, editors. Cardiac mapping, fifth edition. Oxford (United Kingdom): Wiley; 2019. p. 1113–24.

31. Shenasa M, Shenasa H, Rahimian J. Principles of diffusion tensor imaging of the myocardium. In: Shenasa M, et al, editors. Cardiac mapping, fifth edition. Oxford (United Kingdom): Wiley; 2019. p. 1096–112.

32. Schawrtz Y, Ben-Haim SA. Principles of nonfluoroscopic electroanatomical and electromechanical cardiac mapping. In: Shenasa M, et al, editors. Cardiac mapping, third edition. Hoboken (NJ): Wiley-Blackwell; 2008. p. 49–70.

33. Gepstein L, Hayam G, Ben-Haim SA. A novel method for nonfluoroscopic catheter-based electroanatomical mapping of the heart. In vitro and in vivo accuracy results. Circulation 1997;95(6):1611–22.

34. Hindricks G, Weiner S, McElderry T, et al. Acute safety, effectiveness, and real-world clinical usage of ultra-high density mapping for ablation of cardiac arrhythmias: results of the TRUE HD study. Europace 2019;21(4):655–61.

35. Jacobson JT, Afonso VX, Eisenman G, et al. Characterization of the infarct substrate and ventricular tachycardia circuits with noncontact unipolar mapping in a porcine model of myocardial infarction. Heart Rhythm 2006;3(2):189–97.

36. Schlaudecker JD, Bernheisel CR. Gadolinium-associated nephrogenic systemic fibrosis. Am Fam Physician 2009;80:711–4.

37. Kribben A, Witzke O, Hillen U, et al. Nephrogenic systemic fibrosis: pathogenesis, diagnosis, and therapy. J Am Coll Cardiol 2009;53:1621–8.

Moving?

Make sure your subscription moves with you!

To notify us of your new address, find your **Clinics Account Number** (located on your mailing label above your name), and contact customer service at:

Email: journalscustomerservice-usa@elsevier.com

800-654-2452 (subscribers in the U.S. & Canada)
314-447-8871 (subscribers outside of the U.S. & Canada)

Fax number: 314-447-8029

Elsevier Health Sciences Division
Subscription Customer Service
3251 Riverport Lane
Maryland Heights, MO 63043